Development of the Human Dentition

Development of the HUMAN DENTITION

Frans P.G.M. van der Linden, DDS, PhD
Professor Emeritus and Former Chair
Department of Orthodontics
Radboud University Nijmegen
Nijmegen, The Netherlands

quintessence books
Quintessence Publishing Co, Inc
Chicago, Berlin, Tokyo, London, Paris, Milan, Barcelona, Istanbul, Moscow, New Delhi, Prague, São Paulo, Seoul, and Warsaw

Library of Congress Cataloging-in-Publication Data

Names: Linden, Frans P. G. M. van der, 1932- , author.
Title: Development of the human dentition / Frans P.G.M. van der Linden.
Other titles: Gebitsontwikkeling bij de mens. English
Description: Hanover Park, IL : Quintessence Publishing Co., Inc., [2016] |
Translation of: Gebitsontwikkeling bij de mens / F.P.G.M. van der Linden.
Houten : Bohn Stafleu van Loghum, 2010. | Includes bibliographical references and index.
Identifiers: LCCN 2016005916 | ISBN 9780867157253
Subjects: | MESH: Dentition | Maxillofacial Development | Tooth--growth & development | Atlases
Classification: LCC QP88.6 | NLM WU 17 | DDC 611/.314--dc23
LC record available at http://lccn.loc.gov/2016005916

quintessence books

Quintessence Publishing Co Inc
4350 Chandler Drive
Hanover Park, IL 60133
www.quintpub.com

5 4 3 2 1

Editor: Bryn Grisham
Design/Production: Angelina Sanchez

Printed in the United States of America

About the Author

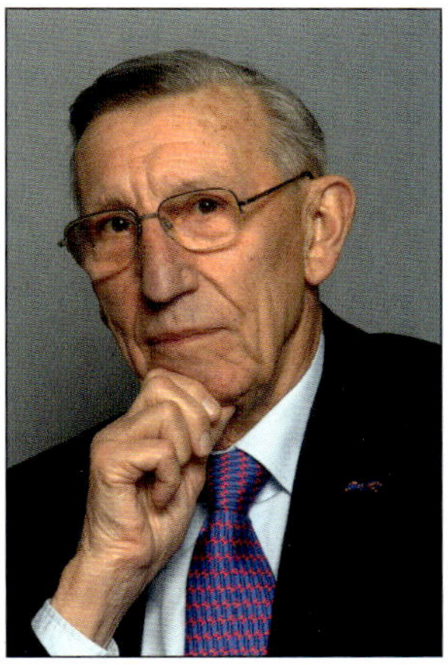

Dr Frans P.G.M. van der Linden

Dr Frans P.G.M. van der Linden received his dental and orthodontic education at the University of Groningen, the Netherlands. In addition he studied orthodontics at the University of Vienna in Austria and the University of Washington in Seattle. From 1962 until 1995 he held the position of Professor and Chairman of Orthodontics at the Radboud University Nijmegen in the Netherlands. In 1969–1970 he served as the Netherlands Visiting Professor at The University of Michigan in Ann Arbor. In 1975 he became the first European to be certified by the American Board of Orthodontics.

Dr Van der Linden has a strong interest in education. He received a grant from the European Union to develop the curriculum with the chairpersons from 15 countries for a 3-year full-time postgraduate course in orthodontics; in 1992, this so-called Erasmus Programme became the international standard in the education of specialists in orthodontics.

Dr Van der Linden is particularly interested in incorporating basic and clinical research results in the theory and practice of orthodontics. He is an internationally recognized lecturer and has published more than 200 papers and a number of books. His main contribution is a series of six textbooks on orthodontics and dentofacial orthopedics. In addition, a practice-oriented book, *Orthodontic Concepts and Strategies* (Quintessence), appeared in 2004. Furthermore, Dr Van der Linden has been Editor-in-Chief and main author of the *Dynamics of Orthodontics* (Quintessence), an international multimedia project that presents the basic aspects of the field of orthodontics in six languages.

Dr Van der Linden's long-lasting activities in research and teaching have been widely recognized, even outside the fields of dentistry and orthodontics. He is the first dentist to be elected, in 1992, to the Royal Netherlands Academy of Arts and Sciences, founded in1808 and consisting of 220 prominent scientists from all fields of arts and sciences. Moreover, in 1993 he received the Professor Lammers Prize from the Faculty of Medical Sciences at the Radboud University Nijmegen for his outstanding contributions in education and teaching. In addition, he received the 1998 Louis Ada Jarabak Memorial International Orthodontic Teachers and Research Award from the American Association of Orthodontists Foundation.

Contents

Video Clips

The contents of this book are accompanied by 50 video clips that are referenced throughout the book. These clips can be accessed at: www.youtube.com/quintbook

Clip	Title	Duration (min:sec)
1	Tooth Development	3:53
2	Formation of Mandibular Molar Crown	0:58
3	Formation of Mandibular Incisor	0:19
4	Formation of Mandibular Canine	0:19
5	Formation of Mandibular Molar	0:24
6	Formation of Mandibular Incisor, Canine, and Molar	0:22
7	Eruption and Transition of Central Incisors with Surrounding Soft Tissues	0:20
8	Transition of Mandibular Incisors with Moderate Space	0:19
9	Transition of Maxillary Incisors with Moderate Space	0:12
10	Transition of Mandibular Incisors with Excess of Space	0:21
11	Transition of Maxillary Incisors with Excess of Space	0:18
12	Transition of Mandibular Incisors with Shortage of Space	0:20
13	Transition of Maxillary Incisors with Shortage of Space	0:21
14	Changes of Maxillary Permanent Incisors After Extraction of Deciduous Canines in Anterior Crowding	0:30
15	Transition of Mandibular and Maxillary Incisors with Moderate Space	0:20
16	Transition of Canines and Premolars with Excess of Space	0:15
17	Transition of Canines and Premolars with Moderate Space	0:16
18	Transition of Canines and Premolars with Shortage of Space	0:17
19	Eruption of Second Permanent Molars	0:15
20	Eruption of Third Permanent Molars	0:18
21	Movements of First Permanent Molars	0:20
22	Rail Mechanism	0:17
23	Eruption Rate and Reduction of Eruption by Force Application	1:43
24	Resorption of Deciduous Molar Associated with Eruption of Premolar	0:14
25	Rotating Overview of Developing Dentition	1:39
26	Cone-Funnel Mechanism	0:49
27	Diagnosing Anterior Forced Bite Component in Mild Class III Malocclusion	0:14
28	Normal Tooth Mobility	0:19

Clip	Title	Duration (min:sec)
29	Excessive Tooth Mobility Caused by Periodontal Breakdown	0:17
30	Radiographic Movie of Swallowing	0:13
31	Eruption and Transition of Central Incisors in Severe Class II/1 with Anterior Soft Tissues and Lip Interposition	0:21
32	Lateral View of Development of Severe Class II/1 Malocclusion	0:51
33	Various Stages Between Normal Occlusion and Severe Class II/1 Malocclusion	0:15
34	Tipping of Central Incisors with Anterior Soft Tissues	0:15
35	Lateral View of Development of Class I Malocclusion with Symptoms of Class II/2 Type A	0:57
36	Overeruption and Tipping of Central Incisors in Class II/2	0:15
37	Frontal View of Development of Class II/2 Type A	0:19
38	Lateral View of Development of Class II/2 Type B	0:48
39	Frontal View of Development of Class II/2 Type B	0:19
40	Lateral View of Tipping of Incisors in Class II/2 Type B	0:17
41	Lateral View of Development of Class II/2 Type C	0:52
42	Eruption and Transition of Central Incisors in Class III with Anterior Soft Tissues	0:20
43	Lateral View of Development of Mild Class III Malocclusion	0:34
44	Lateral View of Development of Severe Class III Malocclusion	0:34
45	Various Stages Between Mild and Severe Class III Malocclusions	0:21
46	Overeruption and Tipping of Central Incisors in Class III	0:14
47	Anterior Forced Bite in Mild Class III Malocclusion	0:17
48	Assessing Maximal Distal Movement in Anterior Forced Bite	0:22
49	Assessing Tongue Position at Rest	1:00
50	Space Creation by Erupting Mandibular Second Premolar	0:16

Preface

Learning about the development of the dentition is an essential part of the education of dentists, orthodontists, pedodontists, and dental hygienists, nurses, and assistants. To be able to determine if development is deviant, one has to be familiar with the variations that lead to an optimal result. Indeed, normal development must be learned before deviations can be understood.

In a dental practice, one is often confronted with the complex aspects of the development of the dentition. These aspects are easier to understand when insight is gained into how certain processes work and why. Such an insight facilitates comprehension of the large diversity typically found in the development of the dentition. In addition, knowledge of interactions between the growth of the face and functions of the orofacial region is essential for understanding the development of the dentition.

This book deals with tooth formation, development of the deciduous dentition, the transition, the changeover to the permanent dentition, and the aging of the dentition. Much emphasis is placed on the relationship and reciprocal influence of the development of the dentition with the growth of the face and with functional factors. Subsequently, the development of orthodontic malocclusions is presented, followed by the effects of untimely loss of deciduous teeth.

For the composition of this book, the work *Development of the Dentition*—published in 1979 in Dutch, in 1983 in English, and subsequently in other languages—served as a model. The information that has become available since its publication is incorporated in this volume. However, new information in this field is scarce. For the last few decades, growth studies involving invasive methods such as radiographs are not allowed. At the same time, analysis of the development of the dentition on skulls has diminished as the export of skeletal material from the Asian countries that previously provided it has been banned. Nevertheless, the picture of the normal and deviating development of the dentition has become quite clear and rather complete. Furthermore, the development of the dentition has not changed over the years and will not do so in the future.

The need for a new edition arose partly from the desire to update the presentation of the information. Two-dimensional illustrations do not adequately represent the spatial conditions or the relationships among the permanent teeth and their predecessors. Furthermore, the relationship between the size of the teeth and the dimension of the surrounding bony structures is not clear, nor are the differences between the maxilla and mandible. To facilitate three-dimensional understanding, digital illustrations have been included, derived from the six-DVD series *Dynamics of Orthodontics*, which was produced by Quintessence under chief editorship of the author. Also derived from this DVD series are the 50 animated video clips that accompany the text and figures to illustrate the development of the dentition. In addition to many line drawings, a large number of photographs of skeletal material are incorporated from the volume *Development of the Human Dentition: An Atlas* (Harper & Row, 1976), co-authored by the author and Herman S. Duterloo.

Acknowledgments

The author was privileged to serve from 1962 until 1995 as the first professor and chair of the Department of Orthodontics of the Radboud University Nijmegen, where excellent conditions were provided to create high-quality education of dentists and orthodontists. Serving as a teacher was a fruitful learning experience, and the contact with students was a continuous source of inspiration and stimulation. In addition, ideal facilities were available for basic and applied research. A national grant made it possible to carry out the Nijmegen Growth Study, a mixed longitudinal study of 486 children, covering the period from 4 to 14 years of age. In addition, more than 100 skulls, which demonstrated the normal development of the dentition as well as the development of malocclusions, could be collected and analyzed. The information obtained from these two investigations served as an important resource for the contents of this book. The results of the University of Groningen School Study and The University of Michigan Elementary and Secondary School Growth Studies, in which the author was involved, also provided a wealth of information.

Several people have contributed to this edition. Drs H. S. Duterloo, J. C. Maltha, G. J. H. Schols, and M. G. Ackermans critically read the manuscript and provided suggestions for improvement. The photographs of the skull material were made by J. L. M. van de Kamp and H. A. W. Bongaerts. The thousands of dental casts of the Nijmegen Growth Study were made by or under the supervision of J. J. W. Siepermann and B. F. Bouwman. Most of the line drawings were made by hand 40 years ago by H. Reckers. More than 550 digital illustrations, derived from the series *Dynamics of Orthodontics*, were adapted by M. Mentz. The material for these illustrations was provided by A. Klebba and M. Hecklinger, who also put together the 50 incorporated animated video clips. M. J. Th. Cillessen-van Hoek took care of the manuscript, and Bryn Grisham edited the English book, while Angelina Sanchez was in charge of its design and production. The author greatly appreciates the professional input and pleasant and constructive cooperation of these individuals.

Author's Note on Terminology

There is large variation in the way teeth are defined. Many authors do not systematically use the same sequence in specifying teeth. In addition, some make use of popular scientific, nonvaluable terms, such as *upper* instead of *maxillary*. The terms *upper* and *lower* should only be used for indicating lips, not teeth. Teeth are placed in a jaw, and thus, the jaw should be specified first. The second differentiation regards the side, *left* or *right*. Third comes the number of the tooth. Finally, *deciduous* and *permanent* should be directly connected with the tooth involved.

So, teeth should be indicated in a standard way that follows a systematic sequence of relevance:

1. Jaw: Maxillary/mandibular
2. Side: Left/right
3. Tooth number: First/second or central/lateral
4. Deciduous/permanent
5. Tooth

Indeed, preference is given to using the correct anatomical descriptions. Therefore, not *upper* or *lower*, but *maxillary* and *mandibular*. Not *cuspid* but *canine* (cuspid is also used for having a cusp). Not *bicuspid* but *premolar* (some premolars have 3 cusps). Not *wisdom tooth*, but *third molar*. Not *primary* but *deciduous* (there are no secondary teeth). *Deciduous* or *permanent* should be placed directly in front of the tooth type because that belongs together and is the most essential specification.

Some examples of the correct tooth terminology used in this book include, maxillary right central permanent incisor, mandibular left deciduous canine, maxillary right second deciduous molar, and mandibular left first permanent molar.

1

Formation of Teeth

Initial Stages of Formation

Teeth arise from the interaction of two germ layers, the ectoderm and the mesoderm. The ectodermal tissue provides the enamel, the mesodermal tissue the dentin.

The first local changes leading to the formation of teeth occur in the 6th week after conception. At that time, the oral cavity is formed and covered with a two-layer epithelium with still-undifferentiated mesenchyme underneath. Between the two layers lies the basal membrane, which facilitates the communication between the two types of tissue.

At the location of the future dental arches, the epithelium thickens, and the dental lamina develops. At every location where a tooth has to appear, the ectoderm of the dental lamina bulges into the mesenchyme. The initial shape of the crown is formed by local differences in mitotic activity (differential proliferation) of the epithelium and mesenchymal tissue. The basal membrane is situated at the future enamel-dentin border. The mesenchymal cells at the inner side of the basal membrane differentiate into odontoblasts; the epithelial cells on the outer side differentiate into ameloblasts. These cells deposit dentin and enamel on the basal membrane and form the crown. Subsequently, the odontoblasts build up the dentin of the root. At the external side of the root, cementum is deposited by cementoblasts, which are differentiated from mesenchymal cells (Fig 1-1).

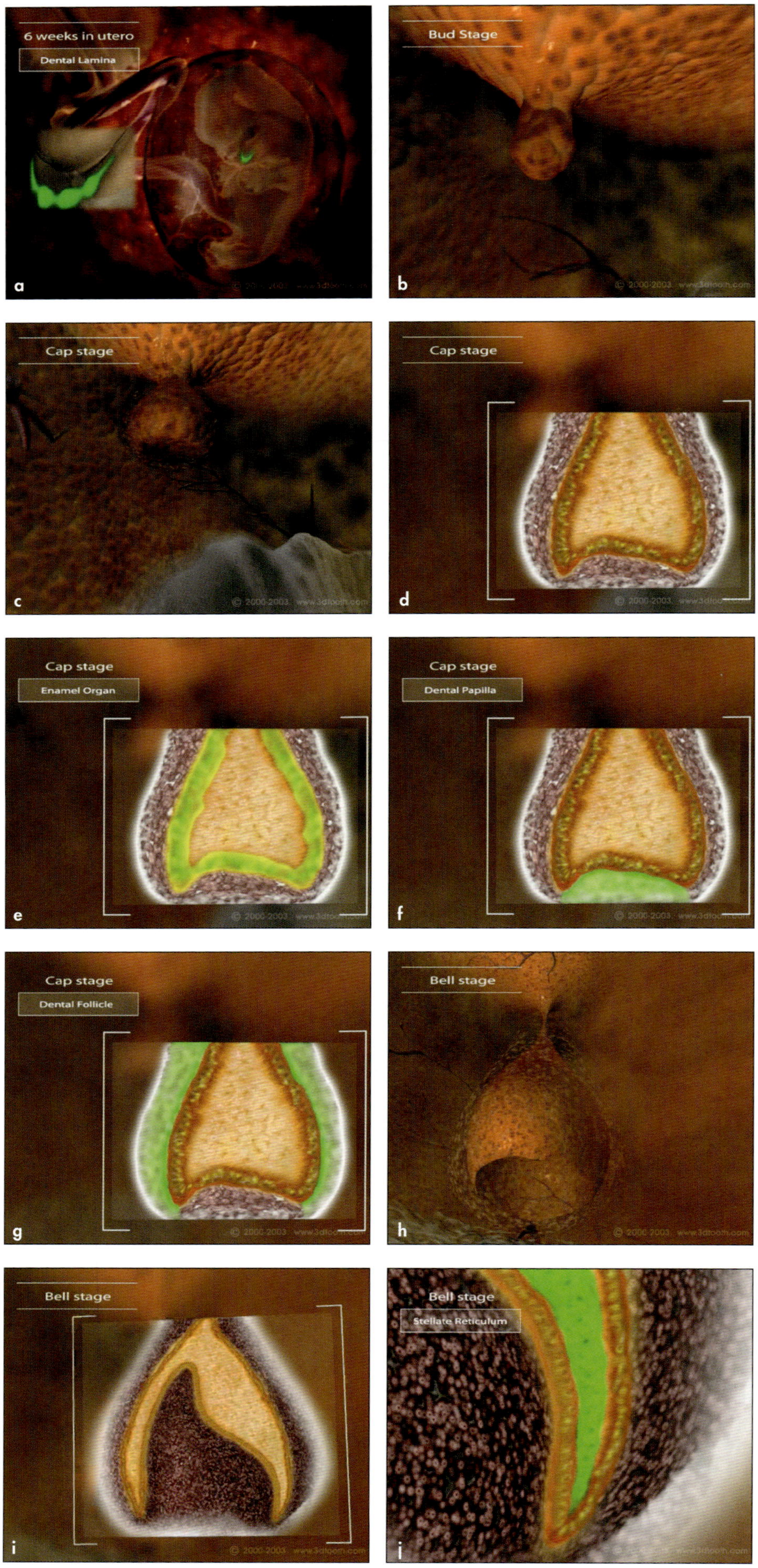

FIG 1-1 The formation of a deciduous incisor. *(a)* In the 6th week after conception, the oral epithelium thickens by differential proliferation at the location where the dental arches will arise. The dental lamina is formed. *(b)* At every location where a tooth has to be formed, the ectodermal tissue bulges into the mesenchymal tissue of the dental lamina, resulting in a tooth bud. *(c)* Extended growth of the epithelium of the tooth bud by differential proliferation results in a cap. *(d)* The cap will partially enclose a cell-dense mass of mesenchymal cells. *(e)* At the inner lining of the epithelial cap, the cells become cylindrically shaped. These are the preameloblasts, the precursors of the cells that later will deposit enamel onto the basal membrane. *(f)* The external surface of the cap continues to consist of cuboidal cells. Within the cap tissue, the stellate reticulum, a loose structure of mesenchymal cells, is formed. The cells at the periphery of the cell-dense mesenchymal mass become arranged along the basal membrane and differentiate into preodontoblasts. These are the precursors of the cells that will deposit dentin at the basal membrane. *(g)* The remaining part of the dental papilla differentiates into the pulp. The mesenchymal cells around the cap form the dental follicle, which later will lead to the formation of the periodontal ligament. *(h and i)* The total structure has attained a bell form. *(j)* Preameloblasts and the stellate reticulum.

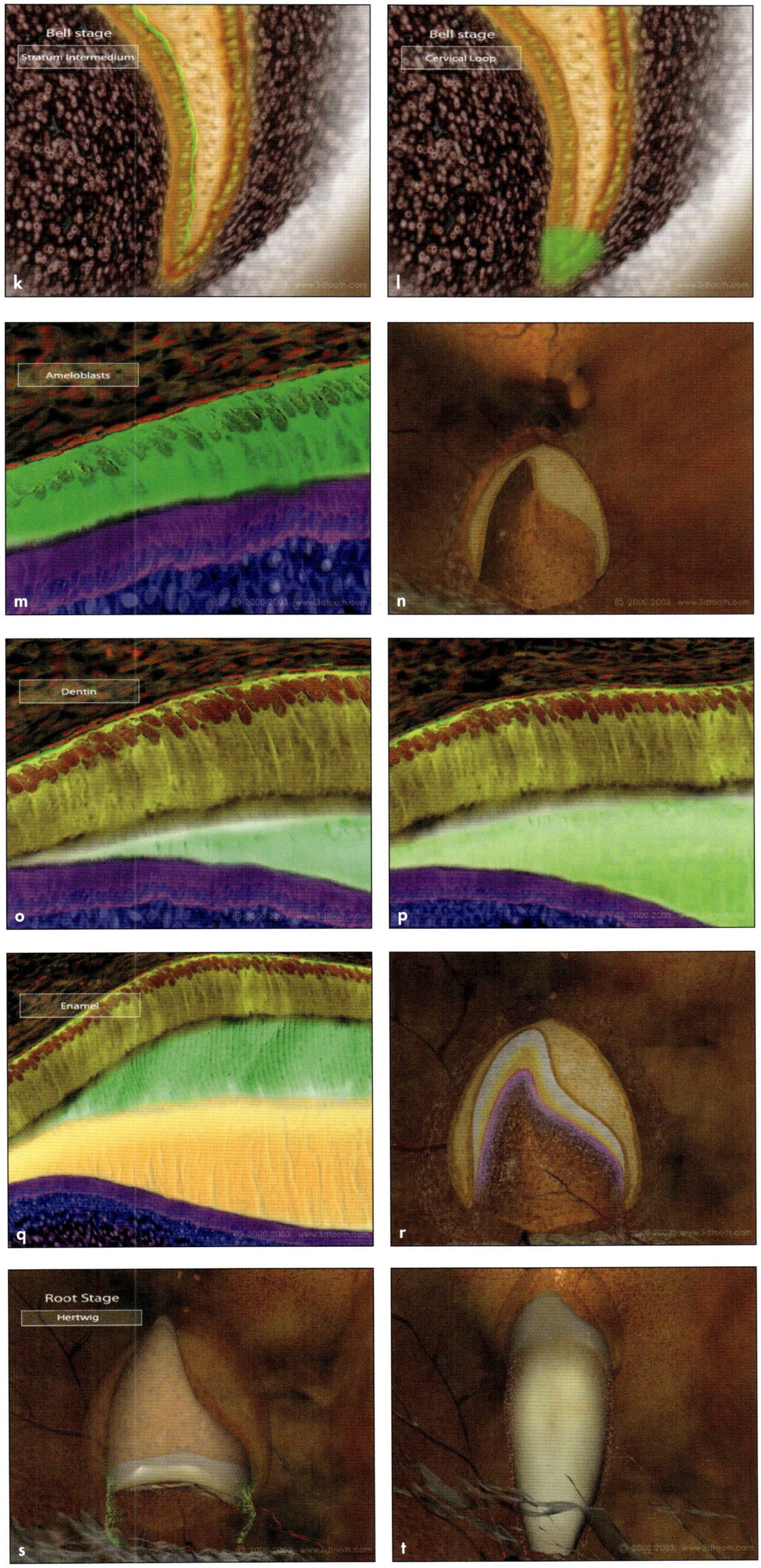

FIG 1-1 *(cont)* *(k)* A separate cell layer, the stratum intermedium, arises between the preameloblasts and the stellate reticulum. *(l)* At the edge of the cap, where the external layer becomes the inner lining, a cervical loop is formed. *(m)* Prior to the deposition of enamel and dentin, the basal membrane together with the preameloblast and preodontoblast layers have attained the form of the future crown. *(n)* Then the crown stage starts. *(o and p)* The preodontoblasts differentiate into odontoblasts that deposit the first dentin at the basal membrane. *(q)* Shortly thereafter, the preameloblasts differentiate into ameloblasts and begin to deposit enamel at the already formed dentin. The dentin is deposited in the direction of the basal membrane. During that process the odontoblasts migrate in the direction of the pulp, leaving odontoblastic processes behind in the dentinal tubules. The ameloblasts deposit enamel also in the direction of the basal membrane but do not leave processes behind. *(r)* The enamel deposition continues until the crown is completely formed. *(s)* After the crown is finished, root formation starts. The tissue of the cervical loop proliferates further in an apical direction and forms the epithelial stocking that is called the *Hertwig root sheath*. *(t)* Pulpal cells become arranged at the inner side of the Hertwig root sheath and differentiate to preodontoblasts and subsequently to odontoblasts, which will deposit the dentin of the root. With the outgrowth of the Hertwig root sheath, gaps appear in its cervical part. Mesenchymal cells of the tooth follicle migrate through these openings to the root surface. Thereafter they differentiate to precementoblasts and further to cementoblasts, which deposit cement against the dentin of the root. See video clip 1. (Printed from van der Linden et al[1] with permission.)

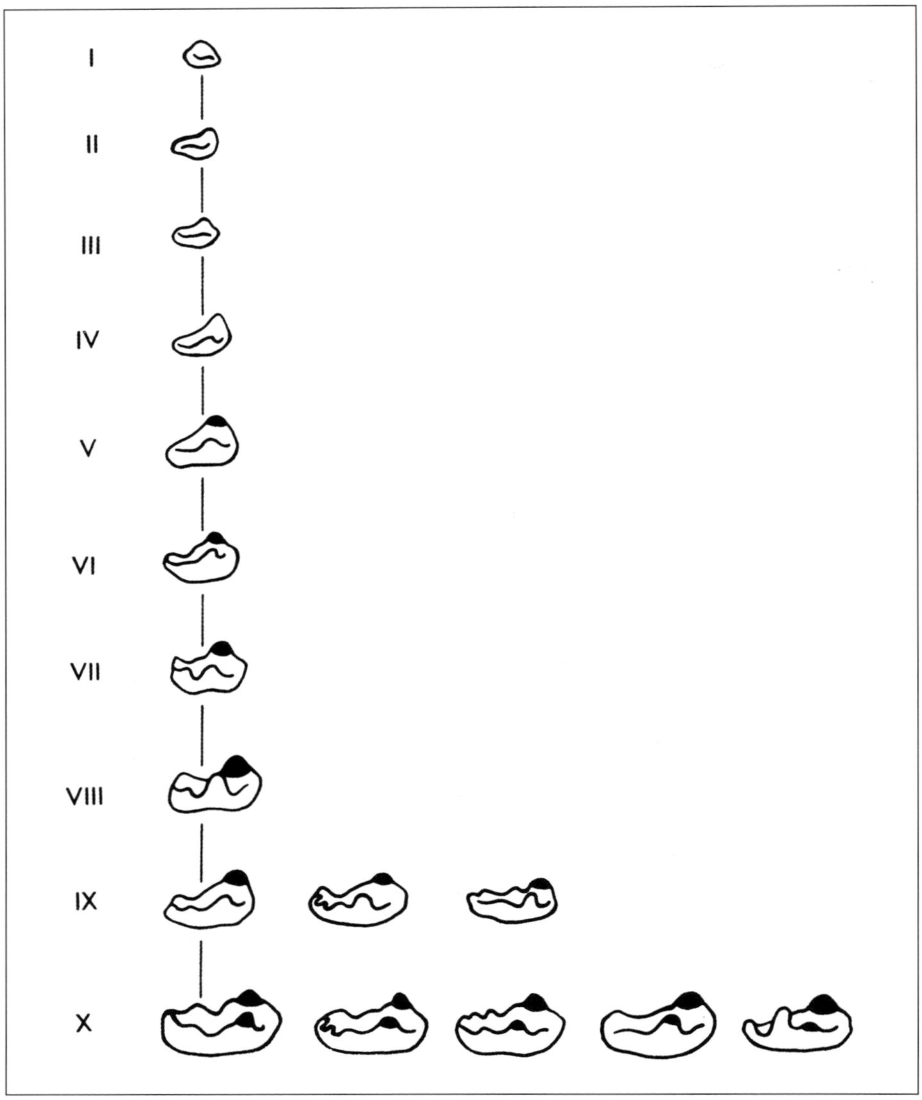

Fig 1-2 Development of the mandibular left first deciduous molar, subdivided in morphodifferential stages. From the first macroscopic indication of the formation of the molar, growth and morphodifferentiation occur (stage I). Mineralization at the first point starts at stage V, at the second point at stage X. Between stages V and X, the size of the future tooth crown increases substantially. The distances between the cusp tips continue to enlarge. From stage IX onward, individual differences in morphodifferentiation occur, resulting in variations in the morphology of the completed crowns. (Reprinted from Kraus and Jordan[2] with permission.)

Morphogenesis of Teeth

The morphogenesis of incisors, canines, and molars is essentially the same. Only the timing and form vary.[2]

Forming molars gradually increase in size by interstitial growth of the inner enamel epithelium. Mineralization starts at one future cusp tip (Fig 1-2). In a genetically determined sequence, ameloblasts and odontoblasts differentiate at other future cusp tips, followed by mineralization. Areas that are not yet mineralized can still increase in size. After the mineralizing fields have become connected (ie, coalescence), the distance between the cusp tips involved cannot increase further. Enamel deposition continues in the valleys between the cusp tips and at the circumference of the crown. After the entire circumference of the occlusal part of the crown is mineralized, only deposition of enamel at the circumference of the crown contributes to the increase in the mesiodistal and buccolingual dimensions (Figs 1-3 and 1-4).

The mineralization of incisors starts almost simultaneously at three locations and spreads horizontally. The mineralization of molars starts at the future cusp tips, one after the other with some time in between, and spreads under a sharp angle with the occlusal surface. Consequently, compared with molars, incisors establish more of their mesiodistal crown dimension at a relatively early stage. Subsequently, they only become wider by approximal enamel deposition.

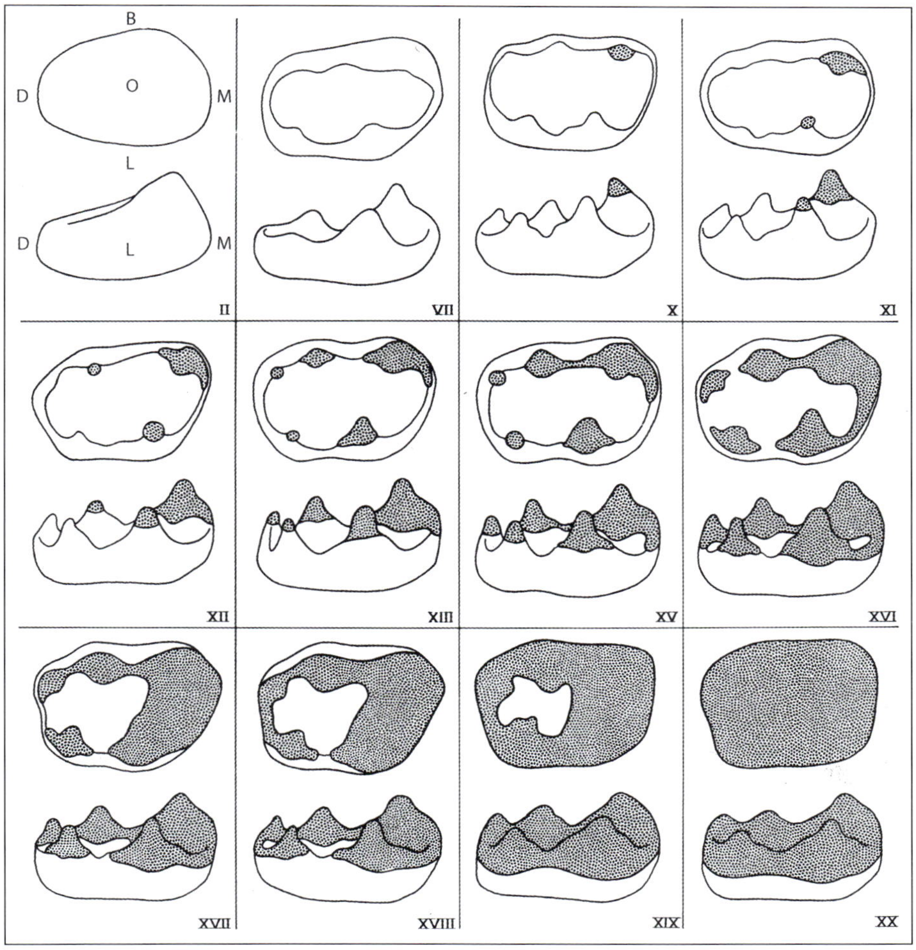

Fig 1-3 Changes in the morphology and the start and extension of the mineralization of a mandibular left second deciduous molar. All stages are presented at the same size, which obscures increases in dimensions (although they are comparable with those of the first deciduous molar in Fig 1-2). Mineralization of the second deciduous molar starts at stage X. In comparison with the first deciduous molar, morphodifferentiation has progressed considerably prior to the formation of predentin and enamel. At stage XV, the first coalescence takes place. At stage XVI, the mesial marginal ridge is established. At stage XVII, the distances between the distolingual, mesiolingual, and distobuccal cusp tips can still increase. At stage XVIII, the coalescence has progressed to the extent that the distances between the cusp tips cannot enlarge anymore. At stage XIX, the coalescence is established around the entire circumference of the occlusal part of the crown. At stage XX, the occlusal surface is fully mineralized. After stage XVIII, the circumference of the crown can increase only by apposition of enamel at its circumference. D, distal; B, buccal; O, occlusal; L, lingual; M, mesial. (Reprinted from Kraus and Jordan[2] with permission.)

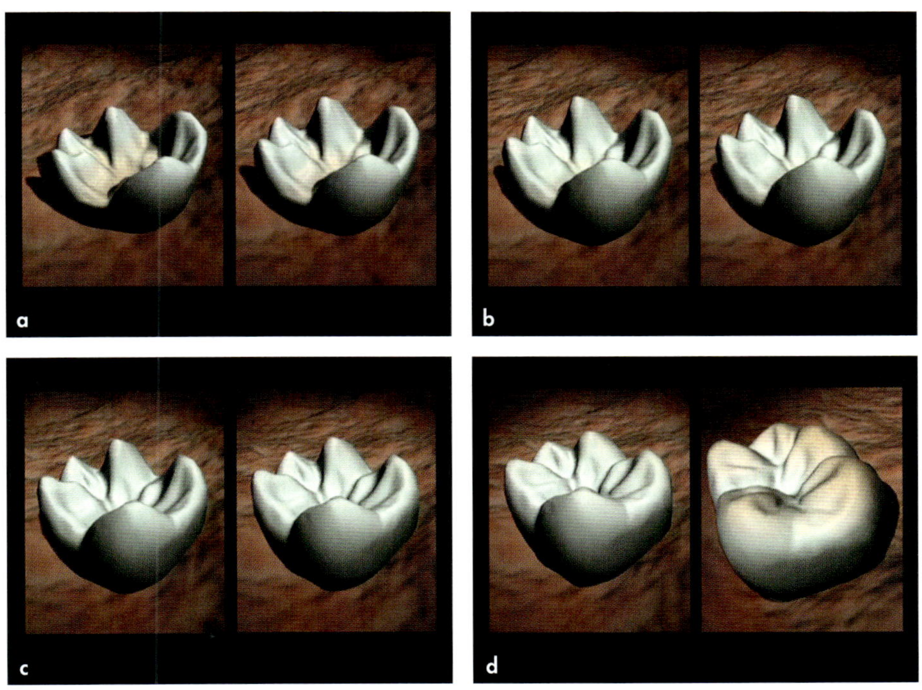

Fig 1-4 Formation of a mandibular first permanent molar observed from different directions. *(a and b)* Mineralization starts at the mesiobuccal cusp, followed successively by the other cusps. In the meantime, the slopes between the cusps become less steep. *(c and d)* Enamel is also deposited at the circumference of the crown, resulting in a slight increase in the mesiodistal and buccolingual dimensions. See video clip 2. (Printed from Van der Linden et al[3] with permission.)

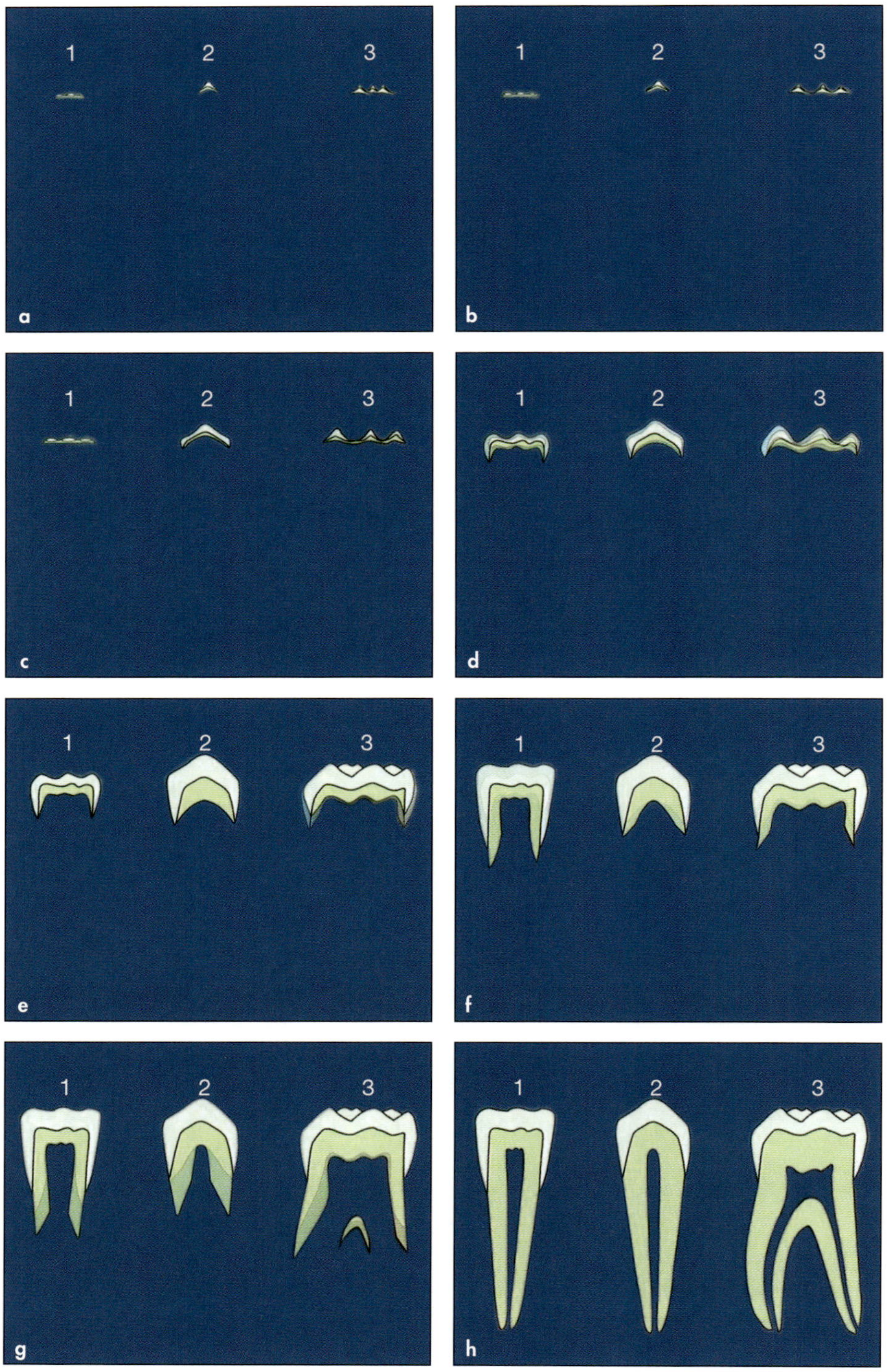

Fig 1-5 Formation of three permanent teeth. *(a and b)* The mineralization of an incisor (1) starts at the middle of the incisal edge and shortly thereafter at two other locations more to the distal and mesial (the future mamelons). *(c and d)* The mineralization spreads parallel with the incisor edge, soon resulting in coalescence. *(e and f)* In that way, a substantial part of the mesiodistal crown dimension is realized early. *(g and h)* After the crown is completed, the root is formed. *(a and b)* The mineralization of a canine (2) starts at one point and spreads under an oblique angle. *(c and d)* A large part of its mesiodistal crown dimension is realized early. *(e and f)* A canine reaches the stage at which the width increase becomes limited to approximal enamel deposition later than an incisor does. The root formation starts. *(g and h)* The pulp cavity becomes smaller by dentin deposition at the pulp chamber and the inner surface of the root. *(a and b)* The mineralization of a molar (3) starts at the mesiobuccal cusp and some time later at the other cusps. *(c and d)* The occlusal dimension of the crown increases until overall coalescence is attained. *(e and f)* The slopes between the cusps become flattened by enamel deposition. The circumference of the crown increases somewhat. *(g and h)* In multirooted teeth, the bi- or trifurcation appears. See video clips 3 to 6. (Printed from Van der Linden et al[3] with permission.)

Mineralization of canines starts at a single point. Their morphodifferentiation and mineralization lag behind that of the incisors and molars. The mineralization of canines spreads under an angle of about 45 degrees with the long axis of the future tooth. The increase in mesiodistal crown width occurs more slowly in canines than in incisors. Due to the differences in crown formation, the mesial and distal demarcations of deciduous molars and canines are reached at about the same time, week 28 after conception; in incisors, this occurs in week 20 (Fig 1-5).

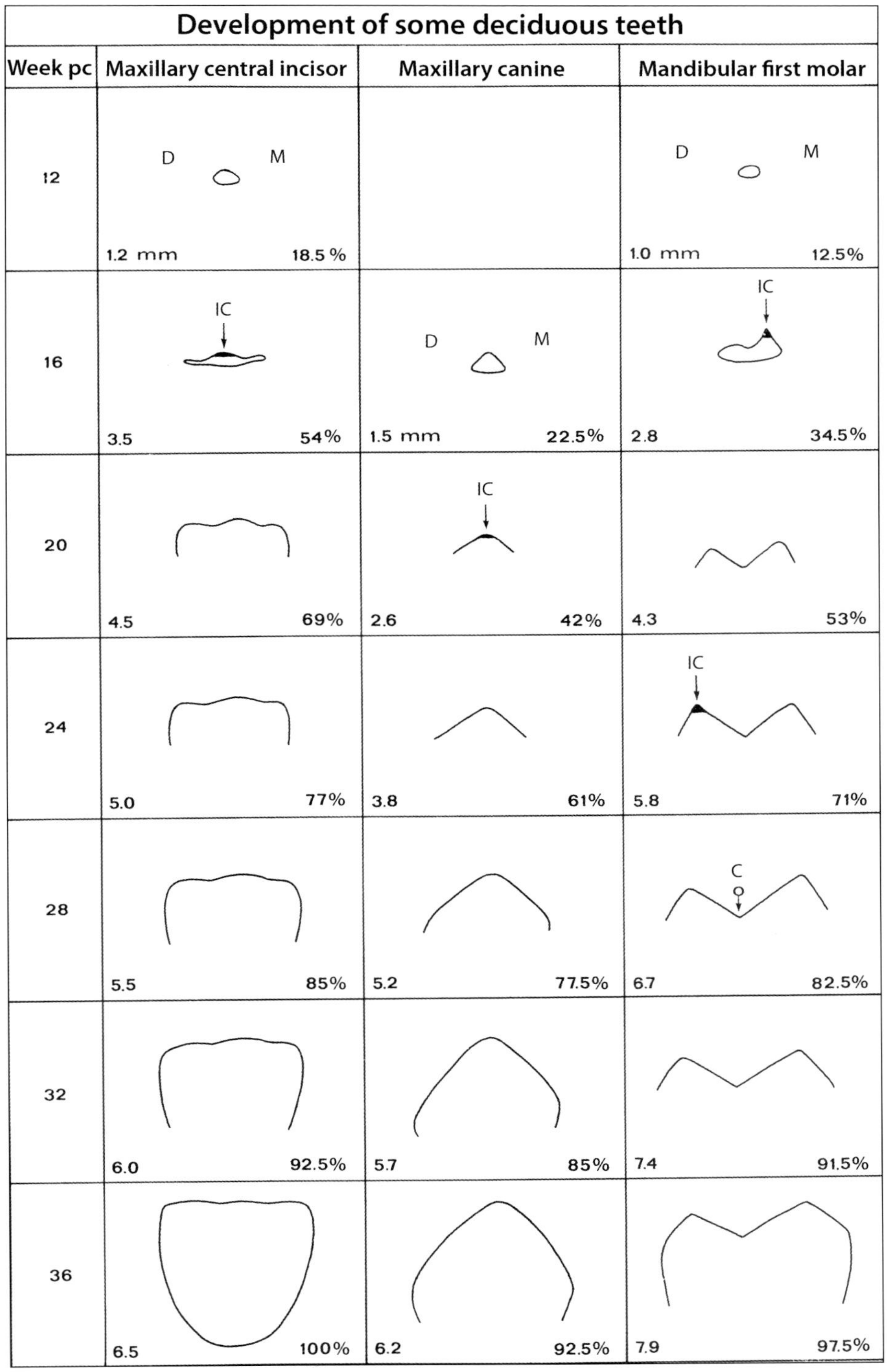

FIG 1-6 Comparison of the enlargement of three deciduous teeth expressed in millimeters and percentages of the final width. The mineralization of the maxillary incisor starts in the 16th week postconception (pc) and is somewhat earlier than that in the mandibular first molar. The mesiodistal dimension of the incisor tooth bud is at that time 3.5 mm, which is 54% of its ultimate size. The corresponding values for the molar are 2.8 mm and 34.5%. In week 20, the formation of the incisor has proceeded to the extent that increase in crown width can only be realized by approximal enamel deposition. The canine starts to mineralize in week 20. Regarding the mesiodistal dimensions, the values reached in week 20 for the incisor, canine, and molar, respectively, are 4.5 mm and 69%, 2.6 mm and 42%, and 4.3 mm and 53%. In week 24, the mineralization starts in the molar at the second point. In week 28, the first coalescence is attained, and the canine has extended to the mesial and distal sides. From that moment on, increase of its crown width is realized only by approximal enamel deposition. D, distal; M, mesial; IC, initial calcification; C, coalescence. (Data from Kraus and Jordan[2] and Van der Linden et al.[4])

The increases in mesiodistal crown dimensions of a maxillary central incisor, maxillary canine, and mandibular first molar of the deciduous dentition are illustrated and compared numerically in Fig 1-6. Development of the incisor is clearly ahead of that of the two other teeth.

The mineralization of the mandibular deciduous teeth in five specimens at increasing developmental stages is presented in Fig 1-7. This figure also shows the relative sizes of the forming teeth within one specimen.

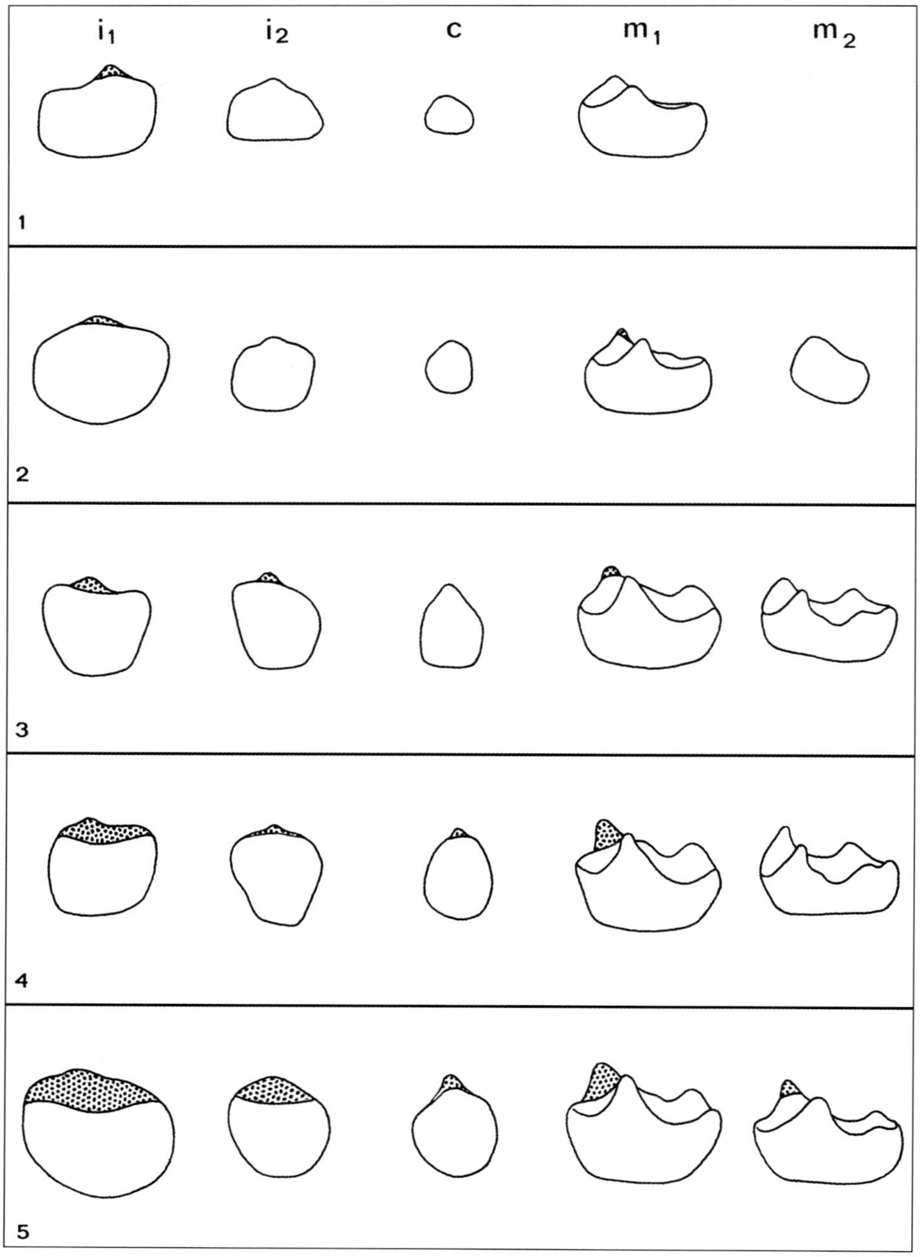

Fig 1-7 Mineralization of mandibular deciduous teeth. This illustration is based on five specimens at successive levels of development. The central incisor (i_1) is the first tooth that starts to mineralize, followed by the mesiobuccal cusp of the first molar (m_1). Subsequently, mineralization begins in the lateral incisor (i_2), the canine (c), and the second molar (m_2). All five teeth are mineralizing prior to the appearance of the second mineralization point in the first molar. The differences in size of the tooth buds in the separate series go back to the differential increase of dimensions in the five teeth. In assessing the five series, one must realize that differences in the ultimate size of corresponding teeth would have come about if their development had not stopped. These differences are not related to the level of development but based on the fact that some children have larger teeth than others. (Reprinted from Kraus and Jordan[2] with permission.)

Basic Properties of Teeth

Teeth have some typical properties. They are composed of the hardest tissues of the body. That applies particularly to the enamel. In comparison with other tissues, enamel and dentin are formed very slowly. For example, the mineralization of the first permanent molar starts before birth. When it emerges at 6 years of age, its root is not yet completely formed.

Deciduous teeth are formed more quickly than permanent teeth. The first deciduous tooth emerges at 6 months of age, the first permanent one at 6 years. A deciduous incisor has only slightly more than 1 year for its formation, while a permanent incisor has almost 7 years (see chapter 17 for details).

In accordance with the differences in time of their formation, deciduous and permanent teeth differ in composition and particularly in the density of enamel. The mineralization level of deciduous teeth is lower than that of permanent ones.[5] They have a whiter color (hence the name *milk teeth*), while permanent teeth have darker and yellower crowns. Because of the lower mineralization level, deciduous crowns are more susceptible to wear than are permanent ones. Deciduous molars lose their sharp cusp tips early.

In contrast to other tissues of the body, teeth cannot repair naturally. The parts of enamel and dentin lost by trauma or decay cannot be replaced. Enamel no longer can be deposited after the crown is completely formed. However, secondary dentin formation can continue on the pulpal side.

Tooth Positions During Development

Insight into the differences in the development of incisors, canines, and molars and of the deciduous and permanent teeth is essential for the understanding of the complex process of the development of the dentition. It is otherwise difficult to comprehend that deciduous and permanent incisors are formed in overlapping positions and that deciduous molars are formed one behind the other, without spatial limitations. On the other hand, second and third permanent molars are formed in a region where not enough space exists prior to the completion of jaw growth for them to be arranged one behind the other; therefore, they overlap.

References

1. Van der Linden FPGM, McNamara JA Jr, Radlanski RJ. Dynamics of Orthodontics: Facial Growth [DVD 2A]. Berlin: Quintessence, 2004.
2. Kraus BS, Jordan RE. The Human Dentition Before Birth. Philadelphia: Lea & Febiger, 1965.
3. Van der Linden FPGM, Radlanski RJ, McNamara JA Jr. Dynamics of Orthodontics: Normal Development of the Dentition [DVD 3A]. Berlin: Quintessence, 2000.
4. Van der Linden FPGM, McNamara JA Jr, Burdi AR. Tooth size and position before birth. J Dent Res 1972;51:71–74.
5. Schumacher GH, Schmidt H. Anatomie und Biochemie der Zähne. Berlin: VEB Verlag Volk und Gesundheit, 1972.

2

Jaw Growth During Formation and Eruption of Deciduous Teeth

Growth of the Body

The form and proportions of the body of a newborn are attuned to the functioning of the systems that are of vital importance. The head, with the neurocranium housing the central nervous system, and the trunk, containing the cardiovascular system and the respiratory and digestive tracts, dominate the other parts of the body. The arms and legs are small; the neck is short. The child grows and learns quickly during the first years of life. The brain operates as that of a scientist and absorbs and digests a tremendous amount of information.[1] The body develops further so it can function on a broader scale. The child learns to walk and speak and acquires many other skills. In the meantime, body proportions alter, which continues at a decreasing rate until adulthood is reached.

In general, the body grows gradually. There is extensive growth during the first years and a growth spurt during the juvenile and adolescent years (Fig 2-1). During puberty, the physical and mental development occurs more in spurts than evenly. Successively, various parts of the body experience a growth spurt, starting with the extremities, with the separate parts of the extremities also experiencing individual growth spurts. For example, the sequence of the short periods of rapid growth for the leg is: the foot, then the lower leg, and finally the upper leg. After the fast growth of the extremities, the hip and chest width increase rapidly, followed by the shoulder width (boys) and finally the rump length and chest depth.[3,4] Last, the mandible experiences a growth spurt, in boys more than in girls.[5,6]

Growth of the Head

Alterations in proportions occur in the head also. In the newborn, the splanchnocranium comprises only a small part of the total head, while the neurocranium, more than any other part of the body, has already realized a substantial portion of its ultimate size. In the first years, the neurocranium grows considerably, and at 6 years of age 90% of the ultimate size is reached. The proportion between the sizes of neuro- and splanchnocranium starts to alter shortly after birth. The splanchnocranium exceeds the neurocranium in growth (Fig 2-2). In the neonatus, the parts of the head that contain the brain and eyes are larger in relation to the structures situated inferior to them than they are at a later stage (Fig 2-3). In a 7-month-old fetus, the neurocranium and eye sockets have attained more of their adult dimensions than the maxilla and mandible. The piriform aperture is still situated mainly between the eyes and the nasal floor that is close to the inferior border of the eye sockets. The morphology of the maxilla and mandible is determined greatly by the tooth buds (Figs 2-4 and 2-5).

As is the case for the body as a whole, the proportions of the neonatal head are based on the functions of vital importance directly after birth—breathing and food consumption. Consequently, within the splanchocranium itself, proportional changes occur also. A nursing child has to be able to breathe and swallow simultaneously, to which the anatomy and physiology is adapted. Erupted teeth are undesirable at that stage because they are a hindrance in breast-feeding. Very rarely (less than 1 in 1,000 births), small mandibular anterior teeth are present at birth, called *natal teeth*. They can also emerge in the following month, in which case they are called *neonatal teeth*. If these teeth damage the tongue of the child or the feeding breast, removal can be considered. This measure has no negative effects on the development of the dentition.[8,9]

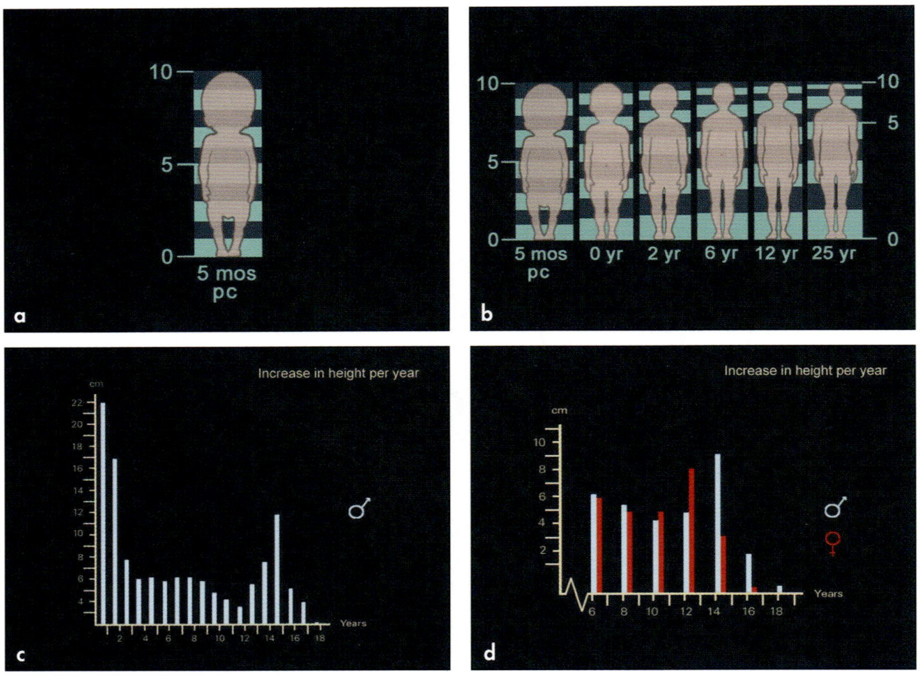

Fig 2-1 Alterations in body proportions and in velocity of growth from the 5th month postconception (pc) until adulthood. *(a and b)* The head of the newborn constitutes about one-quarter of the total body length, the trunk almost half of it. These values are, respectively, at 6 years 16% and 42%, at 12 years 14% and 40%, and in the adult 12% and 33%.[2] *(c)* The increase in the total body length (stature) shows rapid growth in the first year, somewhat less in the second year, and an acceleration during adolescence. *(d)* Boys have a later-occurring adolescent growth spurt and a larger and longer-lasting one than girls.[3]

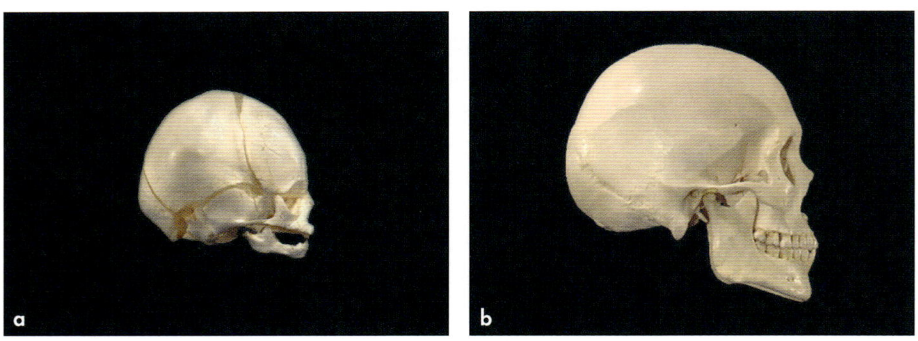

Fig 2-2 Proportional change of the skull. *(a)* In a newborn, the neurocranium is large in comparison with the splanchnocranium. *(b)* In an adult, the splanchnocranium has become much larger, and the neurocranium does not dominate anymore.

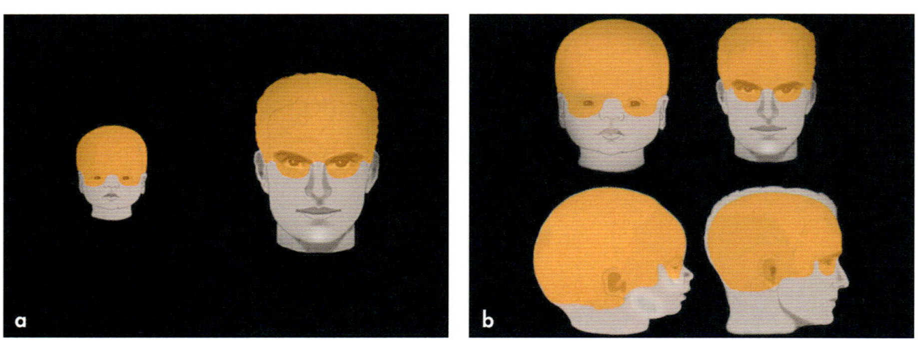

Fig 2-3 Proportional change of the head. In these illustrations, the brain and the eyes are colored orange. *(a)* From birth until adulthood, the face grows more than the rest of the head. Images show actual proportions. *(b)* Head of the newborn enlarged to adult dimensions.

Figure 2-6a shows the reconstruction of the face of a fetus of 9 weeks in which various structures are specified by color. The formation of the splanchnocranium starts early. In week 12 after conception, part of the splanchnocranium is already calcified, and rapid formation of cartilage structures, which later will be transformed into bone, takes place. In contrast to bone, cartilage has the potential for interstitial growth and hence can increase in size rapidly (Fig 2-6b). After calcification has occurred, bone can only increase by apposition at surfaces.

FIG 2-4 Skull of a 7-month-old fetus. *(a and b)* The neurocranium and the eye sockets constitute a large part of the skull. The jaws have developed little. *(c and d)* The mandible has a diminutive ramus and a small ridge at the lower border with a broad portion above that contains the tooth buds.

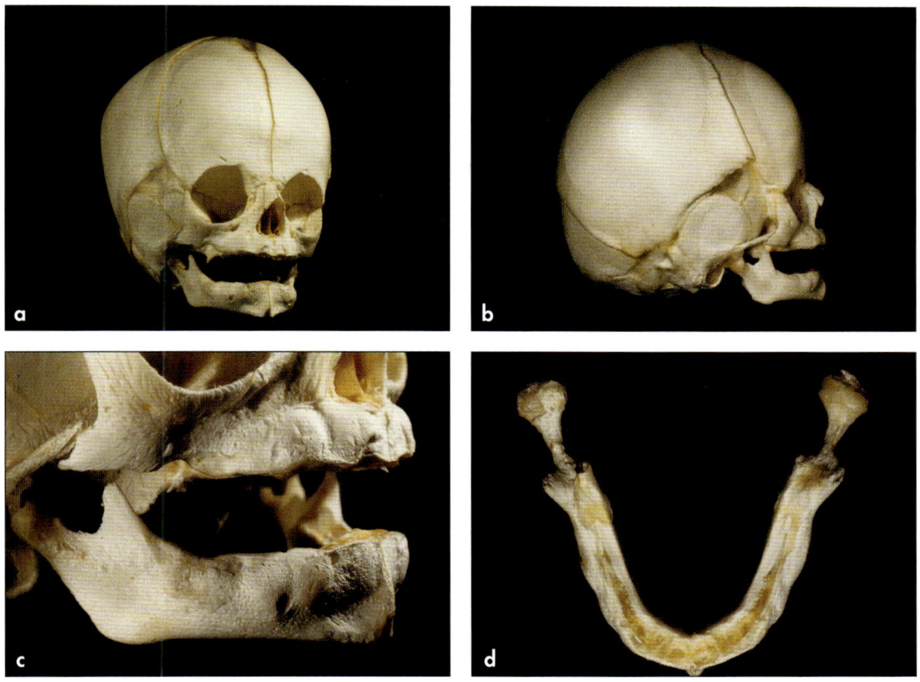

FIG 2-5 Skull of a newborn. The bony structures below the eye sockets have undergone little development. *(a and b)* The floor of the piriform aperture is slightly inferior to the lower ridge of the eye sockets. There is also little vertical development of the jaws. The mandible still exists in two halves, left and right, with the symphysis in between. *(c and d)* The morphology of the tooth-bearing parts of the jaws reflects the location, size, and shape of the tooth buds. In this stage, the jaws do not make contact during swallowing and closing; the tongue lies in between.[7]

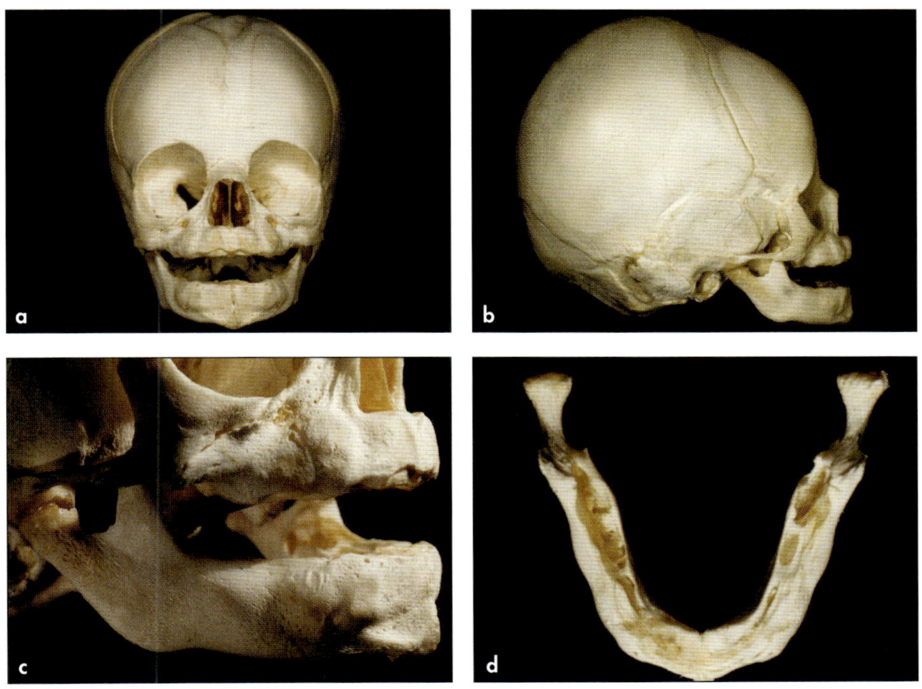

Growth of the Jaws

As previously indicated, the jaws of the newborn are small in comparison with the rest of the head. In addition, the mandible is posteriorly positioned in relation to the maxilla. In the first months after birth, the parts of the jaws that contain the tooth buds grow considerably.

Furthermore, during the first year after birth, the mandible attains a more anterior position than the maxilla. The sagittal relation of the jaws approaches the situation of the complete deciduous dentition.[11–15] More space is available for the formation of the deciduous molars than for the deciduous incisors. The jaws are narrower in the anterior than the posterior regions (Fig 2-7). The deciduous incisors and canines are not formed in the orientation in which they will erupt because the spatial conditions do not allow it.

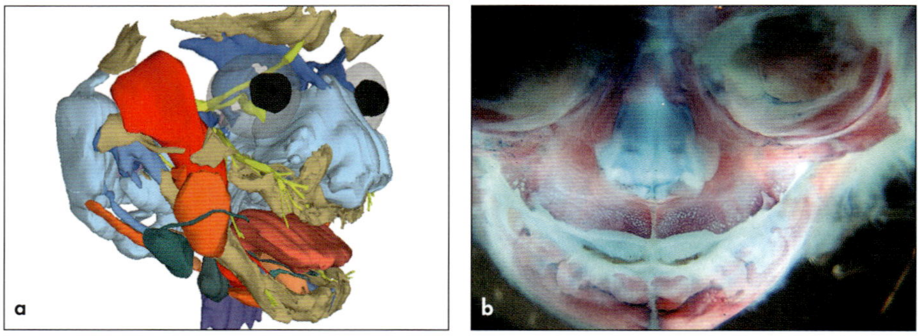

Fig 2-6 Model and specimen showing prenatal facial development. *(a)* Three-dimensional reconstruction of the face of a 9-week-old fetus, based on a series of histologic slides. (Illustration by R. R. Radlanski.) *(b)* In a 22-week-old fetus, bone is colored red and cartilage blue. The bone is more spongeous in the maxilla than in the mandible. (Printed from Van der Linden et al[10] with permission.)

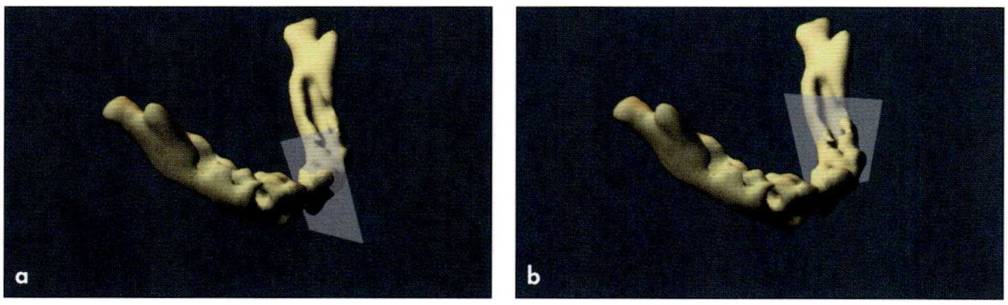

Fig 2-7 The mandible of a 20-week-old fetus. The mandible is narrow in the region where the incisors are formed *(a)* and broad where the molars develop *(b)*. (Printed from Van der Linden et al[10] with permission.)

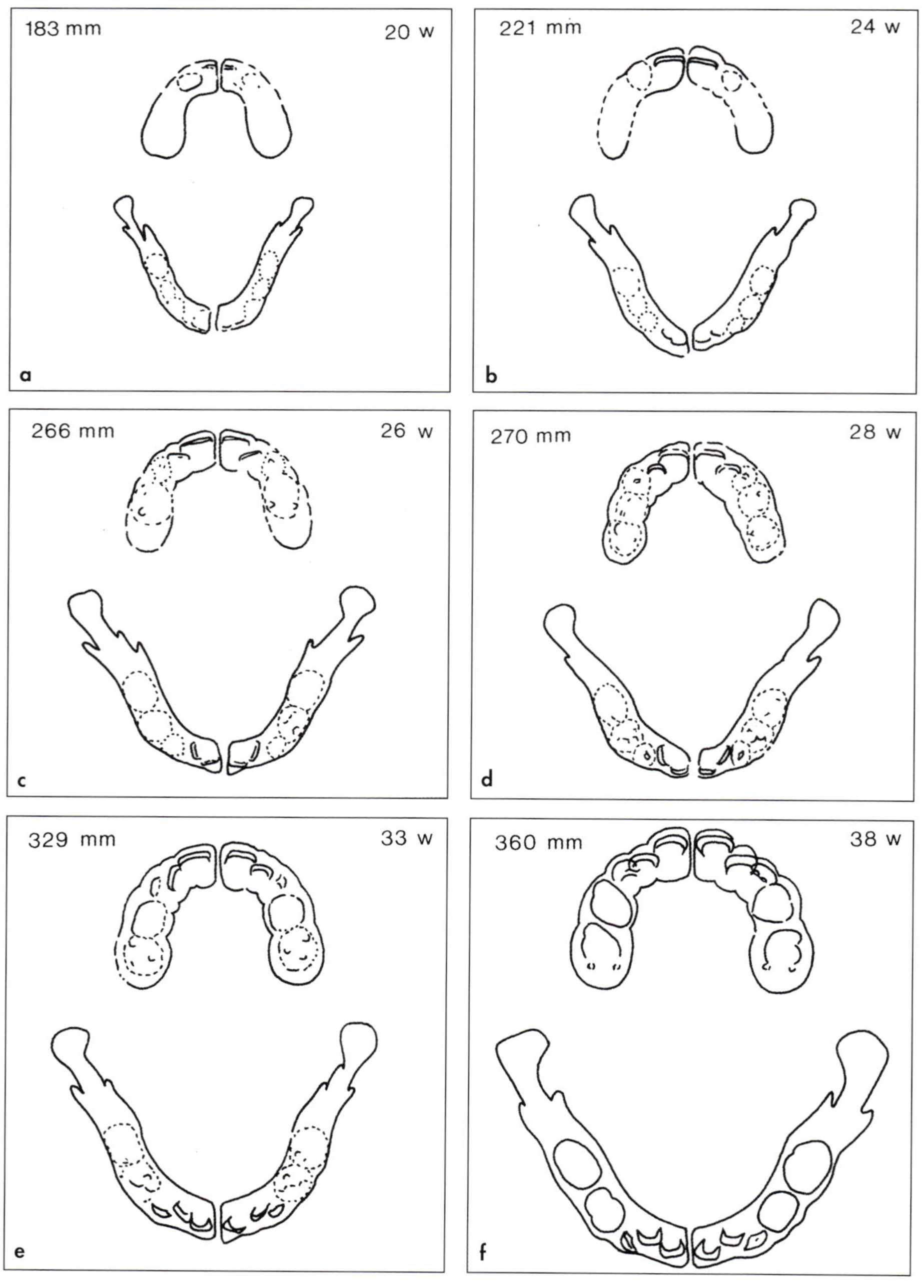

Fig 2-8 Tracings of radiographs of six sets of jaws of fetuses at increasing stages of development. The numbers in the drawings indicate the crown-rump length of the fetus in millimeters (mm) and the estimated age, expressed in weeks (w).[17] The tracings provide insight into the increase in size of the jaws as a whole and of the parts that contain the teeth. In all six specimens, the anterior teeth are rotated or overlap each other. The arrangement of the incisors varies among the jaws. Overlapping of first and second deciduous molars is not seen and does not occur.[18] When evaluating the drawings, one must keep in mind that if these six fetuses had survived, the individuals would have developed teeth and jaws of different sizes. One child will attain larger teeth and jaws than another. Hence, comparison of the dimensions in this figure has some limitations. (Reprinted from Van der Linden et al[16] with permission.)

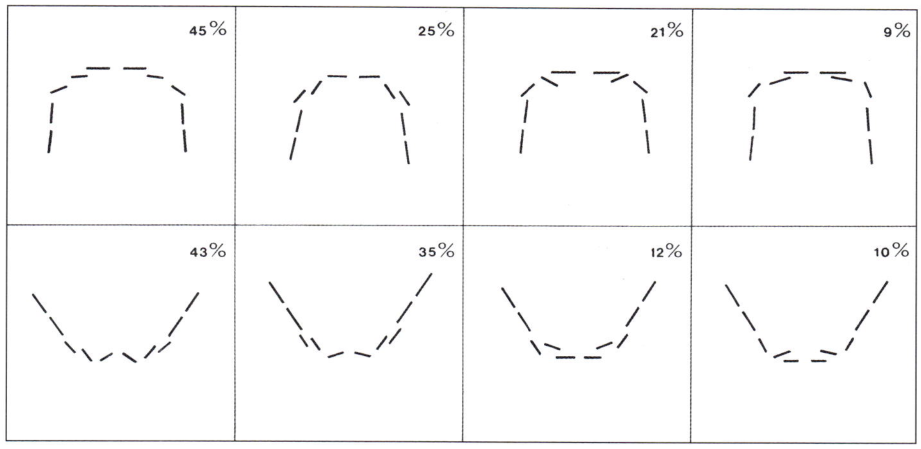

Fig 2-9 Position of teeth prior to birth. A radiographic investigation of the dissected jaws of 28 fetuses revealed for both jaws four patterns of arrangement of deciduous incisors. In all specimens, the maxillary central incisors were oriented perpendicular to the median plane. The frequency of occurrence of the different patterns is indicated in the figure. (Reprinted from Van der Linden et al[16] with permission.)

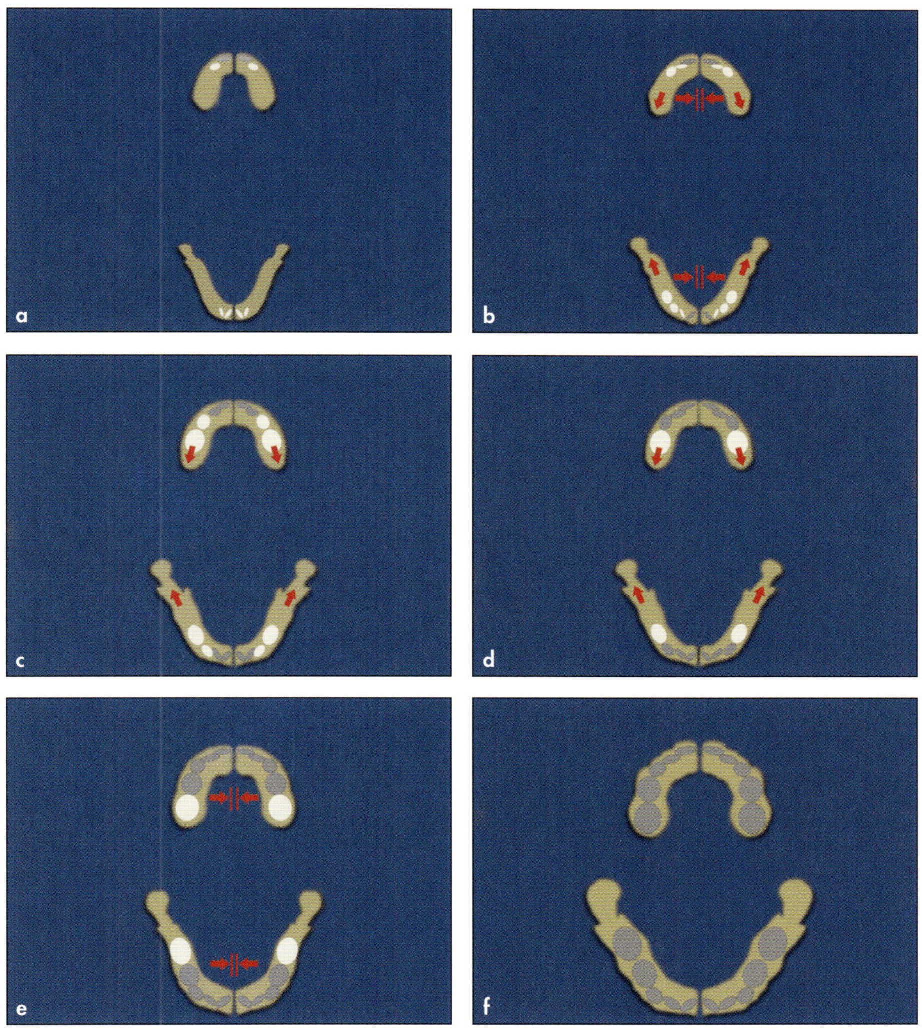

Fig 2-10 Occlusal overview of the relationship between jaw growth and tooth development. *(a)* Twenty weeks after conception, the jaws are small. The maxillary central deciduous incisors and the four mandibular deciduous incisors have started their mineralization. *(b)* The jaws become wider by bone formation in the median regions. *(c and d)* Growth to the posterior provides room for the gradually increasing and locally mineralizing molars. *(e)* The growth in the median regions is insufficient for an improvement in the position of the deciduous incisors. *(f)* In the newborn, the crowns of all deciduous teeth are completely or partially mineralized.

During the prenatal period and also some time after birth, the anterior teeth are rotated or overlapping.[16] Figure 2-8 shows tracings of radiographs of the jaws of six specimens with increasing levels of development. The arrangement of the anterior teeth is not the same in these six specimens. Variations exist in that respect as indicated in Fig 2-9. Prior to birth, the size of the anterior parts of the jaws does not increase much or any more than the sum of the widths of the crowns they contain.[16,19]

It is assumed that the rotated and overlapping arrangement of the anterior deciduous teeth does not change before birth because the space needed for this does not become available. This will occur in the first 6 months after birth (Fig 2-10).

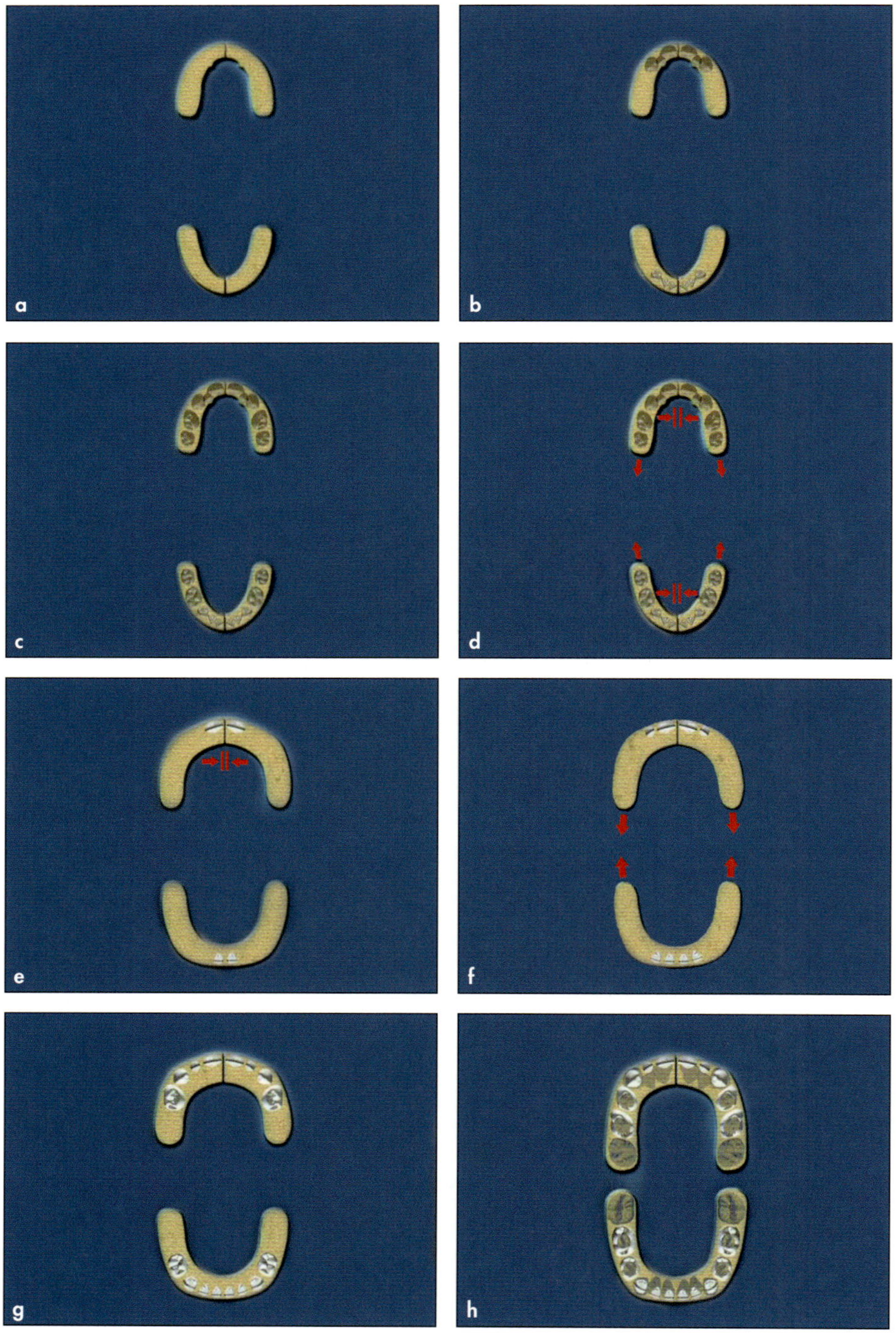

FIG 2-11 Overview of the dentition and jaws from birth to 3 years of age. *(a)* At birth, the jaws are still small. *(b)* In the anterior regions, the tooth buds are rotated or overlap each other. *(c)* Sufficient space is available for the forming deciduous molars. *(d)* From birth to 6 months of age, the jaws grow considerably in the median regions. Prior to emergence, sufficient room becomes available for the deciduous incisors to migrate mesially and attain a good position. *(e)* The mandibular symphysis ossifies prior to the eruption of the mandibular central deciduous incisors. Subsequently, no more transverse growth can occur in the median region of the mandible. The median suture in the maxilla maintains its growth potential until adulthood. *(f)* Both jaws continue to grow posteriorly, resulting in space for distal migration of the gradually developing deciduous molars. The jaws continue to increase in width by bone apposition at the surfaces. *(g)* Subsequent to the incisors, the first deciduous molars emerge, and occlusion becomes established. Some time later the deciduous canines appear. *(h)* In the meantime, the growth of the jaws to the posterior provides space for the second deciduous molars, which emerge about 1 year after the first ones. Further growth to the posterior provides space for the first permanent molars. The permanent incisors overlap each other and will not improve in position prior to emergence. The premolars have sufficient space within the jaws.

The median suture in the maxilla and the symphysis in the mandible provide the largest contribution to the early transverse development of the jaws. In the mandible, the effect is of short duration and terminates with the ossification of the symphysis, which happens 6 months after birth. However, the maxillary median suture continues to contribute to the transverse growth of the maxilla until the development of the dentition is completed.[20] After the deciduous molars have reached occlusion, the transverse growth of the maxilla is adjusted based on the width of the mandible. Indeed, development in the width of the maxilla depends on the shape and size of the mandibular dental arch. The growth potential of the median suture in the maxilla is realized only to a limited extent after the mandibular symphysis is ossified.

The size of the jaws increases to the extent that the deciduous incisors can attain a good position prior to emergence.[21] Indeed, irregular arrangement of deciduous teeth is rare. Sometimes an incomplete correction of a rotated incisor is seen even when sufficient space is available.

The development of the dentition from birth until the complete deciduous dentition stage is presented in Figs 2-11 and 2-12. After emergence, the eruption of deciduous teeth lasts about 6 months, with a rapid period of eruption in the first 3 months.[22] For times of emergence, tooth dimensions, and stages of root development, see chapter 17.

Fig 2-12 Jaw growth and emergence of deciduous teeth. *(a)* At birth, the jaws are relatively small. The deciduous incisors are rotated or overlap each other. The deciduous molars are arranged in the jaw, one after the other, with space in between. *(b)* In the first 6 months after birth, the jaws grow considerably. After calcification of the symphysis, the mandibular central deciduous incisors emerge. *(c)* A few months later, the maxillary central incisors emerge. *(d)* At around 1 year of age, the lateral deciduous incisors emerge, usually first in the maxilla. *(e)* Growth to the posterior provides space for the eruption of the deciduous molars. The first deciduous molars emerge around 16 months of age. *(f)* The deciduous canines emerge around 20 months. After the teeth are fully erupted, they change little in position and in intra-arch relationships. However, the mandibular teeth will gradually attain a slightly more anterior position in relation to the maxillary teeth because of the more forward growth of the mandible compared with the maxilla. *(g)* Between 24 and 30 months of age, the second deciduous molars are the final deciduous teeth to emerge. *(h)* In the overview of the complete deciduous dentition, their successors and the permanent first molars are drawn.

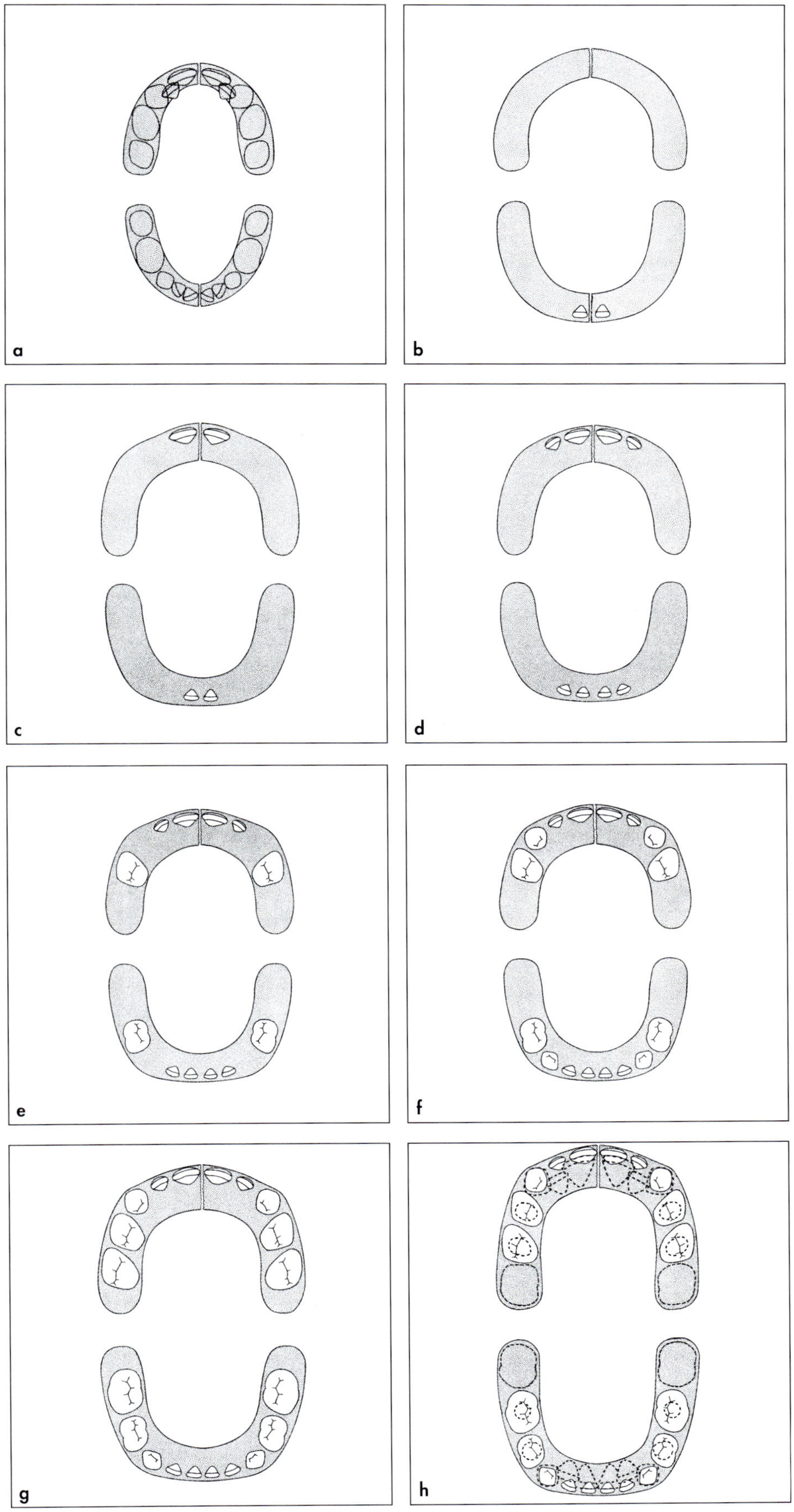

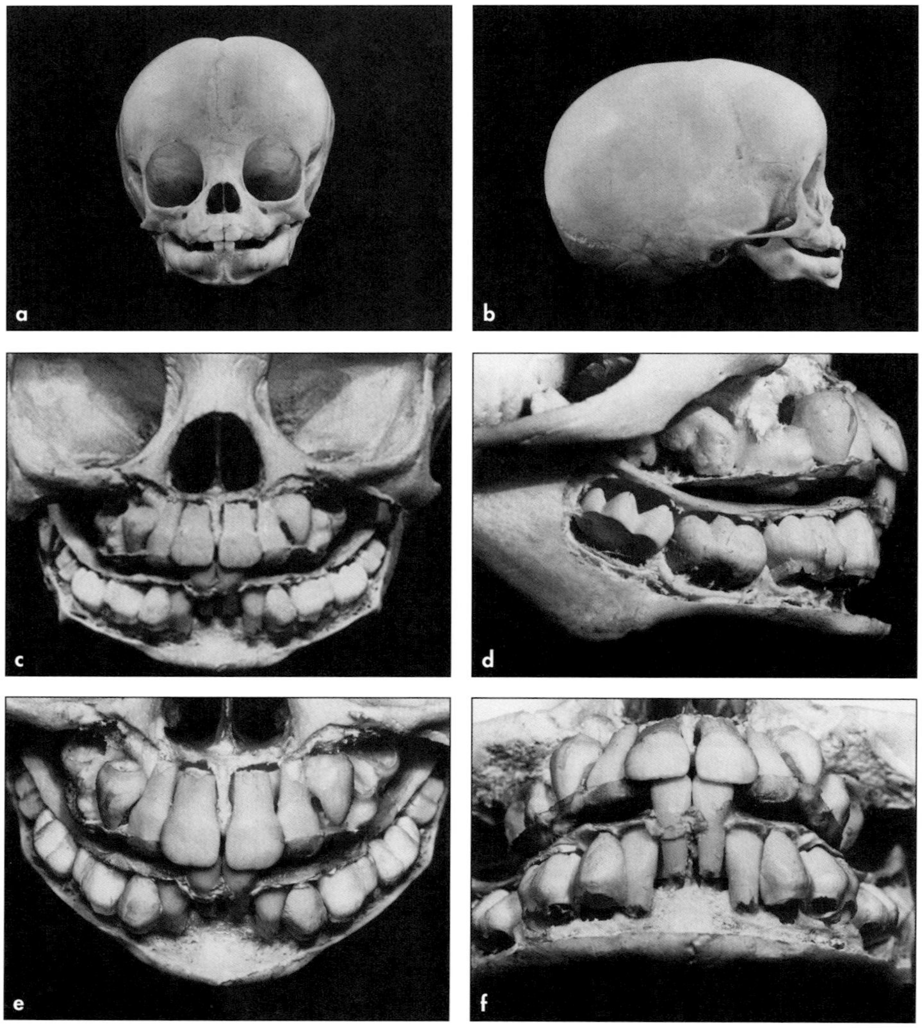

Fig 2-13 Skull at 8 months of age. *(a and b)* In comparison with the neurocranium, the tooth-bearing parts of the jaws are larger than in the prenatal and perinatal period. The ridge at the middle of the mandibular border is narrow. *(c)* The developing dentition completely fills the space between the eye sockets and nasal floor superiorly and the mandibular base inferiorly. The developing parts of the maxillary central deciduous incisors are located close to the nasal floor. *(d)* The occlusal surfaces of the not-yet-emerged mandibular deciduous teeth are oriented as a concave plane. The roots of the first deciduous molars are already partly formed. The crowns of the second deciduous molars are completely formed; those of the first permanent molars are half formed. The latter still have sharp cusp tips. *(e)* The incisal edges of the four maxillary deciduous incisors are at the same level with only the central emerged. The mandibular molars are located at a wider arch, ie, more buccally, than the maxillary molars. *(f)* The root formation of the lateral incisors lags behind that of the central incisors. The crowns of the mandibular molars are inclined lingually.

In Figs 2-13 to 2-15, the spatial orientation of the teeth is demonstrated in an 8-month-old skull. For that purpose, first the buccal alveolar bone is removed, then the anterior deciduous teeth, and finally the permanent teeth. In Figs 2-16 to 2-19, the same procedure is followed in a 6-year-old skull. In addition, the teeth are shown according to the original arrangement, seen from different directions.

FIG 2-14 After removal of the deciduous incisors and canines. *(a)* In the maxilla, the crowns of the central permanent incisors diverge. *(b)* Only a small part of the permanent canine crowns has formed. *(c and d)* In the mandible, the lateral permanent incisors are positioned to the lingual of the central incisors. The latter are at some distance apart. *(e and f)* After removal of the central permanent incisors, the position of the lateral permanent incisors becomes more visible.

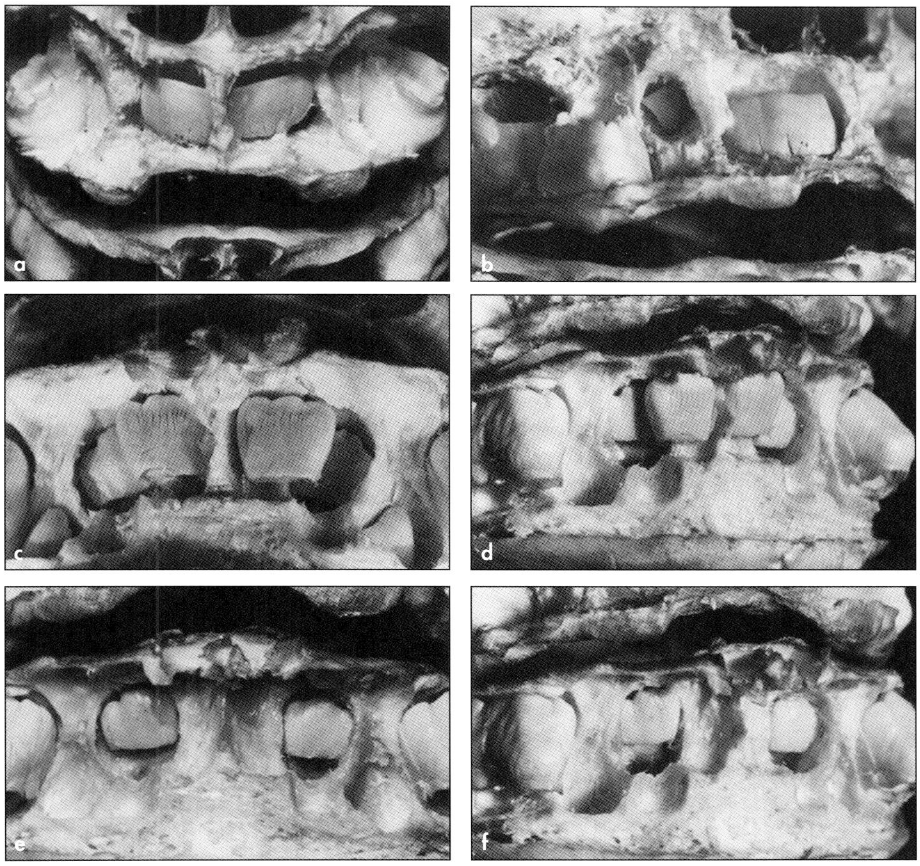

FIG 2-15 After removal of the anterior permanent teeth. *(a to d)* The morphology of the surrounding bone and the local thickness of the lingual walls vary, conforming to the size and position of the teeth they contain.

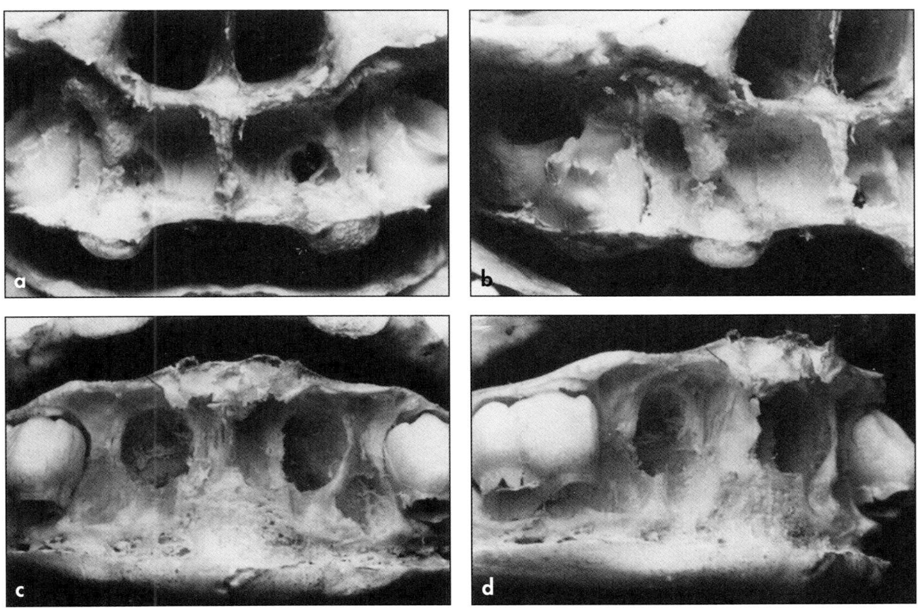

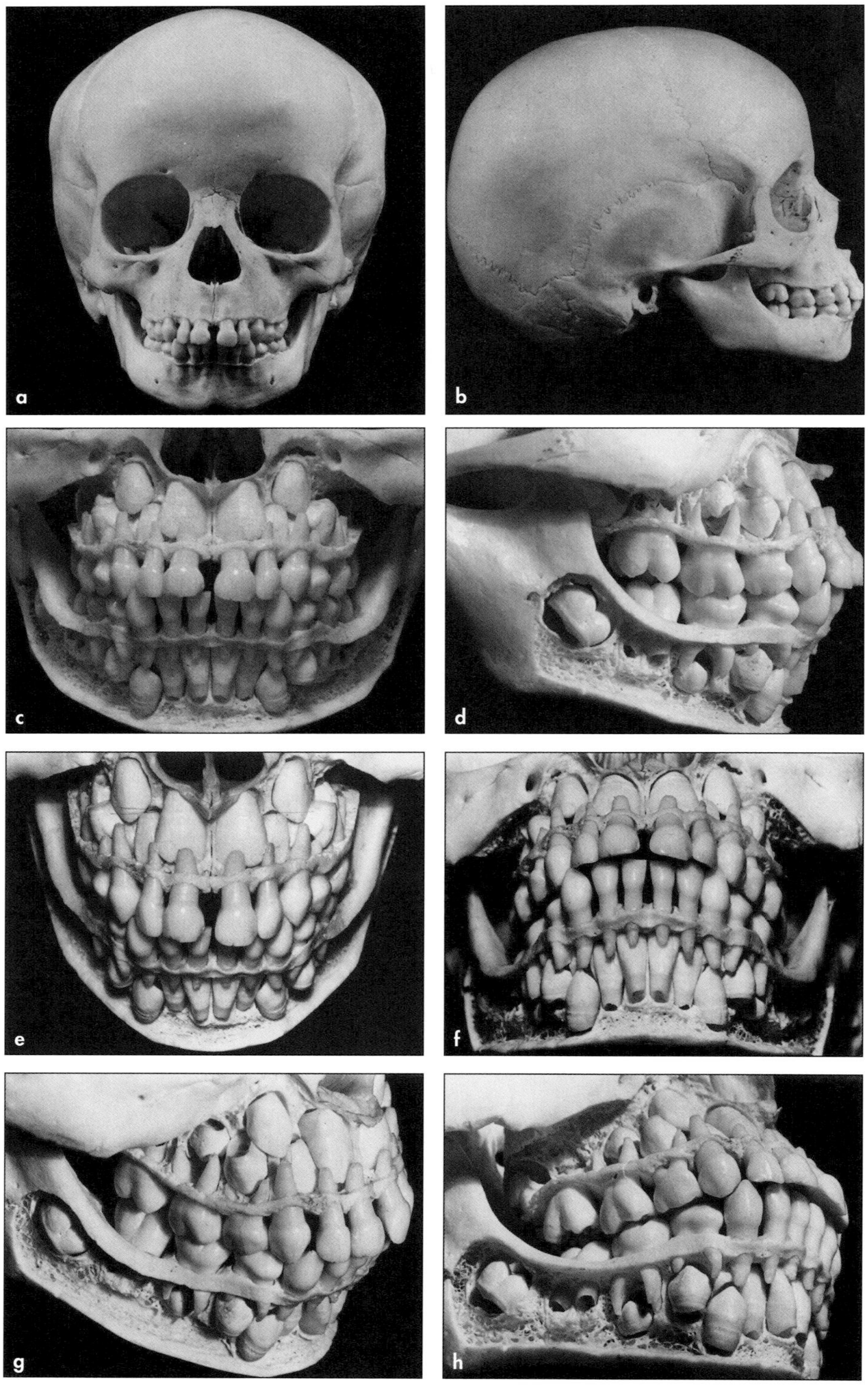

Fig 2-16 Skull at 6 years of age. *(a)* All deciduous teeth and the first permanent molars have emerged. In the preceding years, facial height had increased considerably. A solid broad mandibular border has developed. The nasal floor is now situated inferior to the lower margin of the eye sockets. *(b)* In this specimen, the deciduous incisors are labially inclined. Normally the deciduous incisors are in an upright position, perpendicular to the occlusal plane. *(c)* Also in this skull, the space between the nasal floor and the mandibular base is completely filled with teeth. *(d)* The space available for the permanent canines and premolars is more limited in the maxilla than in the mandible. *(e)* The root ends of the central and lateral deciduous incisors are slightly resorbed. The distoincisal corners of the central permanent incisors are situated close to the roots of the lateral deciduous incisors. *(f)* In the mandible, spaces are present between the deciduous incisors. The crowns of the permanent anterior teeth, except the maxillary central incisors, are close together. *(g)* The resorption pattern of the deciduous incisors reflects the contours of the crowns of their successors. Also, parts of the roots of adjacent deciduous teeth can resorb, as seen here at the maxillary lateral incisors. *(h)* In the mandible, the crowns of the permanent incisors are less labially inclined than in the maxilla. The bone at the cervical regions of the deciduous teeth is also resorbed.

The vertical changes in the jaws are related to the lengthening of permanent teeth, the resorption of the roots of deciduous teeth, and the increase in height of the facial skeleton. The relationship among the crowns of the permanent incisors and the roots of the deciduous incisors varies and depends on the conditions in the anterior parts of the jaws.

The relationship among the crowns of the permanent incisors and the roots of the deciduous teeth alters only little or not at all prior to the start of eruption of the permanent central incisors. The vertical orientation of the forming parts of the maxillary anterior permanent teeth exhibits a uniform pattern. The forming parts of the canines are by far the most superiorly located. Those of the lateral incisors are situated most inferiorly. Those of the central incisors are about halfway between those of the lateral incisors and canines.

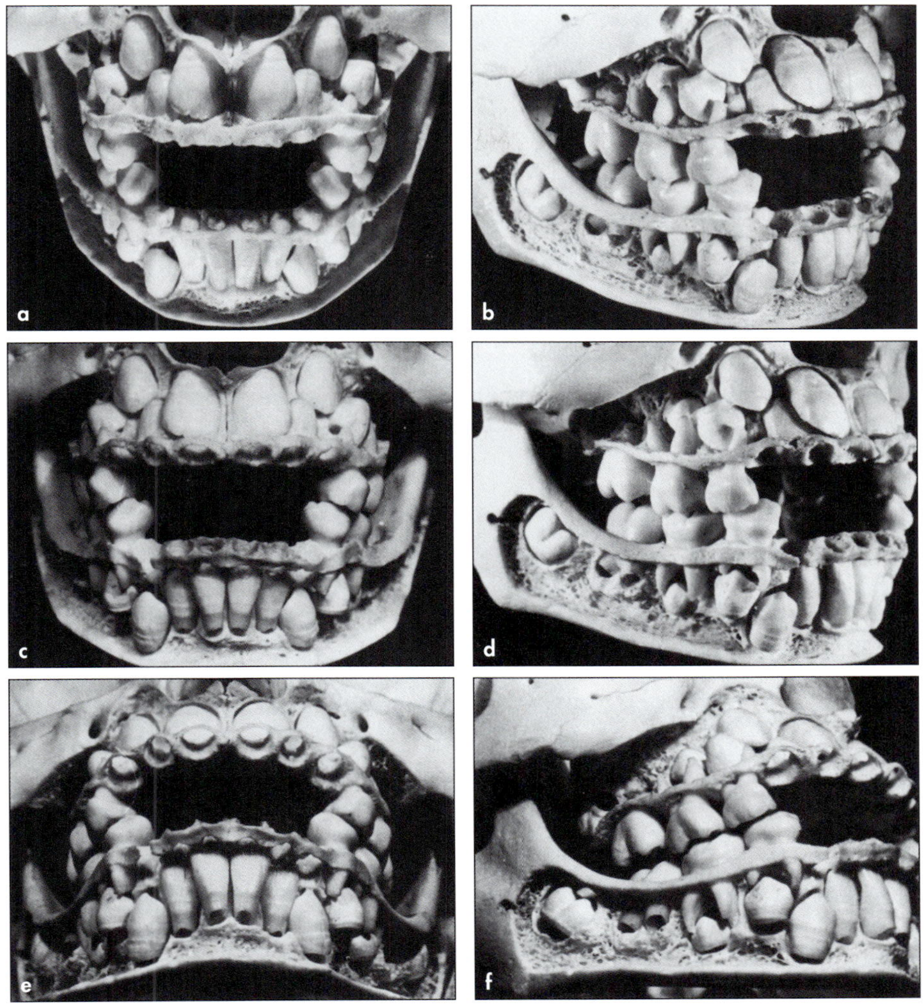

FIG 2-17 After removal of the deciduous incisors and canines. *(a to f)* The position of the permanent incisors and canines is now more visible. It is obvious that the incisal margins of the maxillary lateral incisors are positioned more occlusally than those of the central incisors.

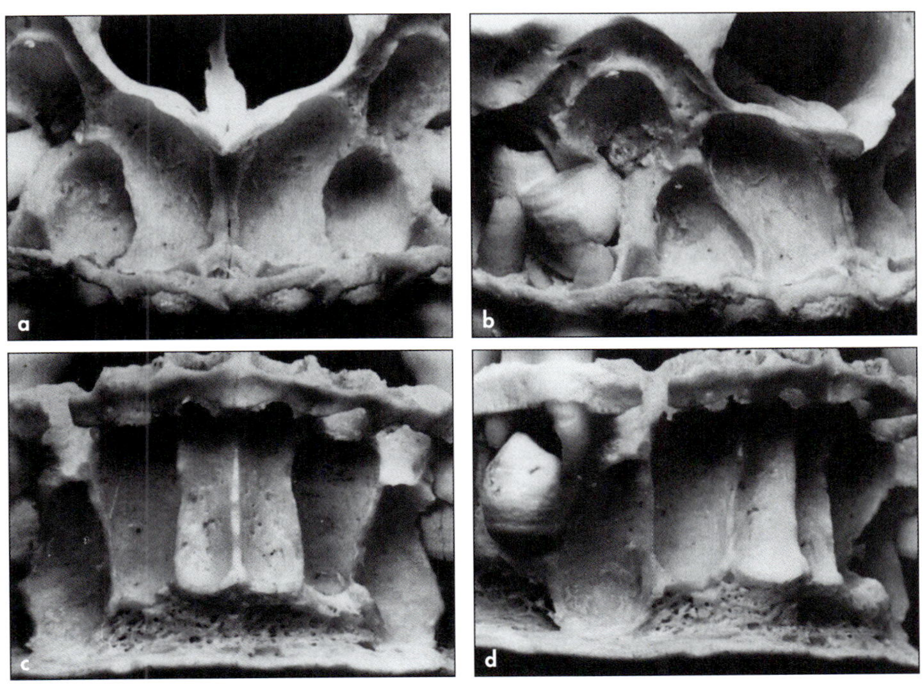

FIG 2-18 After removal of the anterior permanent teeth. *(a to d)* The structure and morphology of the alveolar bone that surrounds the teeth on the lingual side is now visible, as is the relationship between the nasal floor and the bone that surrounds the permanent teeth on the superior side. The difference in height level of the bone at the incisal margins of the mandibular permanent incisors demonstrates that the central incisors are positioned more to the occlusal than are the lateral incisors.

The size, shape, and structure of the mandible vary. That applies also to the mandibular border, the chin prominence, and the space available for teeth. Regarding the last aspect, the location where the formation of the permanent canines starts (which is the eventual location of their apices) is essential.

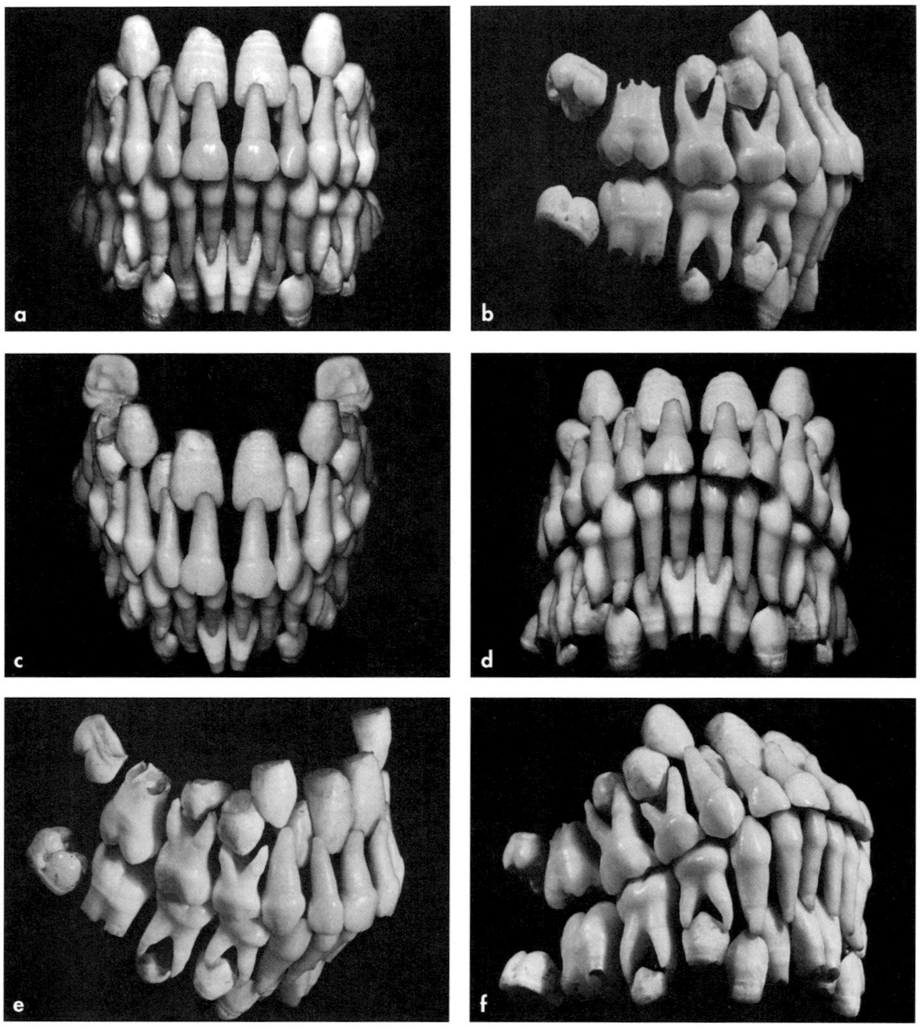

FIG 2-19 The teeth arranged as they were situated in the skull. *(a and b)* The height difference between the incisal margins of the central and lateral permanent incisors is obvious in both the maxillary and mandibular teeth. The proximity of the distoincisal corners of the maxillary central permanent incisors to the roots of the lateral deciduous incisors is clear. The mandibular permanent incisors diverge occlusally. The crowns of the maxillary permanent incisors, canines, and premolars are close together. That is not the case for the distally diverging maxillary central incisors. In both jaws, the permanent canines and premolars are located slightly more distally than their predecessors. In the maxilla, the permanent second molars are buccally inclined and distally angulated; in the mandible, they are lingually inclined and mesially angulated. The frontal view is shown from above *(c)* and below *(d)* and the lateral view from above *(e)* and below *(f)*.

Apical Area of the Jaw

The relationships involved become clearer when they are considered in terms of the concept of the *apical area* as introduced by the author in 1979 and described as follows:

> The apical area in an infant is comprised of the region that contains the forming parts of the deciduous and permanent teeth. In the deciduous dentition, the apical area is constituted of the region in which the apices of the deciduous teeth and the forming parts of the permanent teeth are located. In the mixed dentition, the apical area consists of the region where the roots of the deciduous and permanent teeth and the forming parts of the nonerupted permanent teeth can be located. In the adult state, the apical area is the region where the apices of the fully formed teeth normally can be located.[23]

In both jaws, the apical area can be subdivided into anterior, middle, and posterior sections. The anterior section contains the region between the mesial sides of the forming parts of the permanent canines and that of their apices after complete eruption. The middle section lies between the boundary of the anterior section and the mesial side of the forming part of the first permanent molars and after complete eruption slightly anterior to their mesial apices. The posterior section lies behind the middle section and extends to the posterior side of the maxillary tuberosity and that of the lingual tuberosity in the mandible.[23] Note that the apical area differs from the *apical base* introduced by Axel Lundström in 1925 and defined as "the part of the jaw that includes the apices of the teeth."[24] The concept of the apical area is further explained and illustrated in chapter 9.

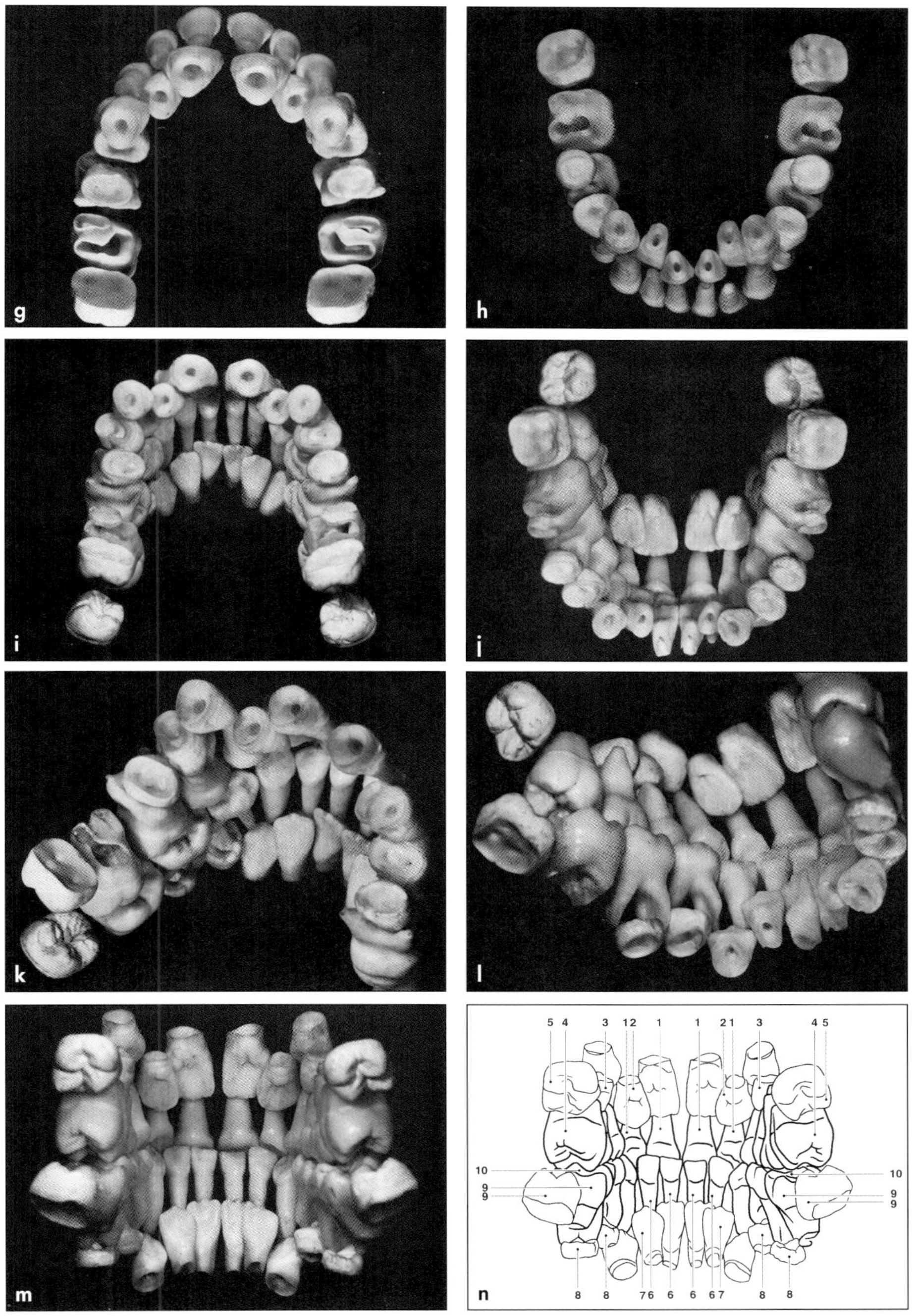

Fig 2-19 *(cont) (g and h)* The apical view shows the various stages of development of the permanent teeth, their arrangement in the dental arch, and symmetry in locations. The forming parts of the teeth are situated on a smaller arch in the maxilla *(g)* than in the mandible *(h)*. The lingual view is shown from above *(i)* and below *(j)*. The lingual lateral view is shown from above *(k)* and below *(l)*. *(m)* The posterior view shows the occlusion and the relationship between the deciduous and permanent teeth at the lingual side. *(n)* For elucidation, a drawing is provided. In the maxilla, the four deciduous incisors (1) are positioned in a tranverse direction nearly perpendicular to the occlusal plane. The lateral permanent incisors (2) are closer to the occlusal plane than the central incisors. The premolars (3) are located above their predecessors. The first permanent molars (4) are oriented perpendicular to the occlusal plane. The second permanent molars (5) are distally angulated and buccally inclined. In the mandible, the deciduous incisors (6) are also oriented perpendicular to the occlusal plane. The central permanent incisors are closer to the occlusal plane than the lateral incisors. The roots of the lateral permanent incisors (7) are shorter than those of the central incisors; later they would have become longer. The partially formed premolar crowns (8) are located under their predecessors. The first and second permanent molars (9) are lingually inclined, with the second molars also mesially angulated. The transverse relation between the opposing permanent molars (10) is normal.

Situation in the mandible

In the mandible, the anterior section of the apical area is bound laterally by the canines and anteroposteriorly by the lingual and labial cortical walls. Early in the development of the dentition, a large amount of tooth material is packed together in that region. As previously indicated, prior to the transition, the roots of deciduous teeth and the forming permanent teeth are arranged in a specific way. The crowns of the permanent teeth are positioned in a manner that optimizes the available space. Depending on the size of that space, the degree to which the permanent lateral incisors are overlapped by the central incisors varies from one-quarter to one-third of the width of the incisal margins of the lateral incisors. The amount that the canines overlap the lateral incisors varies more; they may not overlap at all.

Rotation of permanent teeth prior to emergence is not always a sign of lack of space. Sometimes they are formed in a rotated position and erupt that way. Left and right differences in position among incisors and canines are not uncommon. That also applies to the anteroposterior position, rotation, and degree of overlap. In that respect, the variation is greater in the maxilla than in the mandible.

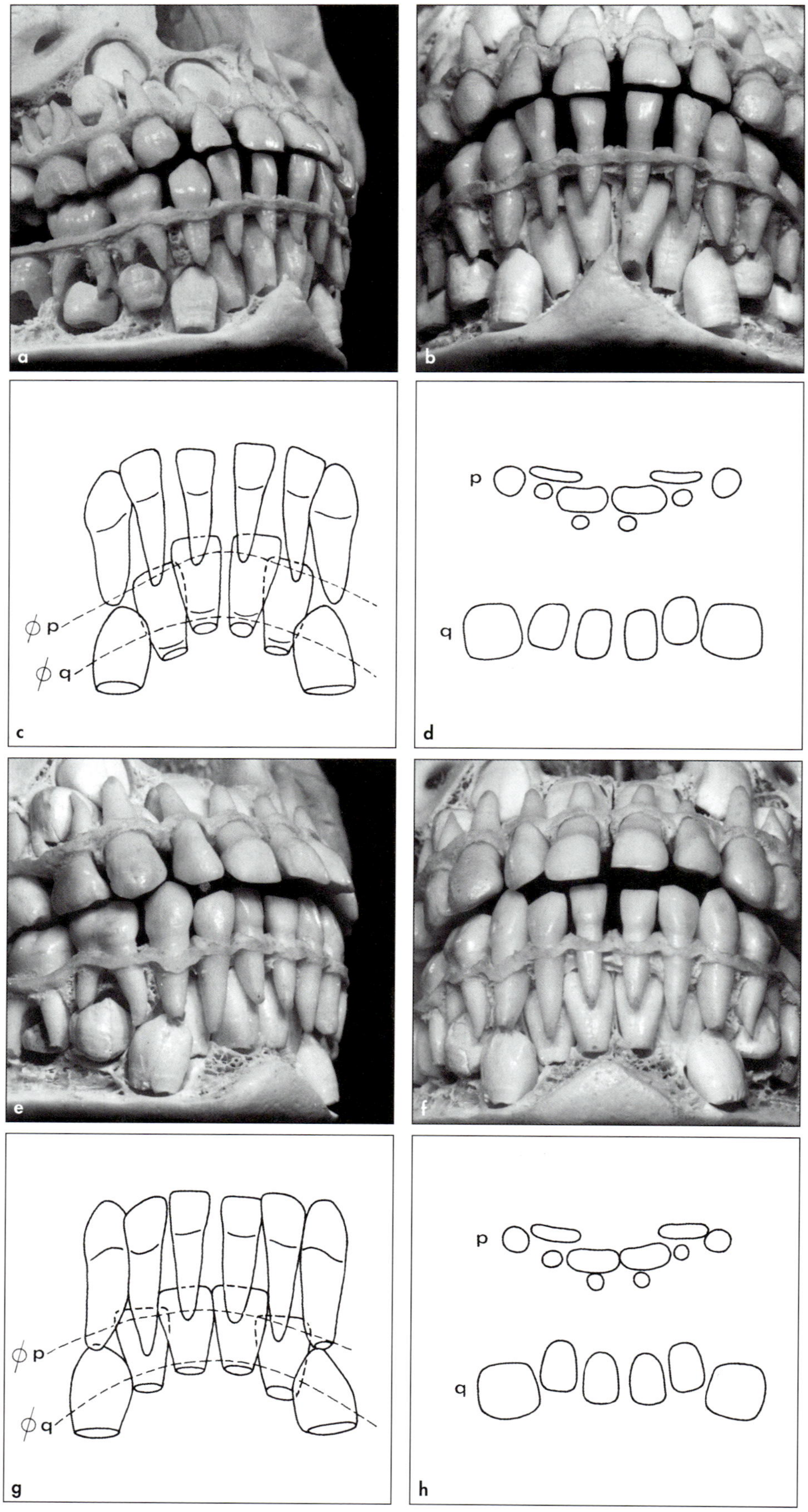

FIG 2-20 Arrangement of the mandibular anterior teeth prior to the transition in relation to the size of the anterior section of the apical area. The first specimen has a large anterior section of the apical area. *(a and b)* There are many and large diastemata. The permanent canines are slightly lingually inclined and mesially angulated. There is space between the central permanent incisors. The crown tips of the permanent canines are situated distally to the apices of their predecessors. *(c and d)* Drawings based on *a* and *b*, with the *dotted lines* in *c* indicating the sectional planes in *d*. There is some space between the central permanent incisors and the roots of the adjacent lateral deciduous incisors. The same applies to the lateral permanent incisors and the deciduous canines. At the level to the incisal margins (p), the lateral incisors are positioned lingually to the central incisors. At the level of the cementoenamel junctions (q), the lateral incisors are located only slightly more lingually than the central incisors, on the left side somewhat more than on the right side. The second specimen has a medium anterior section of the apical area. *(e and f)* There are few and only small diastemata. The permanent canines are lingually inclined and mesially angulated. The crowns of the central incisors and permanent canines overlap the crowns of the lateral permanent incisors. The crown tips of the permanent canines are located close to the roots of their predecessors. *(g)* The distoincisal corners of the lateral permanent incisors are close to the roots of the deciduous canines. The permanent incisor is more mesially angulated and overlaps the lateral permanent incisor more on the left than on the right side. *(h)* At the level of the incisal margins (p), the permanent incisors and deciduous teeth are close together. At the level of the cementoenamel junctions (q), the available space is barely larger than needed.

Fig 2-20 *(cont)* *(i and j)* The third specimen has a small anterior section of the apical area. There are only a few small diastemata. The permanent canines are excessively lingually inclined and mesially angulated. Their crowns overlap those of the lateral permanent incisors. The crown tips of the permanent canines are close to the apices of their predecessors. *(k)* The crowns of the central permanent incisors are close to the roots of the lateral deciduous incisors. *(l)* At the level of the incisal margins (p), the crowns of the permanent teeth and the roots of the deciduous teeth are close together. The distoincisal corners of the lateral permanent incisors are situated lingually to the roots of the deciduous canines. At the level of the cementoenamel junctions (q), the lateral incisors are located lingually to the central incisors and are overlapped by the canine crowns. (Reprinted from Bakker et al[25] with permission.)

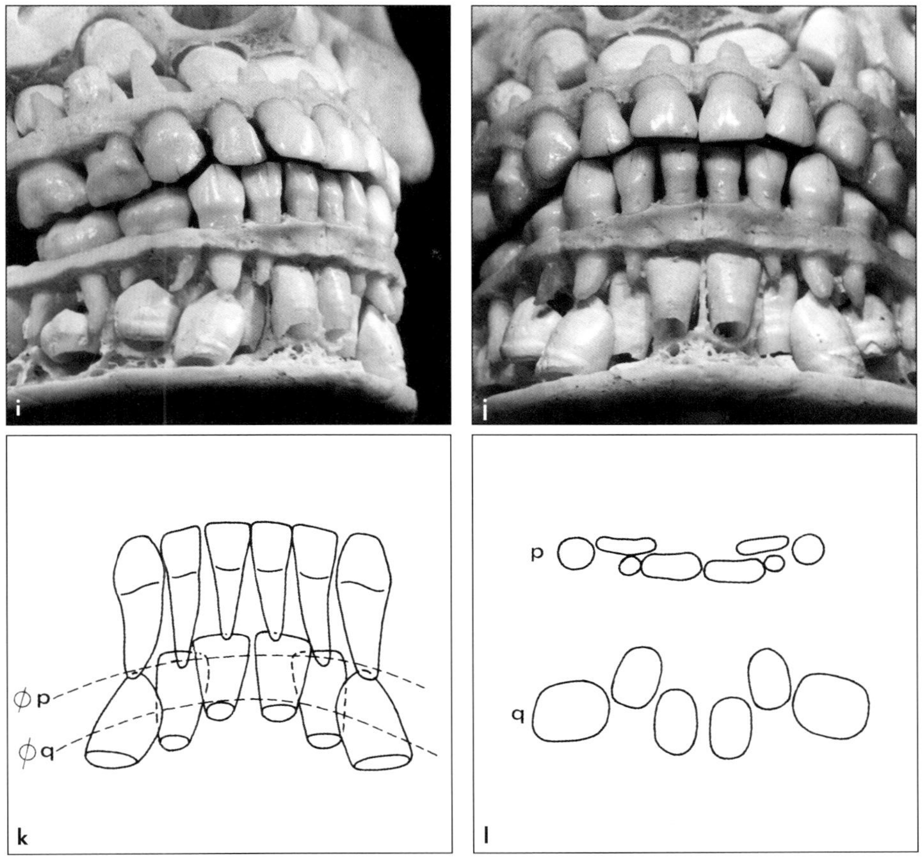

As previously indicated, the arrangement of the mandibular permanent incisors prior to emergence varies depending on the relationship between the available and needed space. This point is illustrated in Fig 2-20, which shows large, medium, and small anterior sections of apical areas. The anterior section of the apical area is considered large when the distance between the permanent canines is relatively great in comparison to the mesiodistal dimensions of the permanent incisors. Such a condition leads to a good transition. In general, the presence of many and large diastemata in the deciduous dentition is a favorable feature; few and small diastemata, or particularly total absence of them, is an unfavorable sign. However, this rule does not always apply. The correlation between the sum of the mesiodistal dimensions of the deciduous incisors and that of their successors is rather small[26] (see chapter 17, Table 17-11). Small crown widths of deciduous incisors do not always correspond with small successors and vice versa. This limitation must be kept in mind when the space needed for the permanent incisors is estimated.

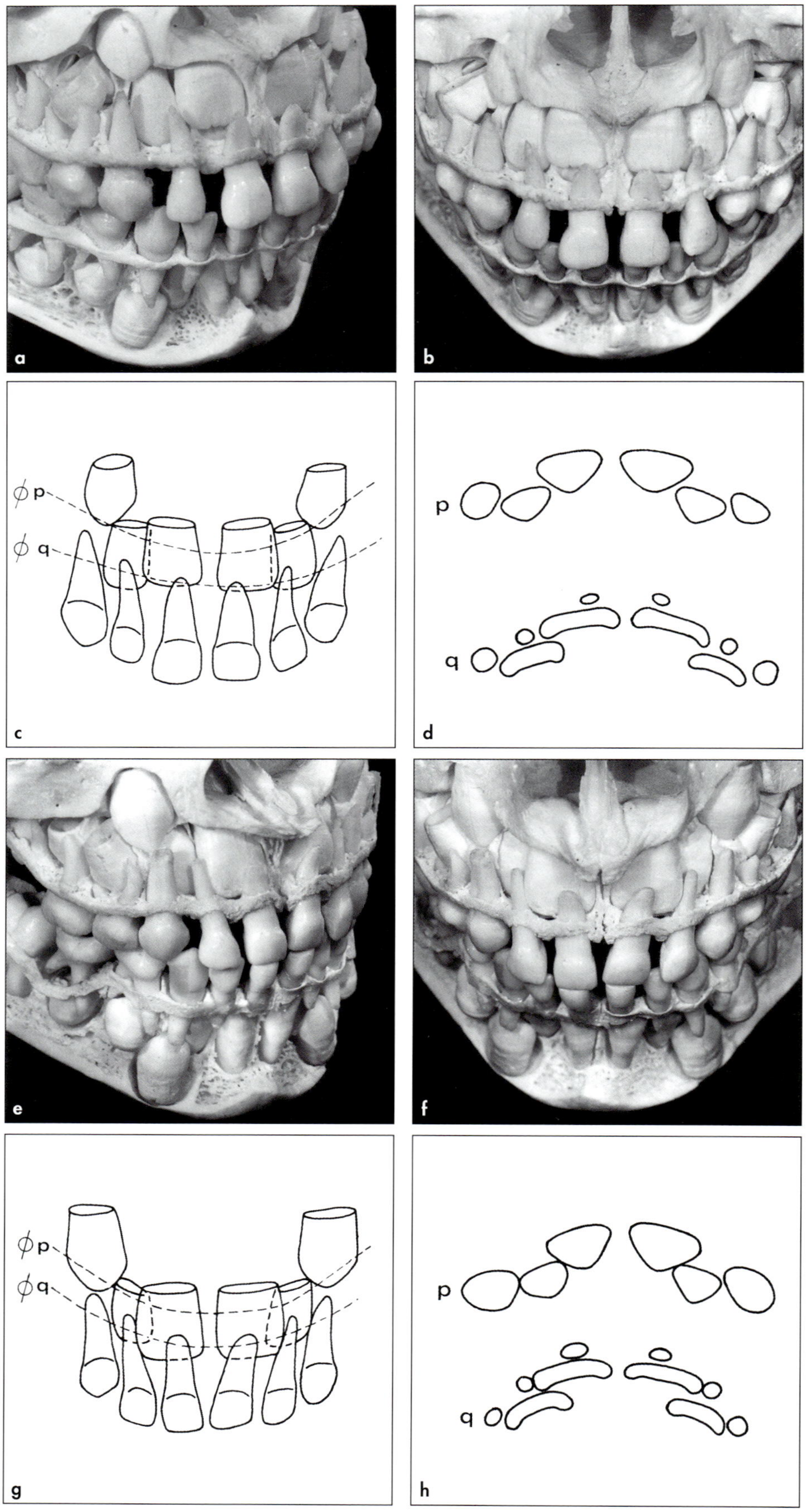

Fig 2-21 Arrangement of the maxillary anterior teeth prior to the transition in relation to the size of the anterior section of the apical area. The first specimen has a large anterior section of the apical area. *(a and b)* There are large diastemata between the deciduous teeth. The piriform aperture is broad, and the distance between the crowns of the permanent canines is large. The central permanent incisors are far apart. They overlap the lateral incisors only slightly. *(c and d)* Drawings based on *a* and *b*, with the *dotted lines* in *c* indicating the sectional planes in *d*. The distoincisal corners of the central permanent incisors are not close to the roots of the lateral deciduous incisors. At the level of the incisal margins (q), spatial conditions are favorable, and the lateral permanent incisors are situated palatally to the central permanent incisors. At the level of the cementoenamel junctions (p), the lateral incisors also are located palatally to the central incisors. The second specimen has a medium anterior section of the apical area. *(e and f)* The diastemata between the deciduous teeth are small. The width of the piriform aperture and the distance between the permanent canine crowns are limited. The central permanent incisors are some distance apart. The permanent canines overlap the lateral incisors only slightly. *(g)* The distoincisal corners of the central permanent incisors are close to the roots of the adjacent lateral deciduous incisors. *(h)* At the level of the incisal margins (q), the crowns of the permanent incisors and the roots of the deciduous incisors are close together. At the level of the cementoenamel junctions of the permanent incisors (p), the teeth overlap each other.

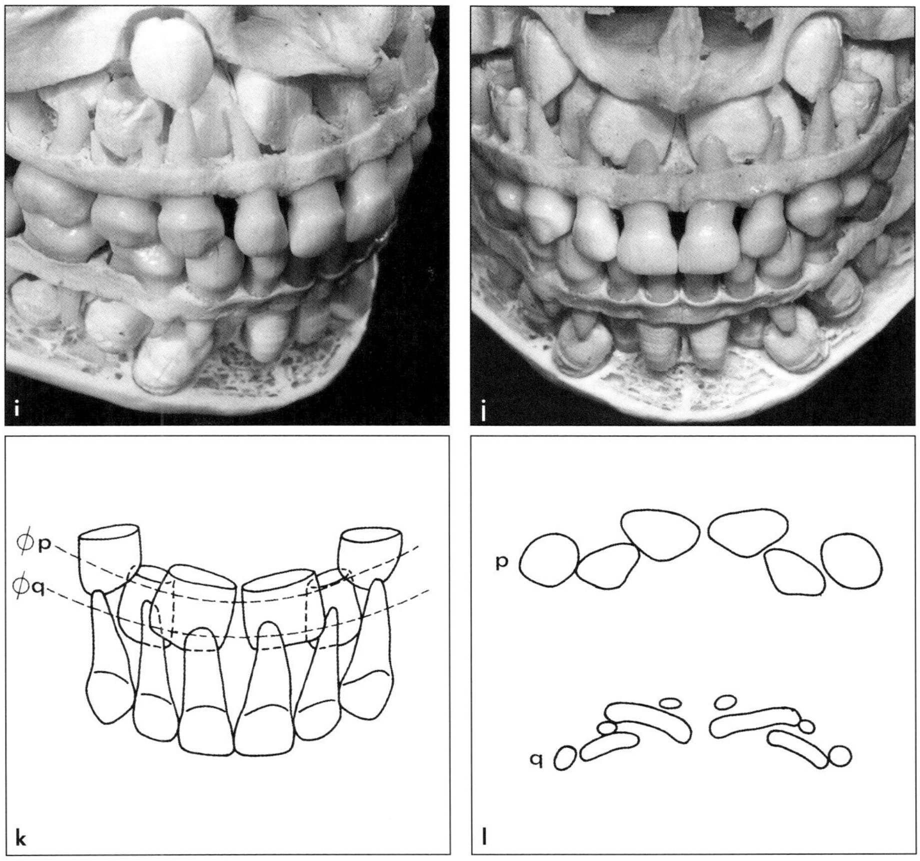

Fig 2-21 *(cont)* *(i and j)* The third specimen has a small anterior part of the apical area. There are no diastemata between the deciduous incisors. The width of the piriform aperture and distance between the permanent canine crowns is small. The distally angulated and mesiopalatally rotated central permanent incisors are close to the nasal floor and median suture. The central permanent incisors overlap approximately half of the width of the lateral incisors. *(k)* The distoincisal corners of the central permanent incisor overlap the roots of the lateral deciduous incisors. *(l)* At the level of the incisal margins (q), the mesioincisal corners of the central permanent incisors are situated palatally. Their distoincisal corners overlap the roots of the lateral deciduous incisors labially. At the level of the cementoenamel junctions (p), the permanent incisors are close together. (Reprinted from Bakker et al[27] with permission.)

Situation in the maxilla

In the maxilla, the relationship between the available and needed space within the anterior section of the apical area also varies considerably. A large anterior section of the apical area corresponds to much space and large diastemata in the deciduous dentition. Few and tiny diastemata indicate a small anterior section of the apical area (Fig 2-21). For maxillary anterior teeth, it also holds true that the correlation between the sum of the mesiodistal crown dimensions of the deciduous incisors and that of the permanent incisors is rather small[26] (see chapter 17, Table 17-11).

Emergence of Teeth into Occlusion

In Fig 2-22, the growth of the jaws and the emergence of deciduous teeth are demonstrated on dental casts obtained monthly from birth until 19 months of age. The measurements carried out on the casts demonstrate that the jaws mainly grow during the first 6 months and little thereafter (Fig 2-23).

Figure 2-24 presents the jaws of five skulls from birth until the complete deciduous dentition stage. These images show the changes occurring in the dentoalveolar bony structures and also the establishment and consolidation of the occlusion in the posterior region.

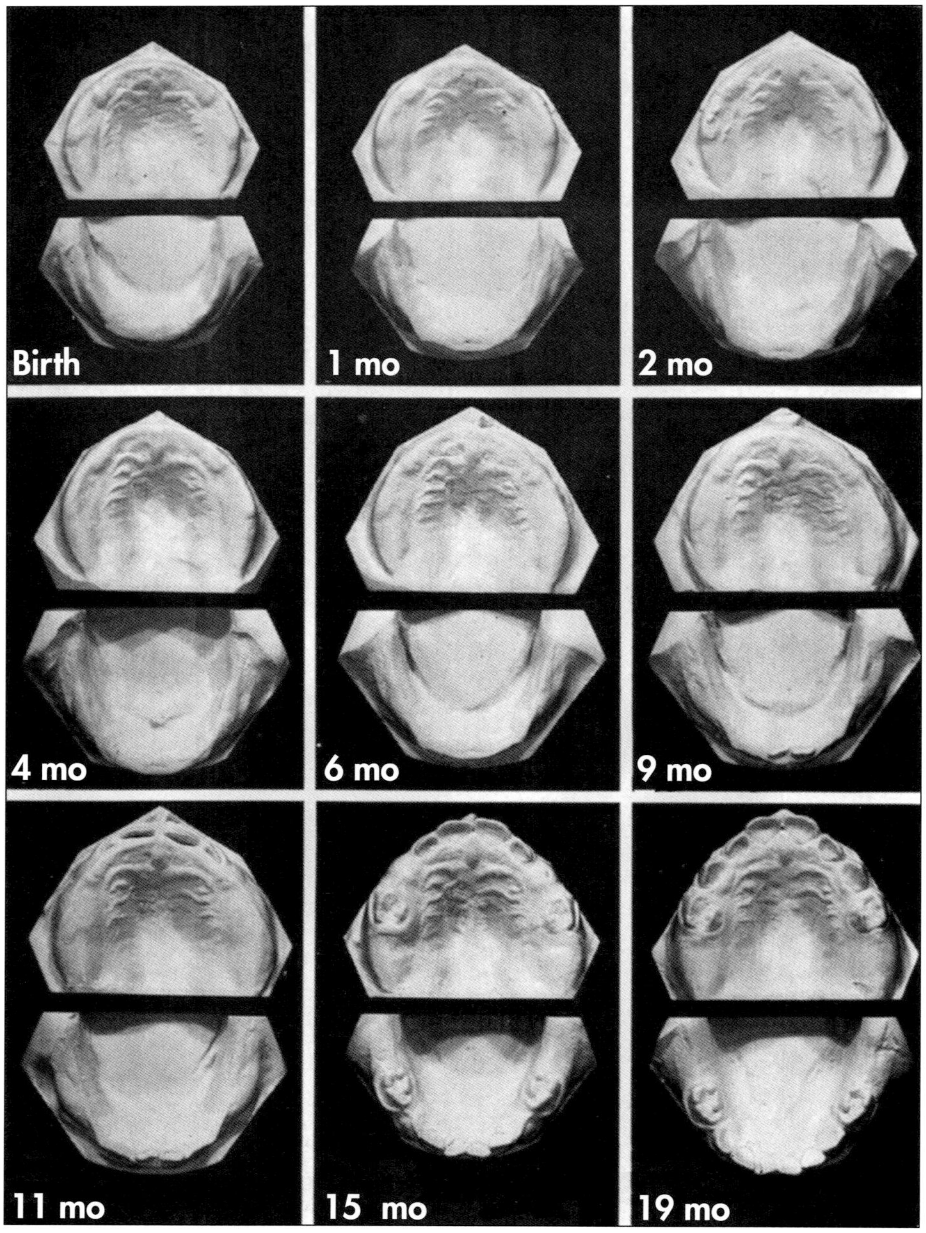

FIG 2-22 Maxillary and mandibular plaster casts of a girl from the day of birth until 19 months of age. The mandible did not grow enough for emergence of the central deciduous incisors in good alignment. They are slightly rotated, which can be traced back to their initial positions within the jaw. In the maxilla, the lateral deciduous incisors are located slightly too palatally. After emergence, the position of the teeth has not improved. (Reprinted from Van der Linden[15] with permission.)

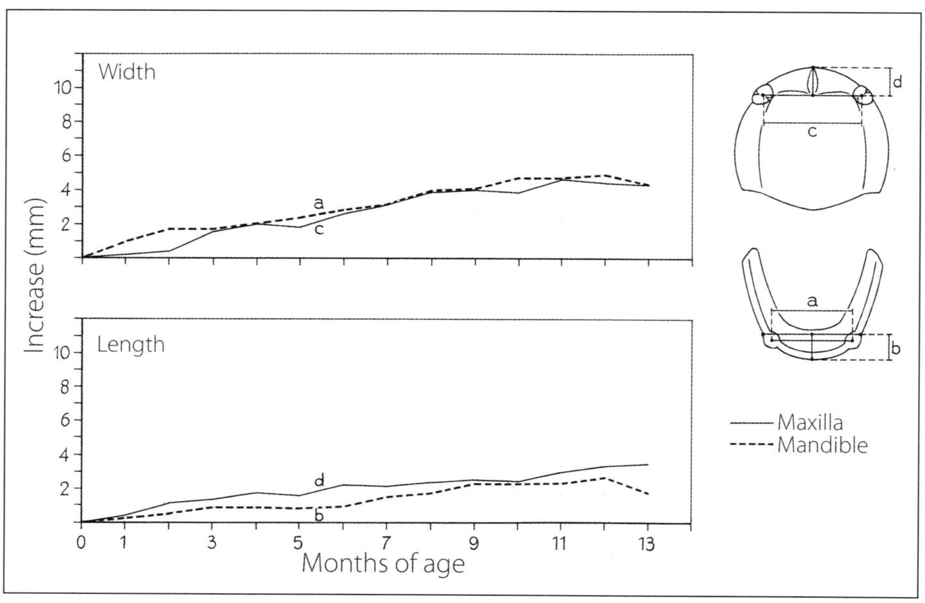

FIG 2-23 Velocity curves of recordings on the monthly collected plaster casts of the girl shown in Fig 2-22. The curves are based on the measurements indicated on the right: the mandibular canine width *(a)*, the labiolingual dimension of the alveolar process in the mandibular median region *(b)*, and the corresponding values in the maxilla *(c and d)*.[15]

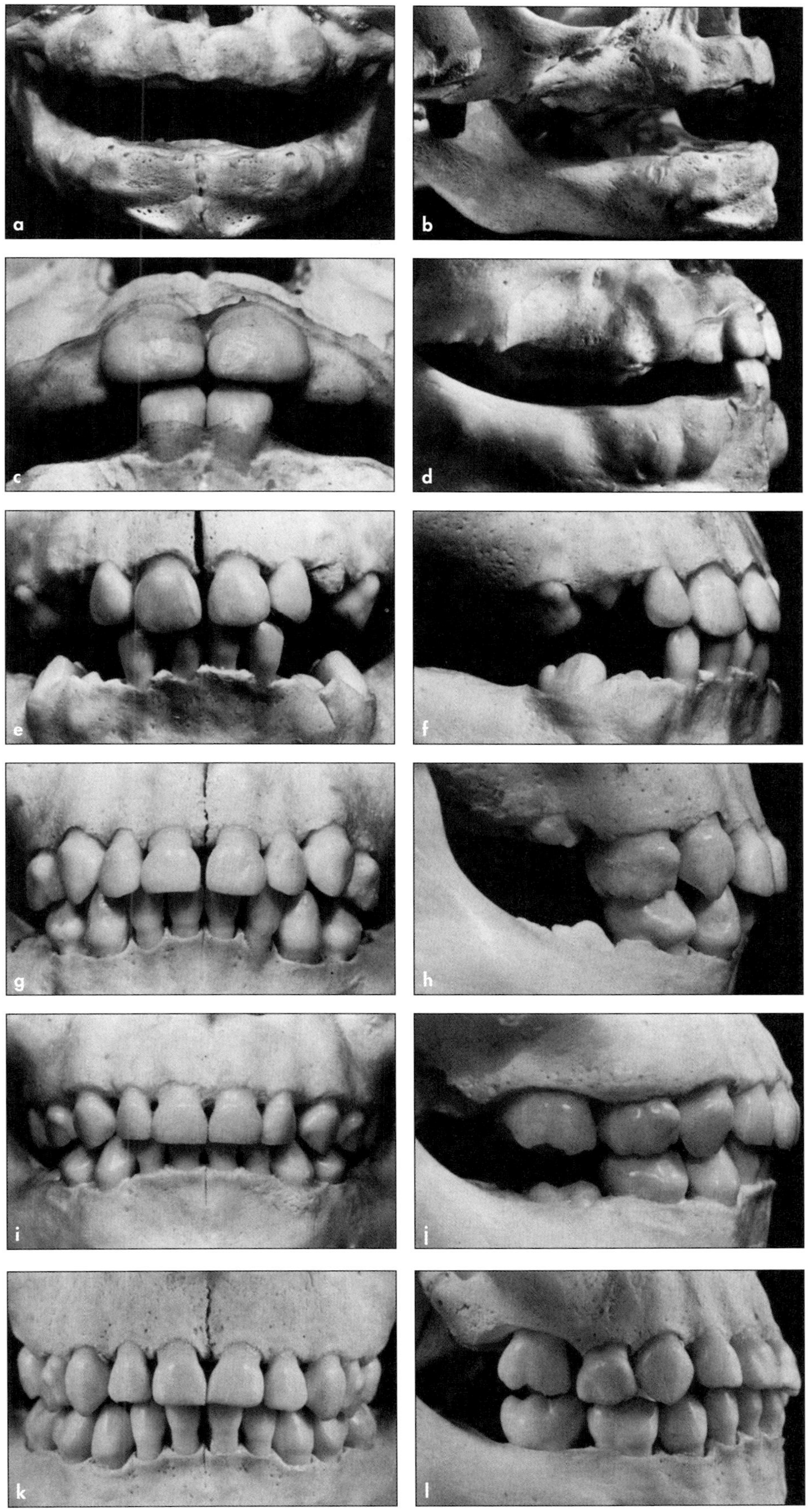

FIG 2-24 Jaws of six skulls to illustrate the development of the deciduous dentition. *(a and b)* In the newborn, the morphology of the jaws is determined predominantly by the tooth buds. *(c and d)* This is even more true at 6 months of age. *(e and f)* Erupting teeth build up their own alveolar process. *(g and h)* After emergence of the first deciduous molars, occlusion is reached for the first time. *(i and j)* Through the cone-funnel mechanism, an optimal intercuspation is attained. *(k and l)* An optimal intercuspation will also be achieved with the second deciduous molars. (Reprinted from Van der Linden and Duterloo[7] with permission.)

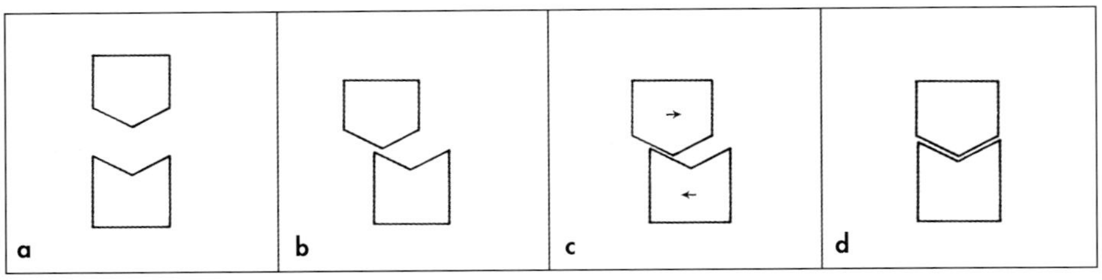

Fig 2-25 The cone-funnel mechanism. *(a)* No displacement is needed when opposing teeth erupt precisely in the right direction, which seldom occurs. *(b)* The cone tip will fall within the funnel. *(c)* Displacement of the maxillary molar and, to a lesser degree, the mandibular molar. *(d)* Final intercuspation.

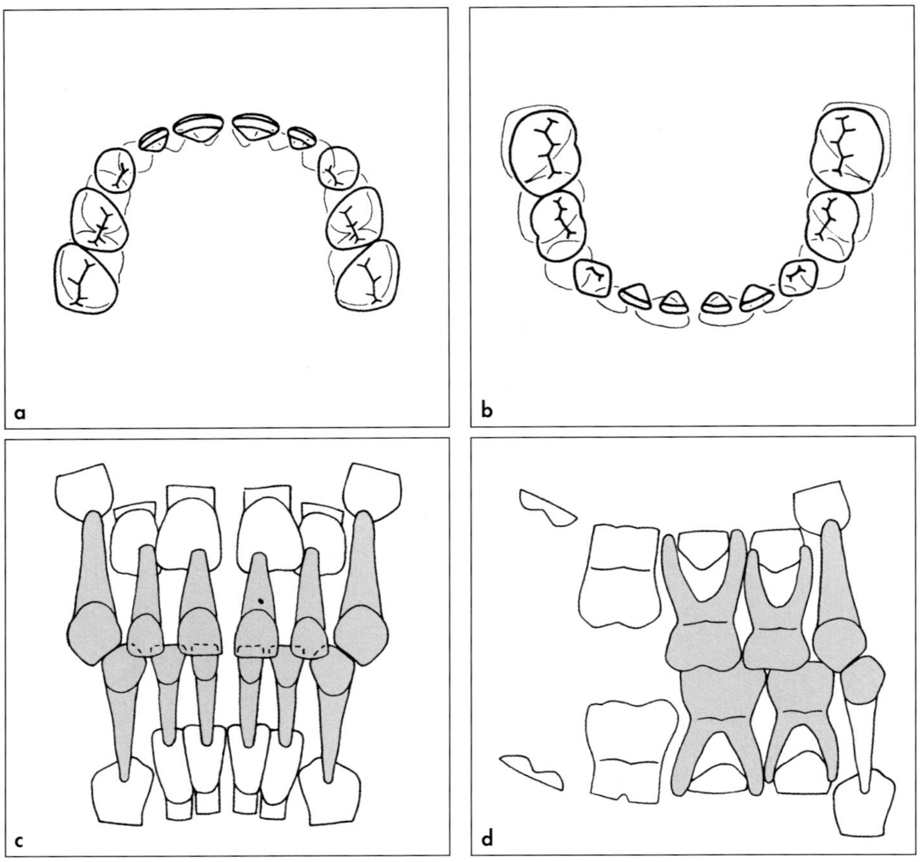

Fig 2-26 Complete deciduous dentition. *(a and b)* Both dental arches have a half-round form. The mandibular dental arch is situated slightly inside the maxillary arch. There are diastemata in the anterior region. *(c)* The opposing incisors have no contact in habitual occlusion. The vertical overjet varies between 0 and 2 mm.[29,30] In the anterior region, the deciduous teeth are oriented perpendicular to the occlusal plane (an imaginary surface that passes through the occlusion of the teeth[31]) in the mesiodistal and labiolingual directions. *(d)* The same applies to the deciduous molars. The mandibular teeth occlude slightly mesially to the corresponding maxillary teeth. The forming parts of the permanent teeth are at the same level with the exception of the canines.

When erupting deciduous and permanent molars as well as premolars attain occlusal contact, they are guided to optimal intercuspation by the cone-funnel mechanism. It seldom happens that antagonists erupt in such a way that no displacement is needed to arrive at good intercuspation. The cone-funnel mechanism acts for the first time when the opposing first deciduous molars touch each other. The eruption movements are guided subsequently by the slope of the central fossa of the mandibular molar. The large palatal cusp of the maxillary first deciduous molar will end up in the bottom of the fossa of the mandibular first molar.[28] The adjustment of the eruption direction occurs more in the maxilla than in the mandible; the morphology of the mandible is less suited for the purpose (Fig 2-25).

At 2½ years of age, the second deciduous molars usually have reached full occlusion and the deciduous dentition is complete (Fig 2-26). Between 2½ and 5 years of age, the position of the deciduous teeth and their occlusion alters little.[30]

References

1. Gopnik A, Meltzoff AN, Kuhl PK. The Scientist in the Crib. Minds, Brains, and How Children Learn. New York: William Morrow, 1999.
2. Medawar PB. The shape of the human being as a function of time. Proc R Soc Lond 1945;132:133–141.
3. Tanner JM. Growth at Adolescence, ed 2. Oxford: Blackwell, 1962.
4. Tanner JM, Whitehouse RH, Marubini E, Resele LE. The adolescent growth spurt of boys and girls of the Harpenden growth study. Ann Hum Biol 1976;3:109–126.
5. Bishara SE, Jamison JE, Peterson LC, DeKock WH. Longitudinal changes in standing height and mandibular parameters between the ages of 8 and 17 years. Am J Orthod 1981;80:115–135.
6. Boersma H, Van der Linden FPGM, Prahl-Andersen B. Craniofacial development. In: Prahl-Andersen B, Kowalsky CJ, Heydendael PHJ (eds). A Mixed-Longitudinal Interdisciplinary Study of Growth and Development. New York: Academic Press, 1979:537–571.
7. Van der Linden FPGM, Duterloo HS. Development of the Human Dentition. An Atlas. Hagerstown, MD: Harper & Row, 1976.
8. To EWH. A study of natal teeth in Hong Kong Chinese. Int J Paediatr Dent 1991;1:73–76.
9. Zhu J, King D. Natal and neonatal teeth. J Dent Child 1995;62:123–128.
10. Van der Linden FPGM, McNamara JA Jr, Radlanski RJ. Dynamics of Orthodontics: Facial Growth [DVD 2A]. Chicago: Quintessence, 2004.
11. Clinch LM. Variations in the mutual relationship of the maxillary and mandibular gum pads in the new born child. Int J Orthod 1934;20:359–372.
12. Clinch LM. An analysis of serial models between three and eight years of age. Dent Rec 1951;71:61–72.
13. Sillman JH. Relationship of maxillary and mandibular gum pads in the newborn infant. Am J Orthod 1938;24:409–424.
14. Sillman JH. Dimensional changes of the dental arches: Longitudinal study from birth to 25 years. Am J Orthod 1964;50:824–842.
15. Van der Linden FPGM. Interrelated factors in the morphogenesis of teeth, the development of the dentition and craniofacial growth. SSO Schweiz Monatsschr Zahnheilkd 1970;80:518–526.
16. Van der Linden FPGM, McNamara JA Jr, Burdi AR. Tooth size and position before birth. J Dent Res 1972;51:71–74.
17. Streeter GL. Developmental horizons in human embryos, description of age groups XV, XVI, XVII and XVIII, being the third issue of a survey of the Carnegie Collection. Contrib Embryol 1948;32:133–203.
18. Ooë T. Human Tooth and Dental Arch Development. Tokyo: Ishiyaku, 1981.
19. Ooë T. Patterns of crowding of the anterior tooth germs in the fetal life. Okajimas Folia Anat Jpn 1968;45:1–9.
20. Knaup B, Yildizhan F, Wehrbein H. Age-related changes in the midpalatal suture. A histomorphometric study. J Orofac Orthop 2004;65:467–474.
21. Ooë T. Changes of position and development of human anterior tooth germs after birth. Okajimas Folia Anat Jpn 1968;45:71–82.
22. Shinji H, Kumasaka S, Matsubara S, Yang J, Ozawa N, Uchimura N. Study on eruption of deciduous teeth. Pediatr Dent J 1998;8:113–118.
23. Van der Linden FPGM. Changes in the dentofacial complex during and after orthodontic treatment. Eur J Orthod 1979;1:97–105.
24. Lundström AF. Malocclusion of the teeth regarded as a problem in connection with the apical base. Int J Orthod Oral Surg Radiogr 1925;11:591–602,724–731,793–812,933–941,1022–1042,1109–1133.
25. Bakker PJMR, Wassenberg HJW, Van der Linden FPGM. Exchange of the lower incisors [in German]. Inf Orthod Kieferorthop 1979;11:144–168.
26. Moorrees CFA, Chadha JM. Available space for the incisors during dental development. Angle Orthod 1965;35:12–22.
27. Bakker PJMR, Wassenberg HJW, Van der Linden FPGM. Change in the upper incisors [in German]. Inf Orthod Kieferorthop 1979;11:239–270.
28. Schwarz AM. Lehrgang der Gebissentwicklung, ed 2. Wien: Urban & Schwarzenberg, 1951.
29. Farsi NMA, Salama FS. Characteristics of primary dentition occlusion in a group of Saudi children. Int J Paediatr Dent 1996;6:253–259.
30. Saitoh I, Hayasaki H, Inada E, Maruyama T, Takemoto Y, Yamasaki Y. Overlap of the primary dentition in children. J Clin Pediatr Dent 2009;33:269–273.
31. Daskalogianakis J. Glossary of Orthodontic Terms. Chicago: Quintessence, 2000.

3

The First Transitional Period: Transition of Incisors and Emergence of First Permanent Molars

Emergence of the First Permanent Molars

Prior to the transition of the incisors, usually at 6 years of age, the first permanent molars emerge: first in the mandible, then in the maxilla. In the preceding years, adequate room was available in the jaws for their development. Continuing posterior growth provided sufficient space for them in the dental arch. They erupt almost perpendicular to the occlusal plane, as the deciduous molars did before them. After their emergence, there is often a surplus of space in the dental arch. Diastemata distal to the second deciduous molars can remain for some time.

The occlusion of the first permanent molars depends on their position in the jaws, the relationship between the mandible and maxilla, and the mesiodistal crown dimensions of the teeth, particularly the mandibular second deciduous molar (Figs 3-1 and 3-2). The width of that tooth varies more than that of any other deciduous tooth. If the mandibular second deciduous molar has a mesiodistal crown dimension that is approximately the same as that of the corresponding maxillary tooth, the terminal plane of the deciduous dentition will have a mesial step. With such a mesial step, the first permanent molars can immediately attain optimal interdigitation (see Figs 3-1a, 3-1b, and 3-2d). However, in most cases the mandibular second deciduous molar is a few millimeters wider than the maxillary second deciduous molar. This results in a flush terminal plane (see Figs 3-1c, 3-1d, 3-2a, and 3-2b). A good mesiodistal occlusion and optimal intercuspation of the first permanent molars cannot occur until the deciduous molars are replaced by the narrower premolars, which have the same crown width. The mandibular first permanent molar then migrates more mesially than the maxillary first molar.

Transition of the Incisors

The replacement of deciduous teeth occurs in two phases. In the first transitional period, the incisors are replaced. In the second transitional period, following an interphase of about 1.5 years (the intertransitional period), the deciduous canines and molars are replaced. Marked differences exist between the two transitional periods, mainly due to differences in spatial conditions between the anterior and posterior regions.

Influence of spatial conditions and perioral soft tissues

The crowns of the permanent incisors and canines are broader than those of their predecessors; this difference is greater in the maxilla than in the mandible. Prior to emergence, the tooth buds are located in the region where later their smaller roots will be situated. For the permanent incisors and canines, the circumference of that region is smaller than the arch segment where their incisal margins will be located (Fig 3-3). Again, this difference is greater in the maxilla than in the mandible. In addition, the anterior area is smaller in relation to the sum of the mesiodistal crown dimensions of the six anterior teeth in the maxilla than in the mandible.[2]

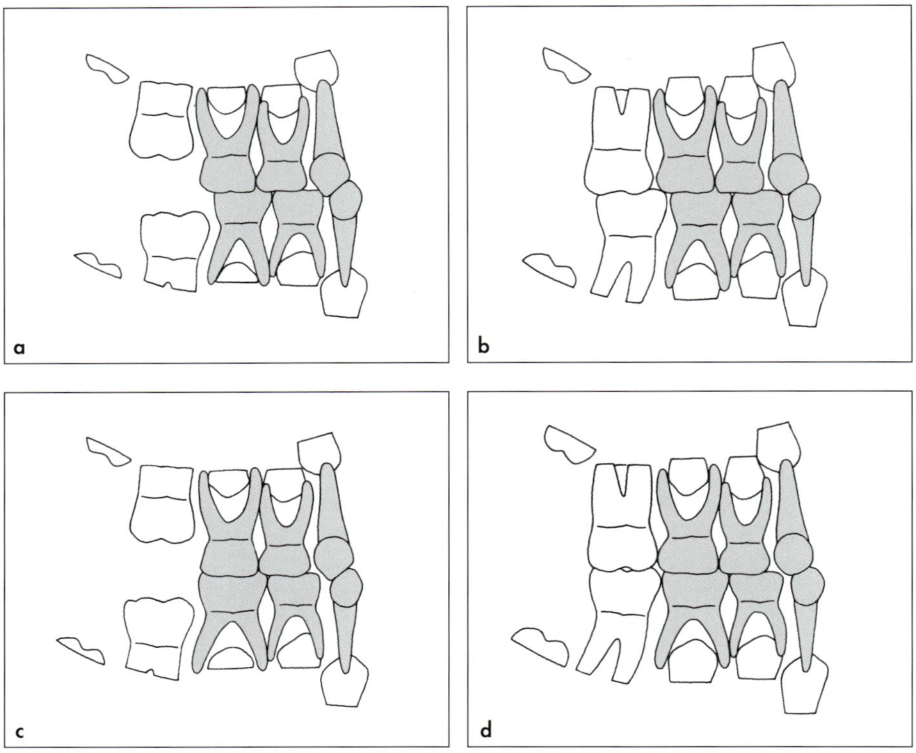

FIG 3-1 Effect of mesiodistal dimensions of second deciduous molars on the occlusion of the first permanent molars. *(a)* In situations of opposing second deciduous molars with equal mesiodistal crown dimensions, the terminal plane of the deciduous dentition has a mesial step. *(b)* After emergence, the first permanent molars can arrive at optimal intercuspation immediately. *(c)* However, in most cases the mandibular second deciduous molar is broader than the opposing maxillary tooth,[1] and as a result the terminal plane is flush. *(d)* Consequently, the first permanent molars erupt with inadequate intercuspation because the cusps are right on top of each other mesiodistally (ie, end-to-end occlusion). However, they do attain an acceptable buccolingual occlusion by means of the cone-funnel mechanism. The maxillary molar is positioned slightly more to the buccal than the opposing mandibular tooth.

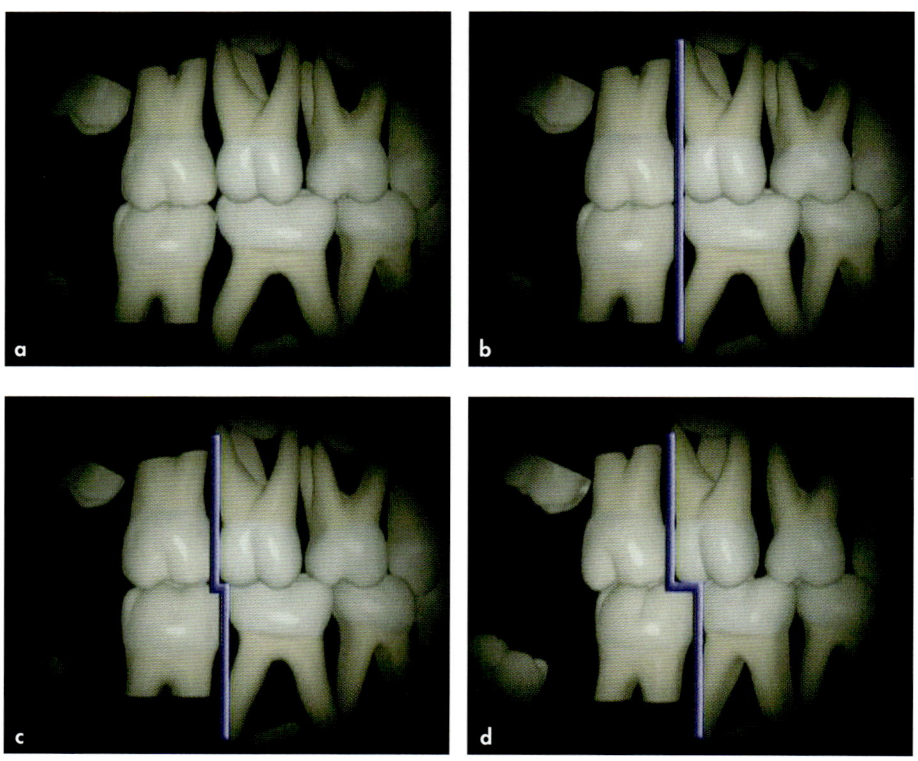

FIG 3-2 Variations in the terminal plane of the deciduous dentition. *(a and b)* The occlusion of the first permanent molars after their emergence depends on the course of the terminal plane *(purple line)*. A large mandibular second deciduous molar results in end-to-end occlusion of the first permanent molars. *(c)* A small mandibular second deciduous molar is correlated with a terminal plane with a small mesial step and corresponding suboptimal occlusion of the first permanent molars. *(d)* In a situation of opposing second deciduous molars with the same mesiodistal crown dimensions, the first permanent molars can immediately attain optimal intercuspation.

Unlike the deciduous incisors, the permanent incisors erupt in the direction in which they are formed.[3,4] Maxillary lateral permanent incisors emerge more labially than the central incisors. After emergence, their labial inclination is reduced through pressure exerted by the lips. In the mandible, the lateral permanent incisors emerge slightly lingual to the dental arch. Subsequently, they migrate labially into alignment with the adjacent teeth through pressure exerted by the tongue. Indeed, the tongue, lips, and cheeks play a major role in the positioning of the teeth. However, local space conditions in the dental arch have the most dominant effect.

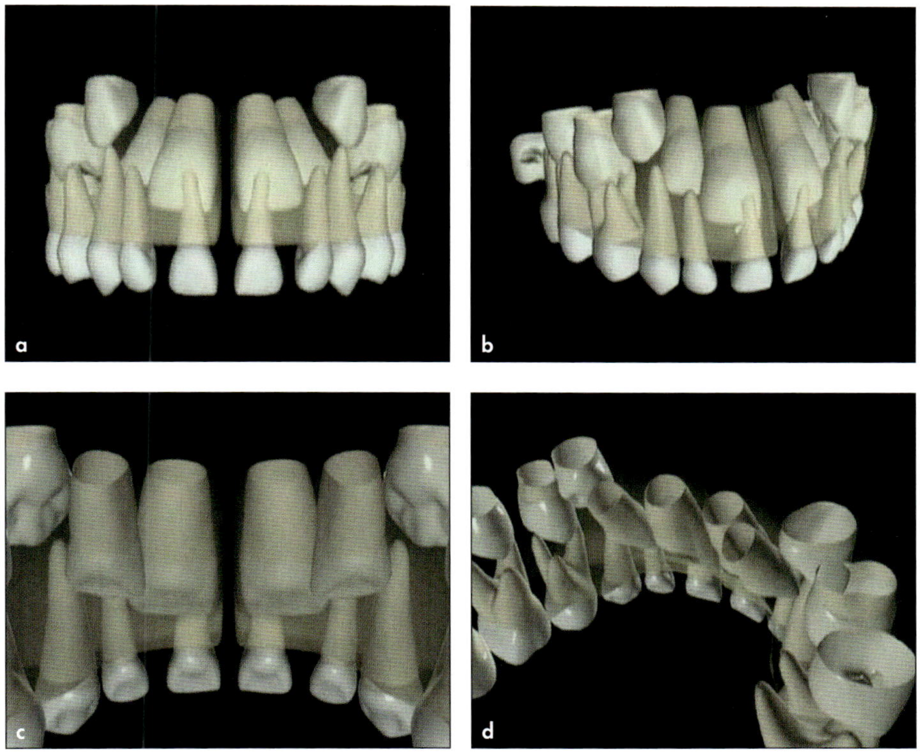

FIG 3-3 Arrangement of maxillary teeth within the surrounding bony structures, some time after the start of eruption of the maxillary central permanent incisors. *(a to d)* Initially, the permanent incisors are arranged within the jaws in such a way that the available space is used maximally. The median suture does not permit proximity of the central permanent incisors. However, their mesial aspects are parallel and close to the median suture, which makes optimal use of the available space. Consequently, these teeth are distally angulated, erupt in a divergent way, and emerge with a central diastema.

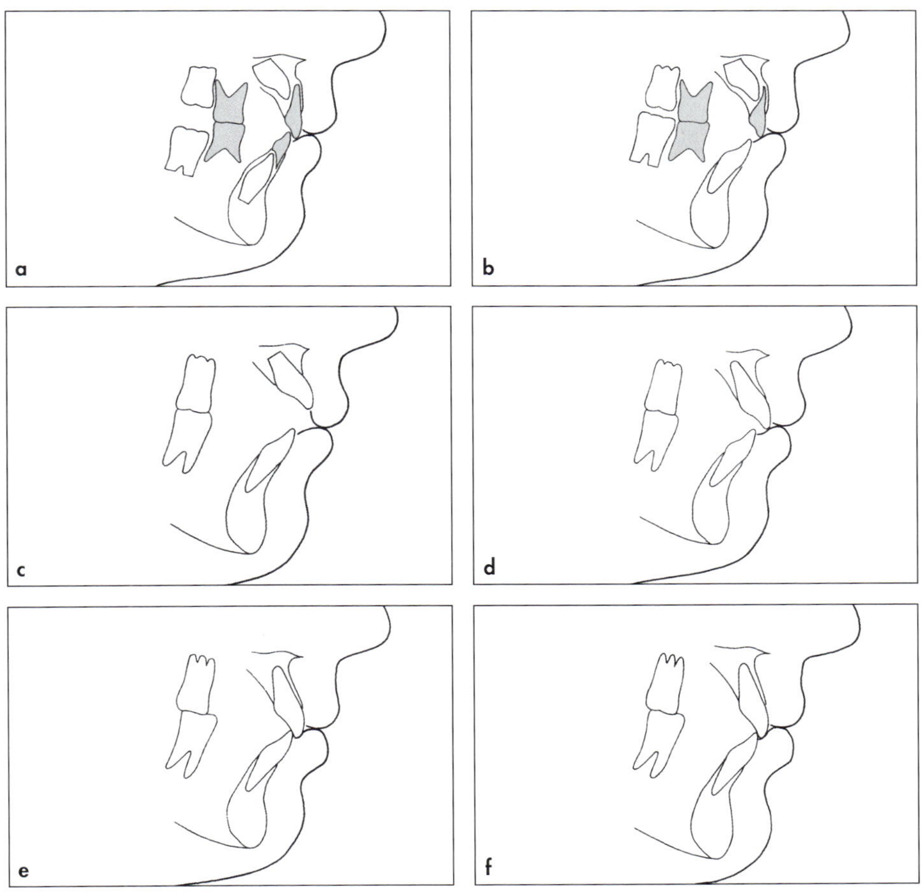

FIG 3-4 Changes in the incisor and molar regions from the complete deciduous dentition stage to adulthood. *(a)* The deciduous incisors are oriented perpendicular to the occlusal plane. The permanent incisors are located lingually to their predecessors and are labially inclined. *(b)* First the mandibular first permanent molar emerges, then the mandibular central incisor. The maxillary central permanent incisor emerges some weeks after the loss of its predecessor. *(c)* In the meantime, the maxillary first permanent molar has emerged. *(d)* The incisors continue to erupt until contact is reached. *(e)* The lower lip touches the incisal margin of the maxillary central incisor and covers 1 to 3 mm of its labial surface. *(f)* Continuing jaw growth and increase of the pressure exerted by the perioral musculature result in a more upright position of the incisors in the adult.

The transition of the incisors lasts almost 3 years, measured from the first associated changes in the deciduous dental arch until the complete eruption of all permanent incisors. The loss of the central deciduous incisors and eruption of their successors is illustrated in Fig 3-4. The second deciduous molars and the first permanent molars are also shown. The changes in relation to the tongue and lips from the complete deciduous dentition stage until adulthood are presented in Fig 3-5.

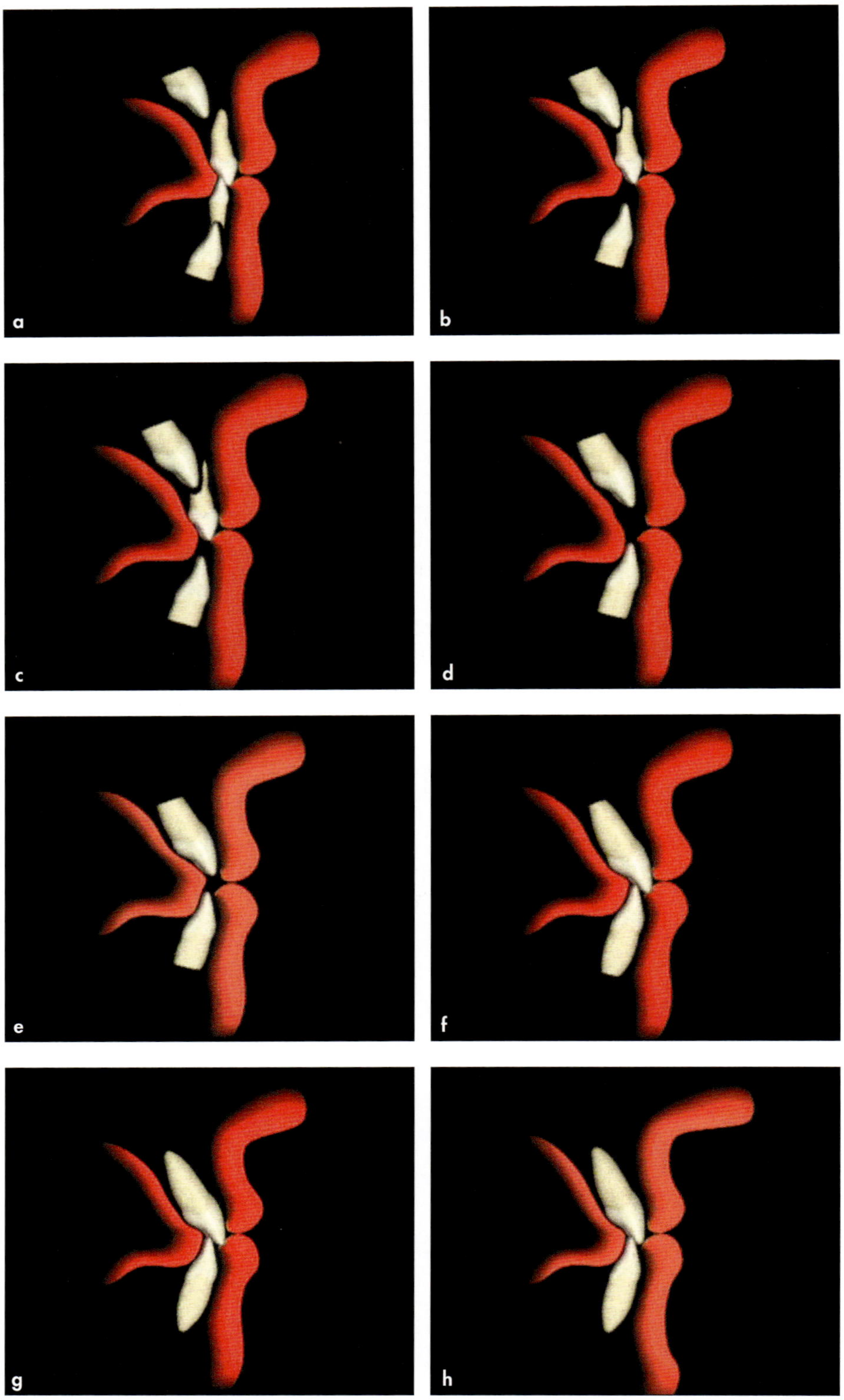

Fig 3-5 Transition of the central incisors in relation to the surrounding soft tissues. *(a)* The upper lip covers the maxillary deciduous incisors, and the lower lip covers the mandibular incisors as well as a small portion of the maxillary incisors. *(b)* After emergence, the mandibular permanent incisors contact the lower lip. *(c)* The incisal margins of the mandibular permanent incisors attain a more labial position than those of the predecessors. *(d)* This phenomenon occurs to an even greater degree in the maxilla. Prior to and following emergence, the maxillary permanent incisors are more labially inclined than the mandibular incisors. *(e)* The pressure exerted by the lips leads to a reduction of the labial inclination. *(f)* The lower lip supports the maxillary incisors vertically together with the mandibular incisors. *(g)* The roots are completed after emergence in the oral cavity. *(h)* The skeleton as well as the soft tissues and the nose continue to grow, resulting in a straighter profile and further uprighting of the incisors, more in the maxilla than in the mandible. See video clip 7. (Printed from Van der Linden et al[5] with permission.)

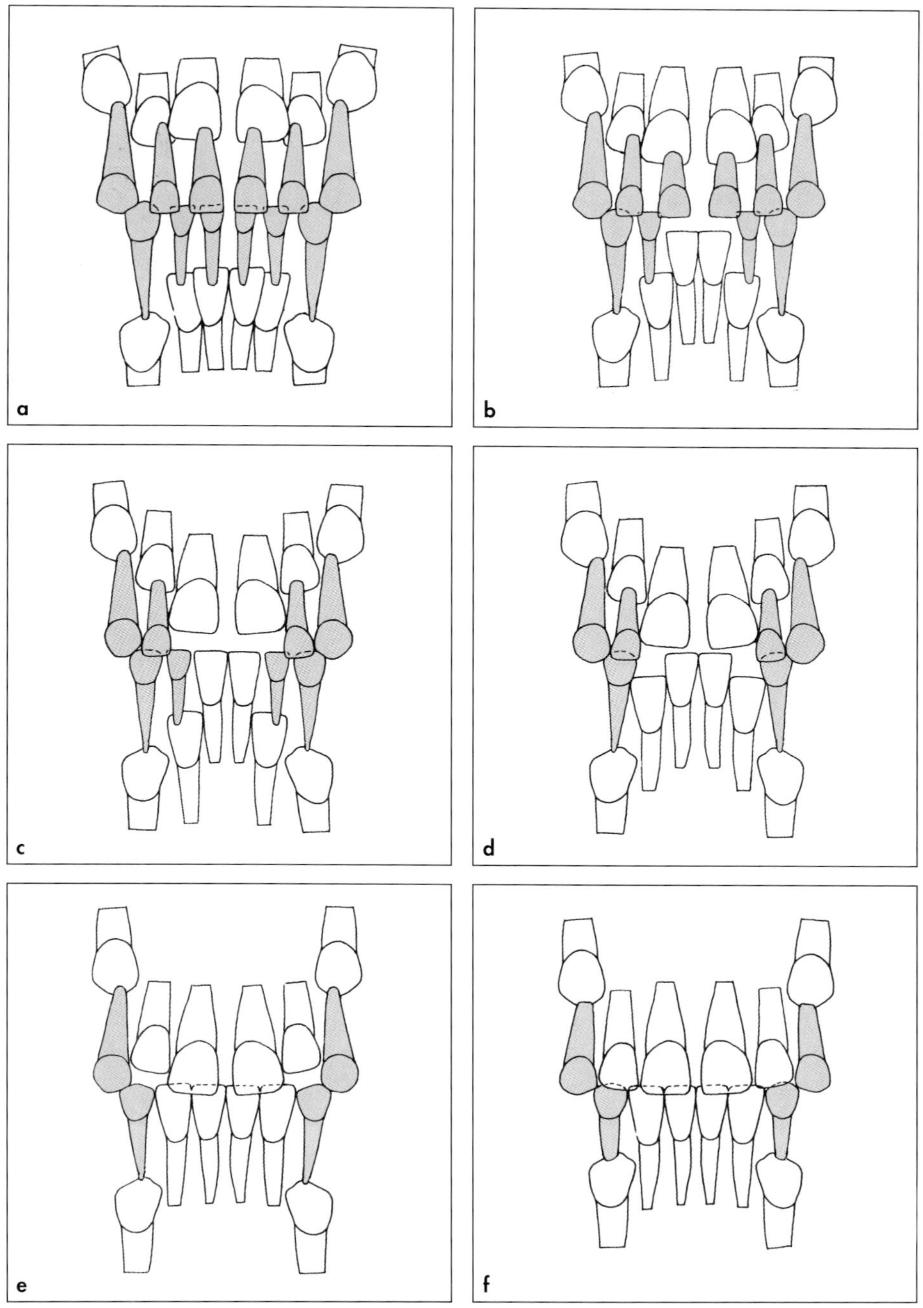

Fig 3-6 The most common mode of transition of incisors. *(a)* At 5 years of age, the eruption of the permanent incisors has not yet started. *(b and c)* First the mandibular central deciduous incisors are lost, followed 1 year later by the maxillary central incisors. The distal displacement of the maxillary lateral deciduous incisors is associated with the eruption of the central permanent incisors, which starts a few months earlier. In the mandible, the eruption of the central permanent incisors is not accompanied by migration of deciduous teeth. *(d)* Shortly before the mandibular lateral permanent incisors emerge, the adjacent deciduous canines move to the distal and buccal. *(e)* The initially more palatally positioned maxillary lateral permanent incisors erupt in a more labial direction than the central incisors. When their crowns come close to those of the central incisors, the central diastema reduces.[6,7] However, that reduction also occurs if this proximity is not reached, as often happens.[8,9] With the eruption of the lateral incisors, more room becomes available for the roots, allowing those of the central incisors to move distally. Their mesiodistal angulation alters, and the crowns move toward each other. *(f)* The maxillary lateral permanent incisors are the last to reach the level of the occlusal plane. There are diastemata in the maxillary anterior region and quite often also in the mandibular region. The roots of the lateral incisors are near the crowns of the permanent canines.

Transition of the incisors in a medium anterior section of the apical area

The most common mode of transition of incisors (ie, in a medium anterior section of the apical area) is illustrated in Fig 3-6. The mandibular central deciduous incisors are the first to be lost. Some weeks later their successors emerge, and the overlapping of the lateral incisors reduces. The proximity of the distoincisal corners of the maxillary central permanent incisors to the mesial aspects of the roots of the lateral deciduous incisors causes the latter to migrate distally. This leads to a reduction of the diastemata mesial to the maxillary deciduous canines and to more space for the central permanent incisors. With their further eruption, the deciduous canines migrate distally and buccally.

In the mandible, the distoincisal corners of the erupting lateral permanent incisors are in close proximity to the roots of the deciduous canines, which move distally and buccally. Due to the fact that the distal displacement of the deciduous canines occurs in both jaws at about the same time, the increase in intercanine distance usually happens simultaneously.[10–15]

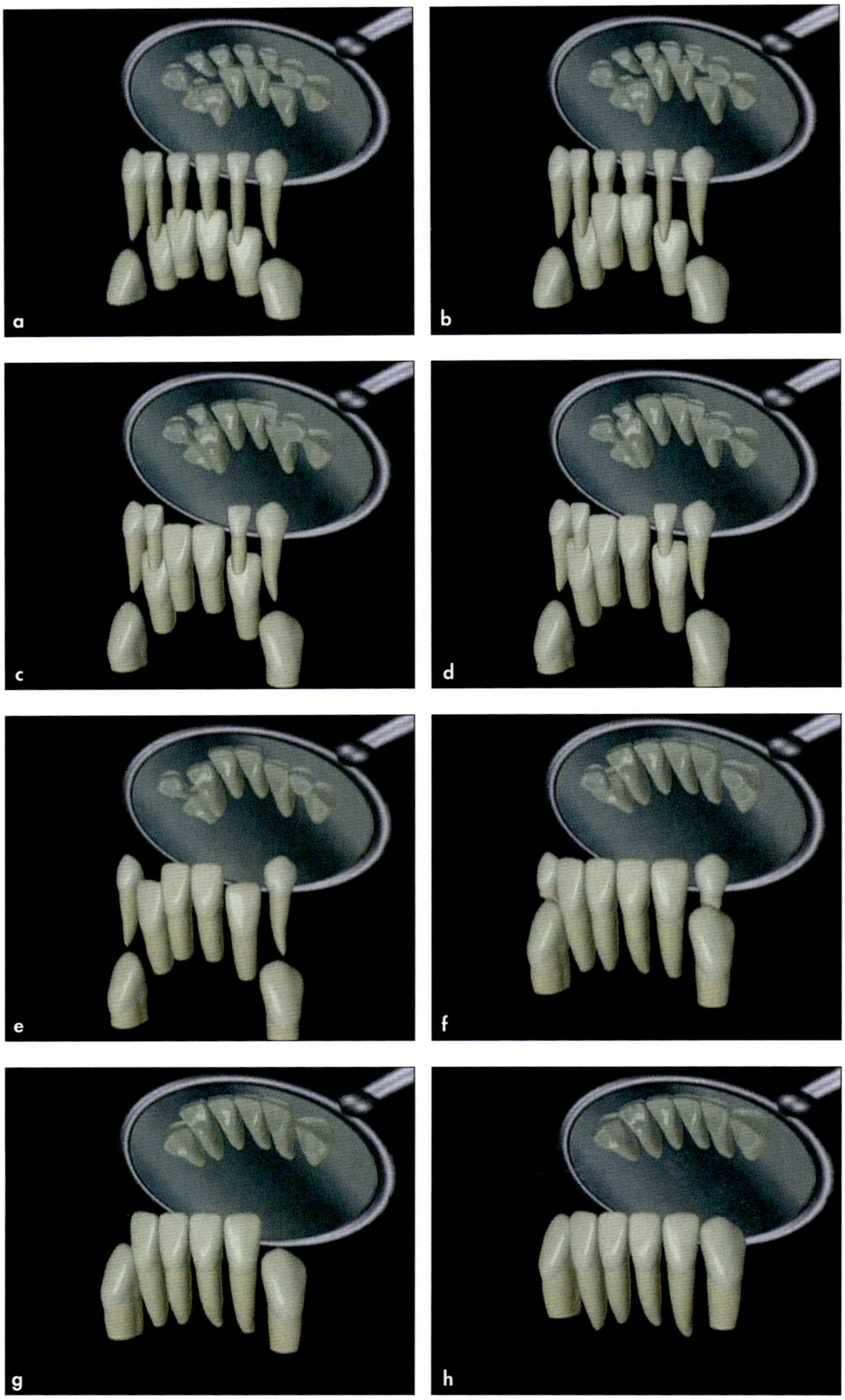

FIG 3-7 Transition of the mandibular incisors in a medium anterior section of the apical area. *(a)* As indicated, the central permanent incisors are initially located more occlusally than the lateral incisors. They are in close proximity. *(b)* The roots of the deciduous incisors resorb primarily on the lingual aspect. *(c)* The central deciduous incisors are lost, and their successors erupt further. *(d)* They are not in close proximity to the lateral deciduous incisors; as a result, these are not displaced, nor are the deciduous canines. *(e)* The eruption of the lateral permanent incisors is accompanied by distal and buccal displacement of the deciduous canines. *(f)* As the lateral permanent incisors reach the occlusal level, no or only small diastemata are present among the anterior teeth. *(g)* The apices of the lateral incisors are situated more lingually than those of the central incisors. This corresponds with their positions at formation. *(h)* The lateral incisors are slightly more labially inclined than the central incisors. After emergence, their crowns are moved labially through pressure exerted by the tongue, making them well aligned in the dental arch. See video clip 8. (Printed from Van der Linden et al[5] with permission.)

In both jaws, the lateral permanent incisors emerge about 1 year after the central permanent incisors. The mandibular lateral incisors emerge at about the same time as the maxillary central incisors. Following its emergence, it takes about 8 months for a crown of a maxillary central permanent incisor to become fully exposed.[16] (For times of emergence and other statistical data, see chapter 17.)

The modes of transition described above occur when some extra space is needed for adequate eruption and arrangement in the dental arch (ie, a medium anterior section of the apical area). This development is illustrated for the mandible in Fig 3-7, for the maxilla in Fig 3-8.

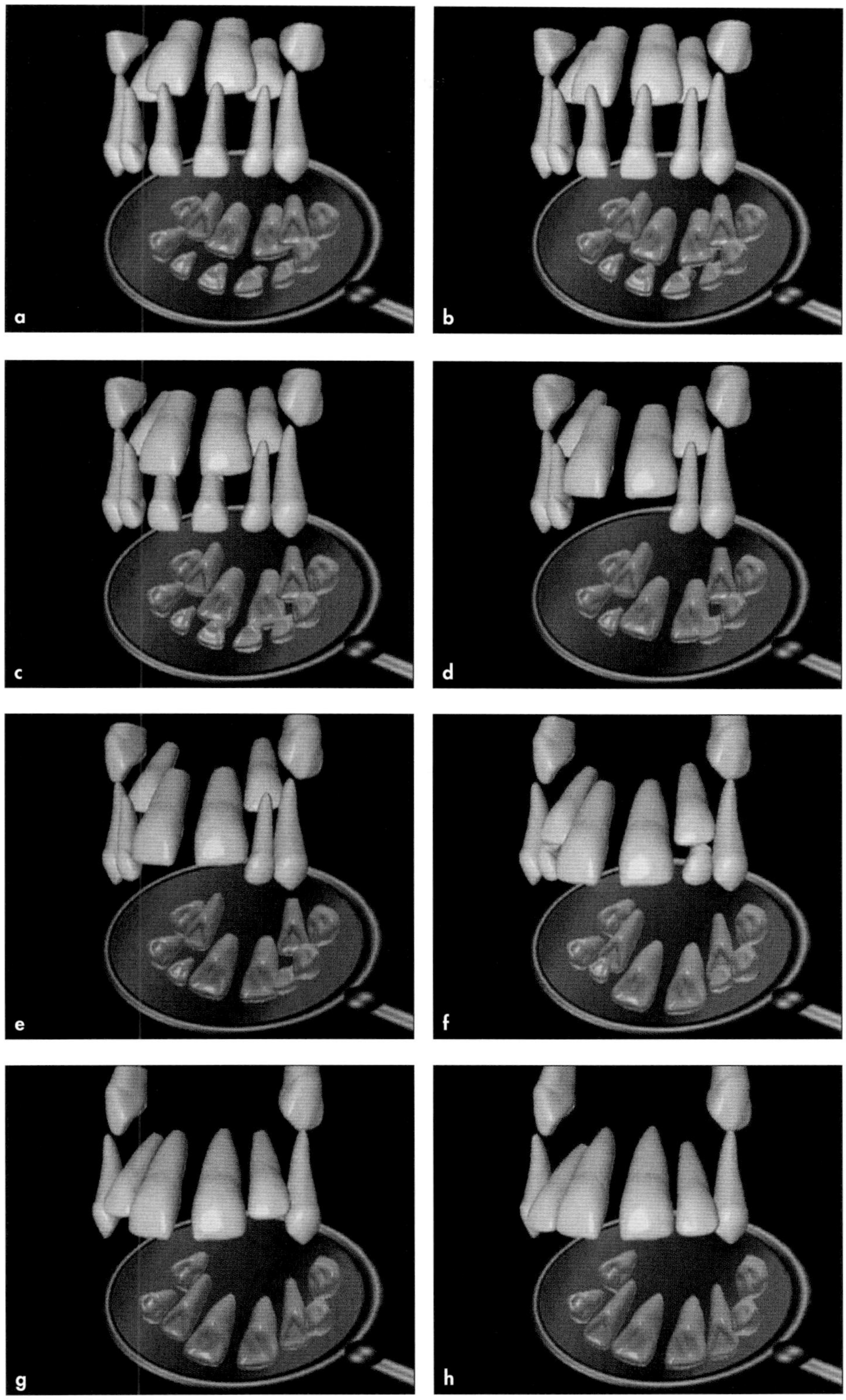

Fig 3-8 Transition of the maxillary incisors in a medium anterior section of the apical area. *(a)* The incisal edges of the maxillary central permanent incisors are more superiorly located than those of the lateral incisors. *(b)* The central incisors erupt and pass the lateral incisors. *(c)* The roots of their predecessors resorb gradually. This breakdown corresponds in speed, amount, and shape with the displacement and morphology of the approaching successors. The deciduous incisors resorb from the palatal aspect, resulting in a thin and sharp labial end. At the time the deciduous incisors are shed, their roots are almost completely resorbed. *(d)* The central permanent incisor moves occlusally alongside the lateral deciduous incisors, which migrate distally. *(e)* When the lateral deciduous incisor approaches the deciduous canine, the latter will also migrate distally and buccally. Through these migrations, sufficient space becomes available for the emergence of the central permanent incisors. *(f)* Subsequently, the lateral incisors descend, for which sufficient room has become available. In erupting, they do not contact the central incisors. *(g)* In accordance with the positions at initial formation, the apices of the fully erupted lateral permanent incisors are located more palatally and also more occlusally than those of the central incisors. *(h)* The permanent incisors are distally angulated, and there is a large central diastema. See video clip 9. (Printed from Van der Linden et al[5] with permission.)

Asymmetric transition of the incisors

Corresponding left and right incisors do not always emerge at or even near the same time. There is usually a marked difference if a deciduous incisor (in most cases a maxillary central incisor) has experienced trauma. Its successor usually emerges considerably later than its counterpart, but sometimes earlier. The displacement of the maxillary lateral deciduous incisor and canine then does not occur on both sides at the same time because their displacement is related to the eruption of the central permanent incisor in the involved quadrant. Such an asymmetric transition is demonstrated in Fig 3-9.

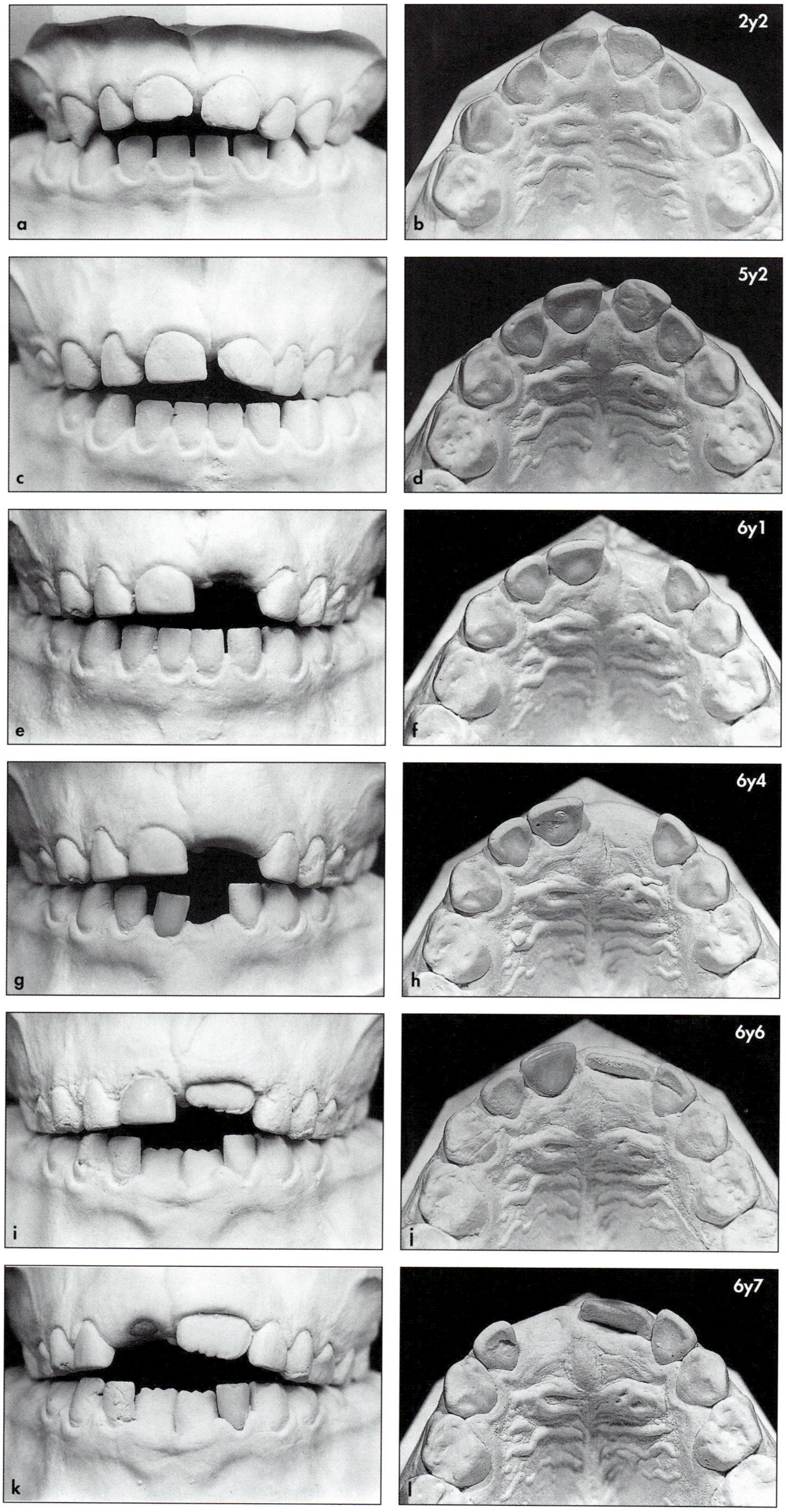

Fig 3-9 Asymmetric transition of maxillary incisors. This series of dental casts, from a girl with a Class II, division 1 malocclusion, covers the period from 2 years 2 months to 7 years 6 months of age and shows the changes during the transition of the maxillary incisors. She had sucked her thumb until the emergence of the maxillary central permanent incisors and had an anterior open bite for many years. At the age of 4 years, the crown of the maxillary left central deciduous incisor was fractured by trauma, and the tooth migrated distally and became discolored. *(a and b)* At the age of 2 years 2 months, large diastemata were present in the maxillary dental arch, and the tooth positioning on the left side was similar to the positioning on the right side. *(c and d)* Three years later, little had changed on the right side. On the left side, where the trauma had occurred, both deciduous incisors had migrated, and the diastemata had closed. *(e and f)* At the age of 6 years 1 month, the left central deciduous incisor was exfoliated; the right one had moved distally and was in contact with the lateral deciduous incisor. *(g and h)* Three months later, the situation had not changed. *(i and j)* After 2 more months had passed, the left central permanent incisor had emerged. The right central deciduous incisor was lost in the process of impression taking and saved for incorporation in the plaster cast. The diastemata distal to the right lateral deciduous incisor and canine had decreased only slightly or not at all. *(k and l)* One month later, these diastemata were closed, and the involved teeth had moved distally.

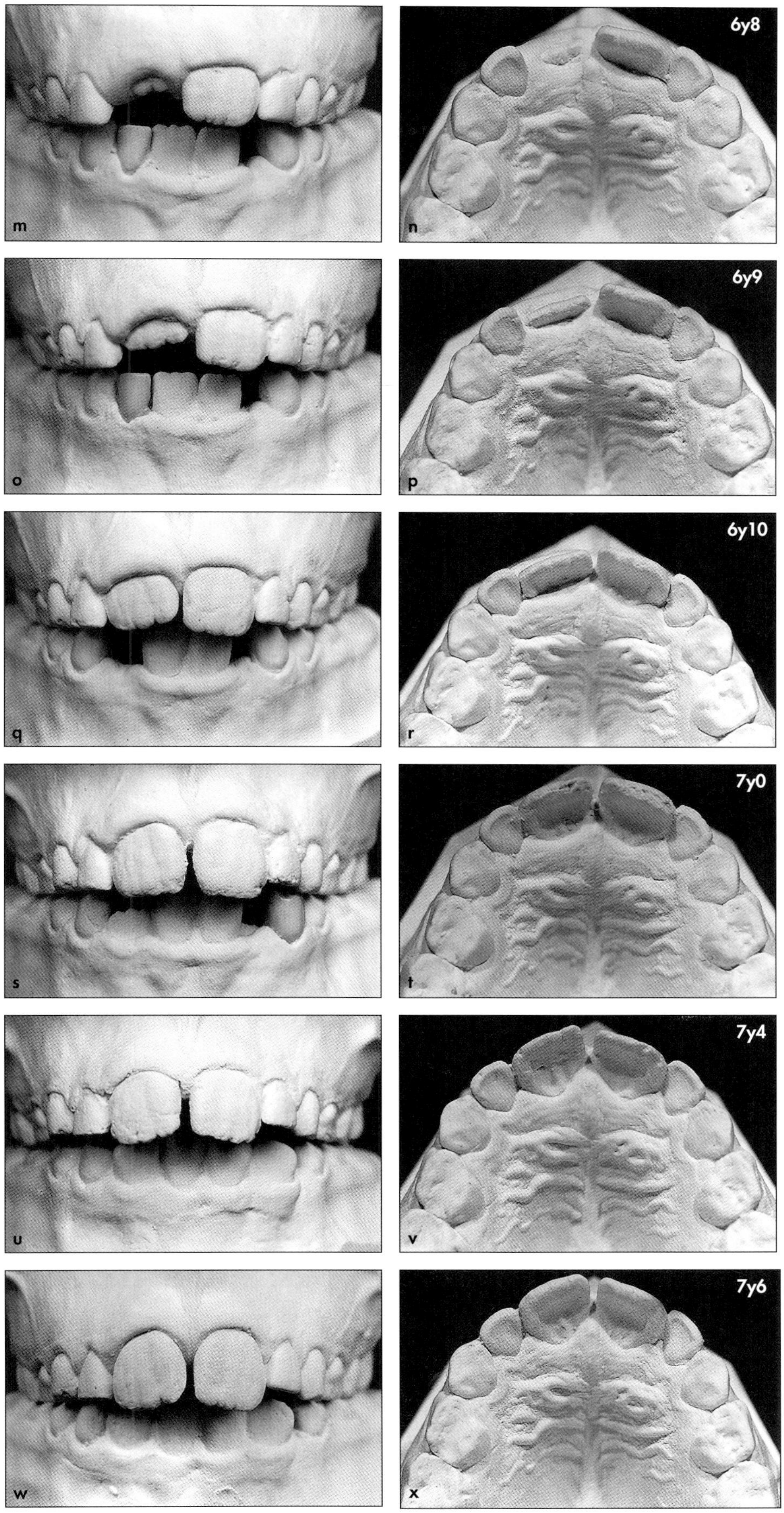

Fig 3-9 *(cont) (m and n)* One month later, the right central permanent incisor emerged with sufficient space, 2 months after its predecessor was shed. *(o and p)* In the ensuing month, the right central permanent incisor erupted further, and the space increased slightly because of the buccal movement of the deciduous canine. *(q and r)* At the age of 6 years 10 months, the incisal edge of the right central permanent incisor, 3 months after emergence, had almost reached the level of the incisal edge of the left central incisor. *(s to x)* In the 8 months following, few changes took place. The central diastema and the angulation of the incisors stayed more or less the same. This series demonstrates that the gain in space needed for the larger permanent incisors, realized by the displacement of adjacent deciduous teeth, is a unilateral phenomenon related to the time of emergence of the largest of the two permanent incisors on one side. (Reprinted from Van der Linden[17] with permission.)

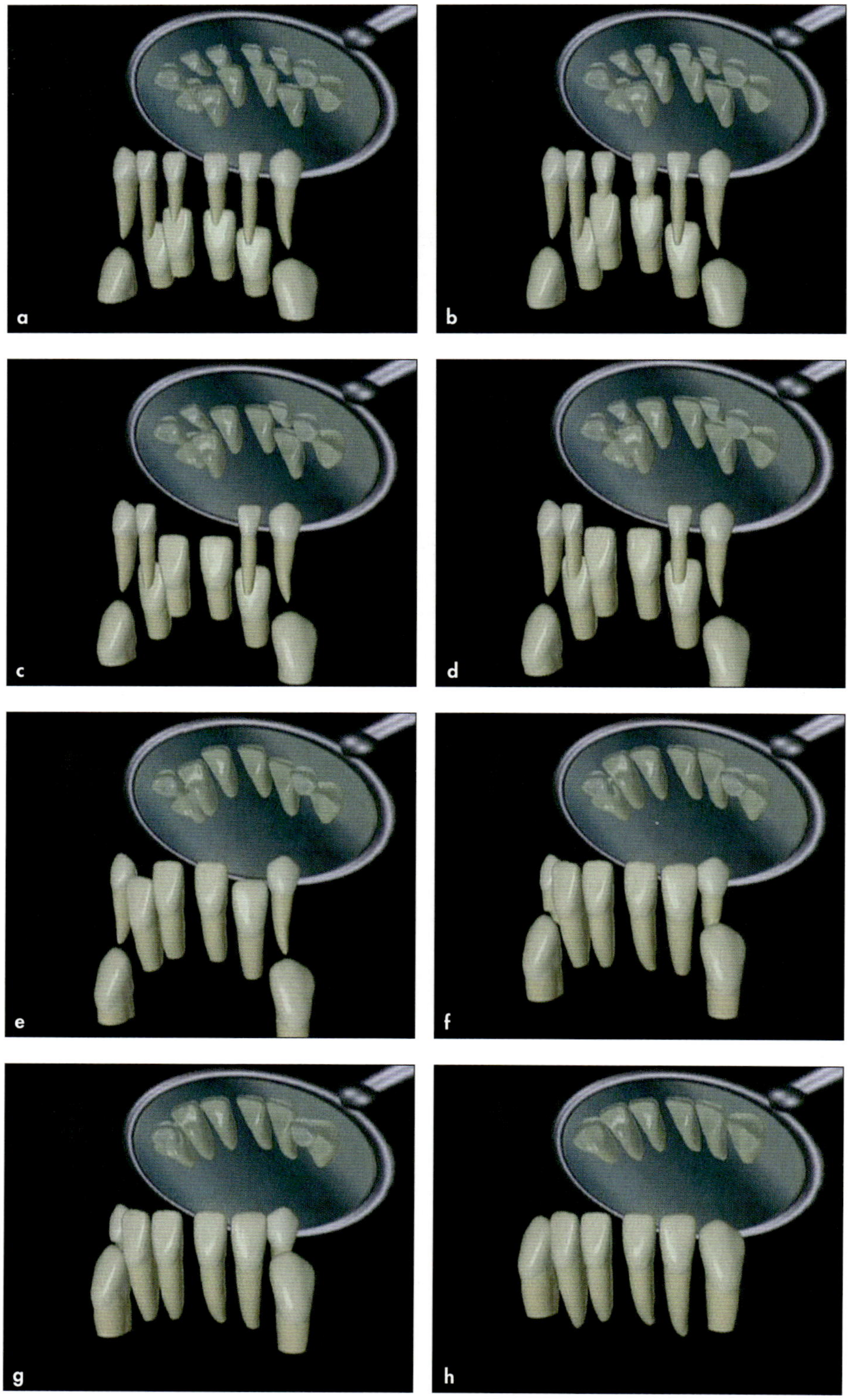

FIG 3-10 Transition of the mandibular incisors in a large anterior section of the apical area. *(a to d)* There is so much room that the permanent incisors can erupt without displacement of the deciduous canines. *(e to h)* After all permanent incisors have completed their eruption, multiple diastemata remain among the anterior teeth. See video clip 10. (Printed from Van der Linden et al[5] with permission.)

Transition of the incisors in a large anterior section of the apical area

In situations with excess space, the transition takes place without displacement of deciduous teeth. If there is a severe shortage of space, adjacent deciduous teeth resorb and are lost prematurely. In both situations, the intercanine distance does not increase during the transition of the incisors.[12,18–20]

Indeed, in cases with excess space in the jaws, migration of deciduous teeth is not needed to provide extra room for the emergence of the maxillary central permanent incisors and mandibular lateral incisors. This mode of transition is illustrated for the mandibular incisors in Fig 3-10 and for the maxillary incisors in Fig 3-11.

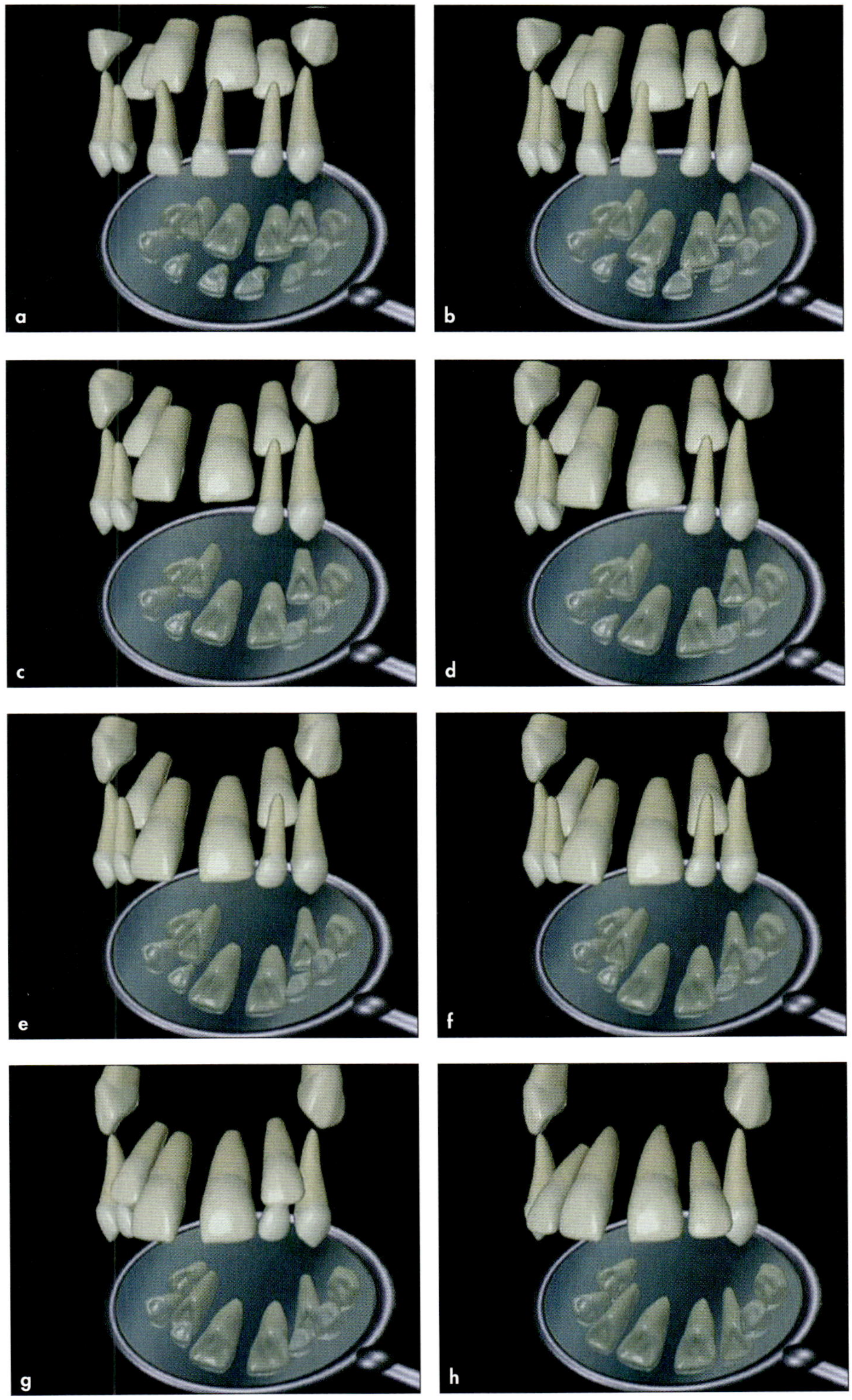

Fig 3-11 Transition of the maxillary incisors in a large anterior section of the apical area. *(a to d)* With excess space, the erupting central permanent incisors will not come in close proximity with the roots of the lateral deciduous incisors, which will not move distally. *(e to h)* In turn, the deciduous canines also will not be moved distally. See video clip 11. (Printed from Van der Linden et al[5] with permission.)

Transition of the incisors in a small anterior section of the apical area

In situations with a severe shortage of space in the mandible, the eruption and emergence of the central permanent incisor is preceded not only by loss of its predecessor but also by premature loss of the adjacent lateral deciduous incisor. With the eruption of the lateral permanent incisor, the deciduous canine exfoliates. Subsequently, the four permanent incisors can become well aligned. However, the space remaining in the dental arch for the permanent canine is too small (Fig 3-12).

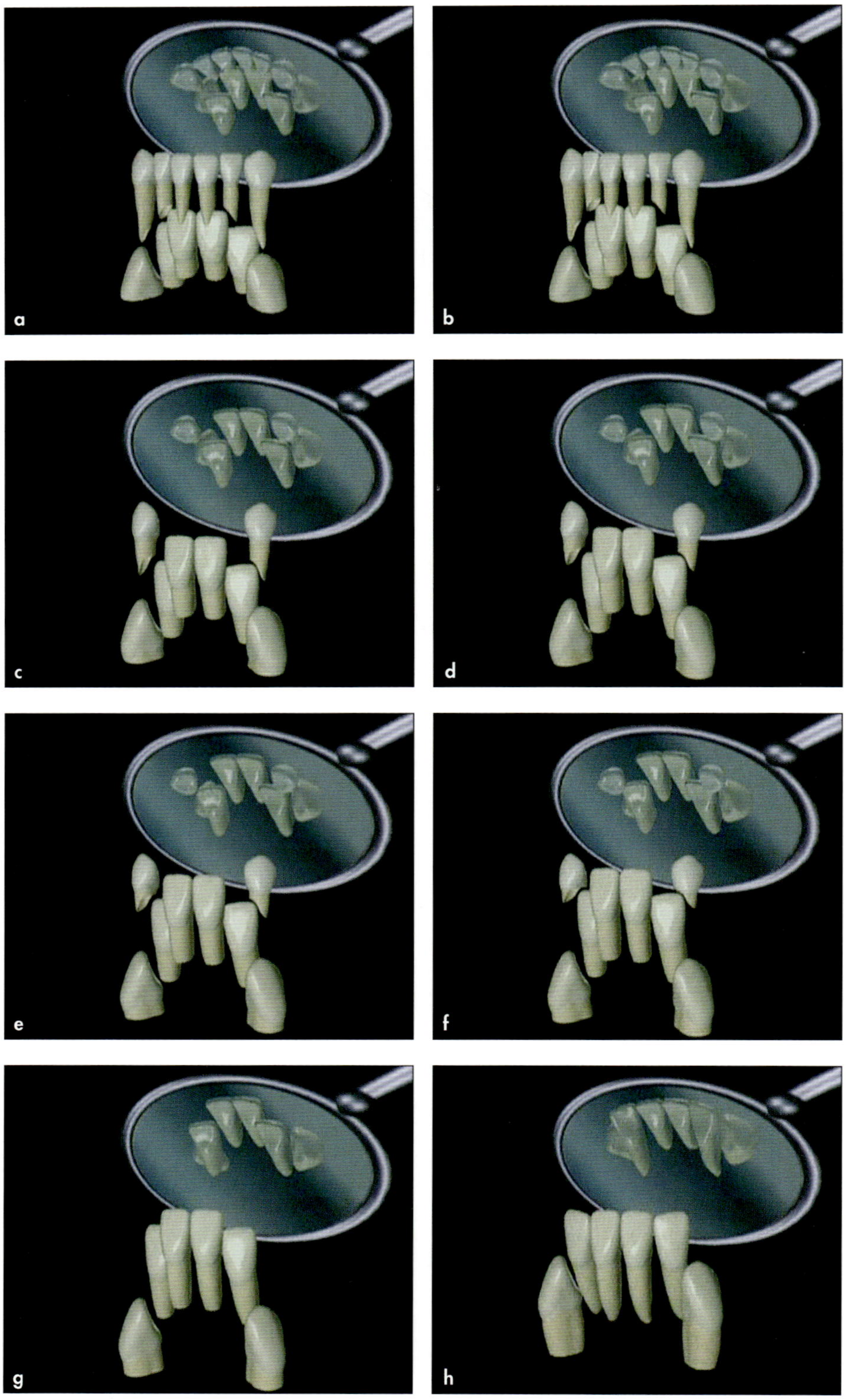

Fig 3-12 Transition of the mandibular incisors in a small anterior section of the apical area. Note that in this figure, as in the preceding ones, the transitional process is presented symmetrically. However, that is often not the case, particularly in the mandible, where the teeth can cross the median plane prior to emergence. It happens quite often that a deciduous canine is lost prematurely only on one side, and the process described below occurs unilaterally. *(a)* The absence of diastemata in the anterior region of the complete deciduous dentition is a sign of lack of space. Within the jaw, the permanent teeth overlap each other extensively. *(b)* With the eruption of the central permanent incisors, the roots of their predecessors as well as those of the adjacent lateral deciduous incisors become resorbed. *(c)* The central deciduous incisors exfoliate first. *(d)* Shortly thereafter, the lateral incisors exfoliate. *(e)* Insufficient space remains for the lateral permanent incisors. *(f)* When they move occlusally, the roots of the deciduous canines resorb prematurely. *(g)* They exfoliate prior to the emergence of the lateral permanent incisors. *(h)* This provides space for them to attain a better position in the dental arch. This happens at the cost of the space that remains for the permanent canines. They will later erupt in a buccal position. See video clip 12. (Printed from Van der Linden et al[5] with permission.)

In situations with a severe shortage of space in the maxilla, the eruption of the maxillary central incisor usually results in premature resorption and loss of the adjacent lateral deciduous incisor. The extra space that would otherwise become available with the distal and buccal displacement of the deciduous canine is not gained. The lateral permanent incisor will then erupt palatally (Fig 3-13). This can occur on both sides but also on one side only, in which case the other incisors and the midline of the dental arch will migrate to the side of the loss. However, the roots cannot move through the median suture, which blocks further migration. In the mandible, not only the crowns but also the roots can pass the median plane. Hence, an asymmetric transition occurs more frequently with one-sided premature loss of a deciduous tooth in the mandible than in the maxilla.

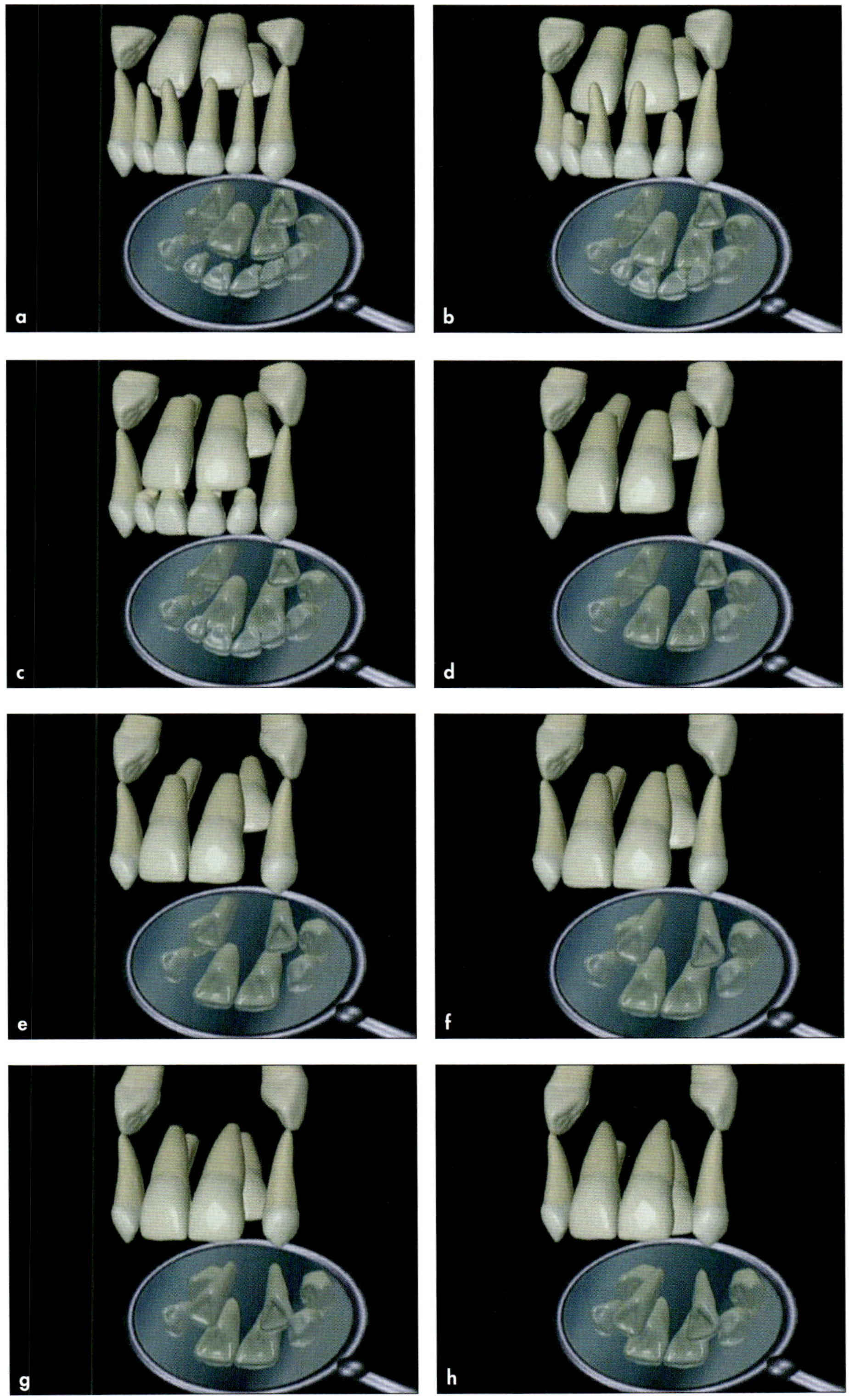

Fig 3-13 Transition of the maxillary incisors in a small section of the apical area. *(a)* In a deciduous dental arch with no or only small diastemata in the anterior region, not enough room is available in the jaws for adequate transition of the incisors. *(b)* The width of the piriform aperture is small, as is the distance between the forming parts of the permanent canines. The incisal margins of the central permanent incisors are in close proximity with the roots of the central and lateral deciduous incisors. *(c)* First, the central deciduous incisors exfoliate. *(d)* Soon thereafter, the lateral deciduous incisors exfoliate. *(e)* Subsequently, the central permanent incisors descend further, without distal and buccal displacement of the deciduous canines. Hence, additional space is not created in the dental arch. *(f)* After the central permanent incisors have emerged, the lateral incisors start to descend. However, they cannot move labially and emerge palatally to the central permanent incisors and deciduous canines. *(g)* They may end up in negative overjet with the mandibular incisors. *(h)* Severe shortage of space in the dental arch results. This is due to initial shortage of space and the lack of displacement of the deciduous canines. Both aspects can be traced back to a discrepancy between the size of the anterior maxilla and the mesiodistal dimensions of the permanent teeth. See video clip 13. (Printed from Van der Linden et al[5] with permission.)

In situations with a severe shortage of space in the maxilla, not only lateral deciduous incisors but also deciduous canines can be lost prematurely (see Fig 16-2). The transition process is comparable to the one illustrated for the mandibular incisors in Fig 3-12. See video clip 14.

Anatomical Considerations in the First Transitional Period

Transition of the incisors

Every deciduous incisor and canine has a small opening at the lingual side of the alveolar bone. This is the oral side of the gubernacular canal that runs to the crypt of the successor. Initially, the gubernacular canal contains the gubernacular cord, which consists of epithelium of the dental lamina. The epithelium gets lost, and a connective tissue strand remains but successively disintegrates further.[21,22] The oral opening of the gubernacular canal enlarges gradually with the eruption of the permanent tooth. The gubernacular canal probably has a function in guiding the eruption of incisors and canines to the openings at the alveolar bone, where emergence will take place. Indeed, permanent incisors and canines emerge through the alveolar bone at the location of the oral opening of the gubernacular canal, which is lingual to the location of their predecessors (Fig 3-14).

The loss of deciduous teeth is caused by resorption of their roots and the surrounding bone. Both processes start early. At 4 years of age, part of the roots of the mandibular and maxillary central deciduous incisors is already resorbed, as is the bone at the cervical margin. When a deciduous tooth is shed, the bone that surrounds the root is lost. With the eruption of the successor, the alveolar process is built up again as the erupting tooth constructs its own alveolar process by osteogenic activity of the periodontal ligament.[24]

Some weeks pass between the loss of a deciduous incisor and the emergence of its successor. During that interval, the gingival defect caused by the loss of the tooth is repaired, and a new opening in the gingiva is created. In the meantime, the alveolar process is built up.

One or two months between the time of emergence of corresponding left and right incisors is not uncommon. Such asymmetry occurs more in the maxilla than in the mandible.

Permanent teeth start to erupt shortly after root formation has begun and emerge in the oral cavity when three-quarters of the root length is complete.[25,26]

Emergence of the first permanent molars

The posterior morphology and extension of the maxilla and mandible allow sufficient space to become available for the first permanent molars (Figs 3-15 and 3-16). As indicated previously, these teeth are initially mesiodistally oriented perpendicular to the occlusal plane (Fig 3-17).

The first permanent molars are the largest teeth and provide important support to the occlusion. The large mesiopalatal cusp of the maxillary first molar has to coincide with the central fossa of the mandibular first molar. Angle has called the maxillary first permanent molar the "key to occlusion."[27]

The posterior extension of the tooth-bearing parts of the jaws that precedes the emergence of molars is reflected in so-called molar fields behind the last tooth in the posterior region.[28] These molar fields are visible and palpable in the mouth, most clearly in the maxilla where the morphology of the tuber is easy to assess. It is more difficult to specify the posterior border of the alveolar process in the mandible. Molar fields develop prior to the emergence of deciduous and permanent molars. They can be too small for the second or third permanent molars if the preceding posterior jaw extension has been insufficient. This topic is discussed in detail in chapter 6.

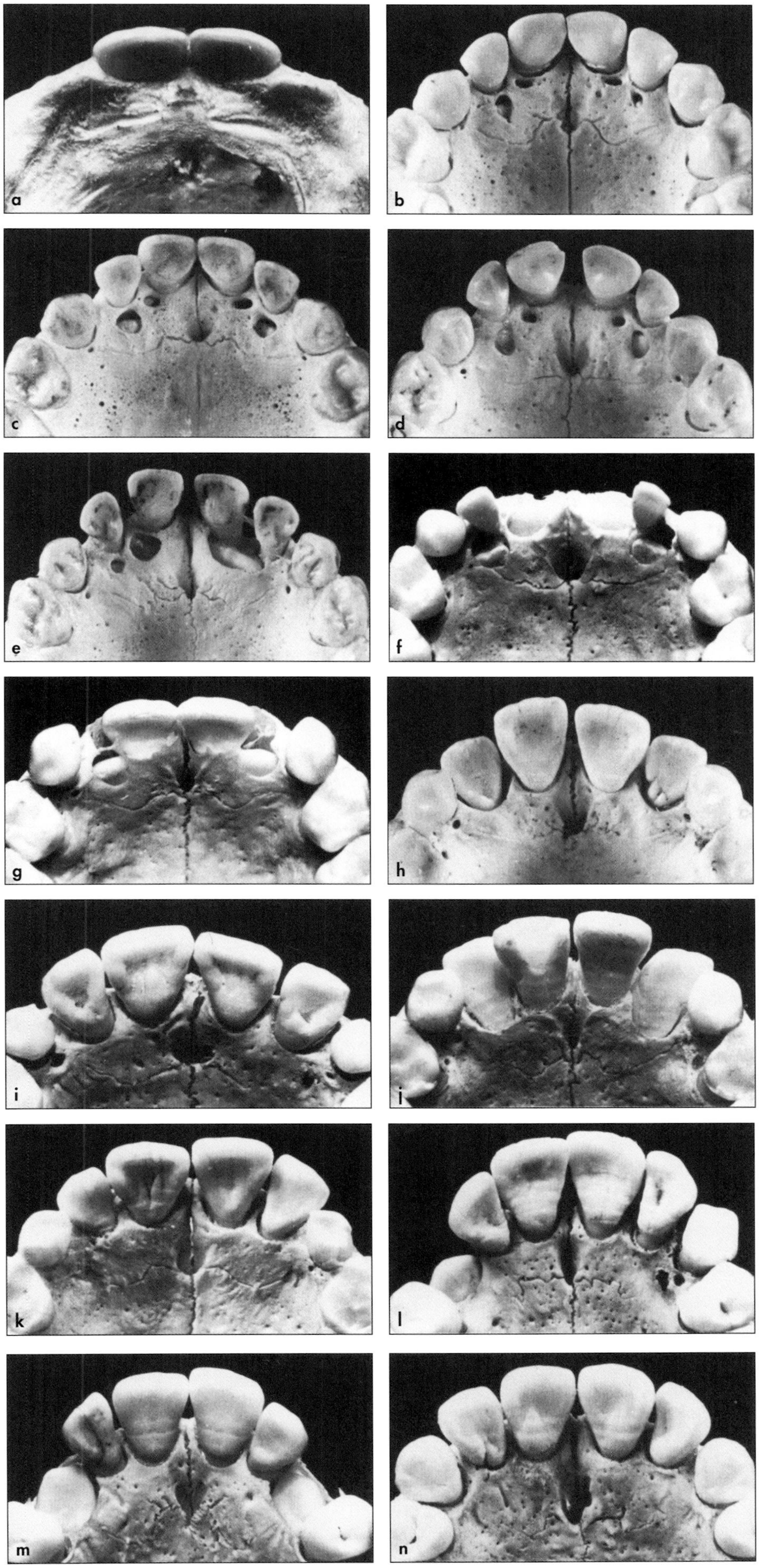

Fig 3-14 Gubernacular canals and the eruption and emergence of the maxillary permanent incisors. *(a to h)* The gradually increasing openings in the alveolar bone, located palatal to the deciduous incisors and canines, are the ends of the gubernacular canals, which run between the crypts of the permanent teeth and the palatal bone surface. These canals contain the gubernacular cord, a connective tissue strand that connects the tooth follicle with the lamina propria of the gingiva.[23] They are present in both jaws where permanent teeth will replace deciduous teeth and also at the permanent molars. The gubernacular canals become wider through the resorption that precedes eruption. The permanent teeth pass the bone surface through the gradually enlarging openings at the end of the gubernacular canals. *(i to n)* Various situations after the emergence of permanent incisors.

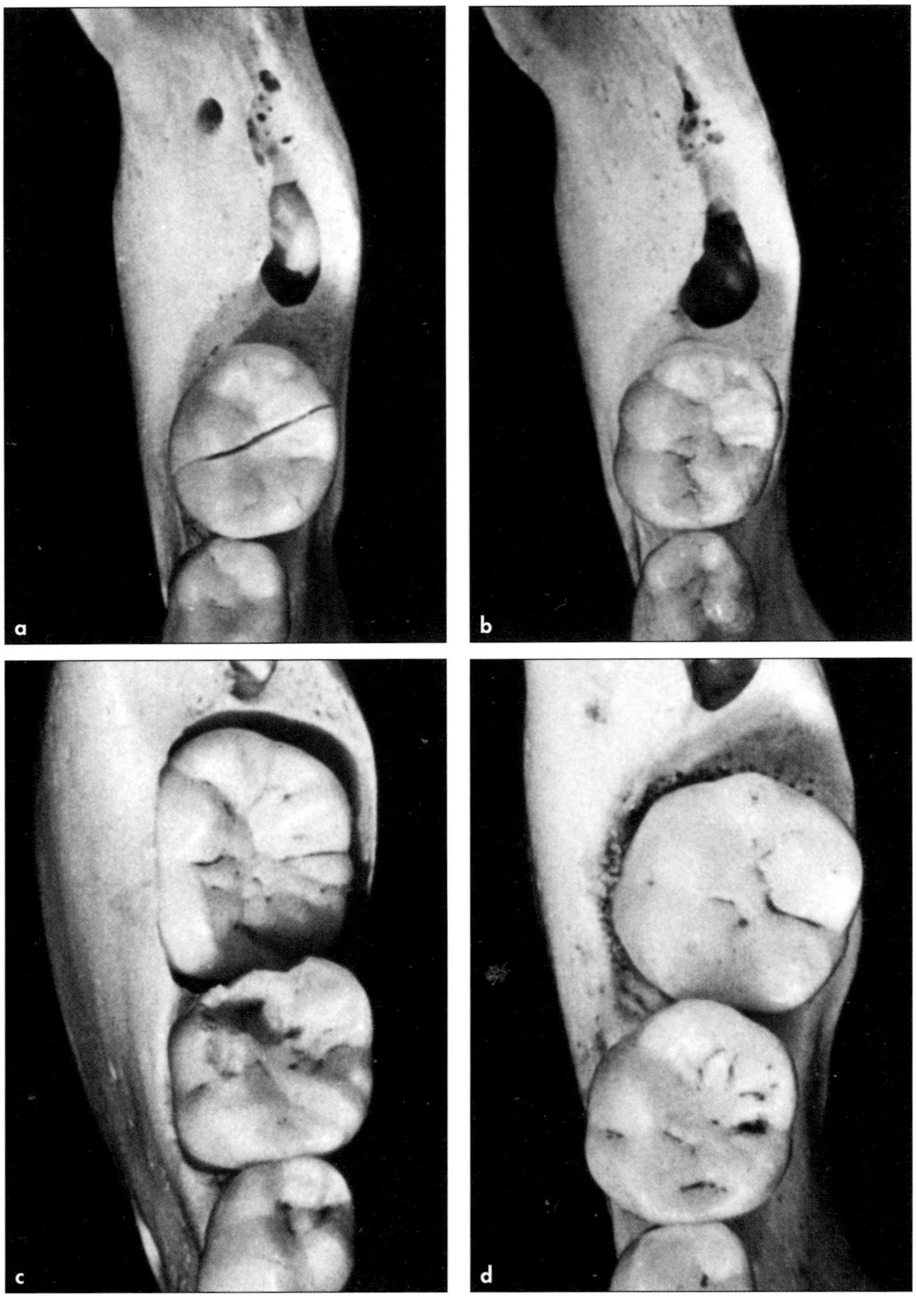

FIG 3-15 Emergence of mandibular first permanent molars, demonstrated in four right jaw fragments. *(a)* Initially, the crown of the first permanent molar is situated in the mandible directly mesial to the obtuse lateral angle. *(b)* The opening of the gubernacular canal enlarges gradually. *(c)* Sufficient bone is resorbed for the emergence of the crown. *(d)* During the eruption following emergence, alveolar bone is built up in the cervical region.

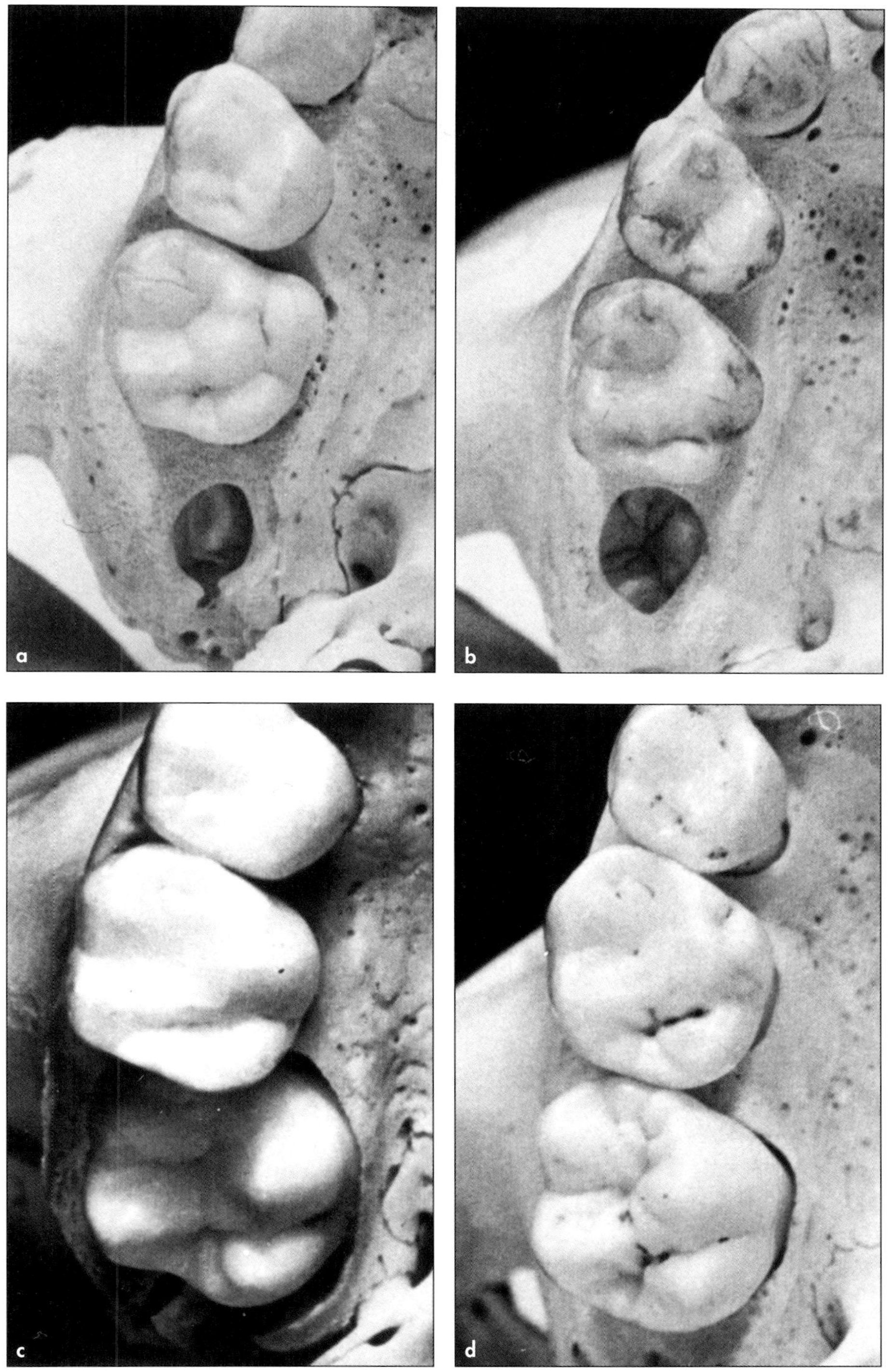

FIG 3-16 Emergence of maxillary first permanent molars, demonstrated in four right jaw fragments. *(a)* Initially, the gubernacular opening is small. *(b)* With progressing eruption, the size of the opening increases. *(c)* Sufficient bone is resorbed for the emergence of the crown. *(d)* Subsequently, the alveolar bone in the cervical region is built up.

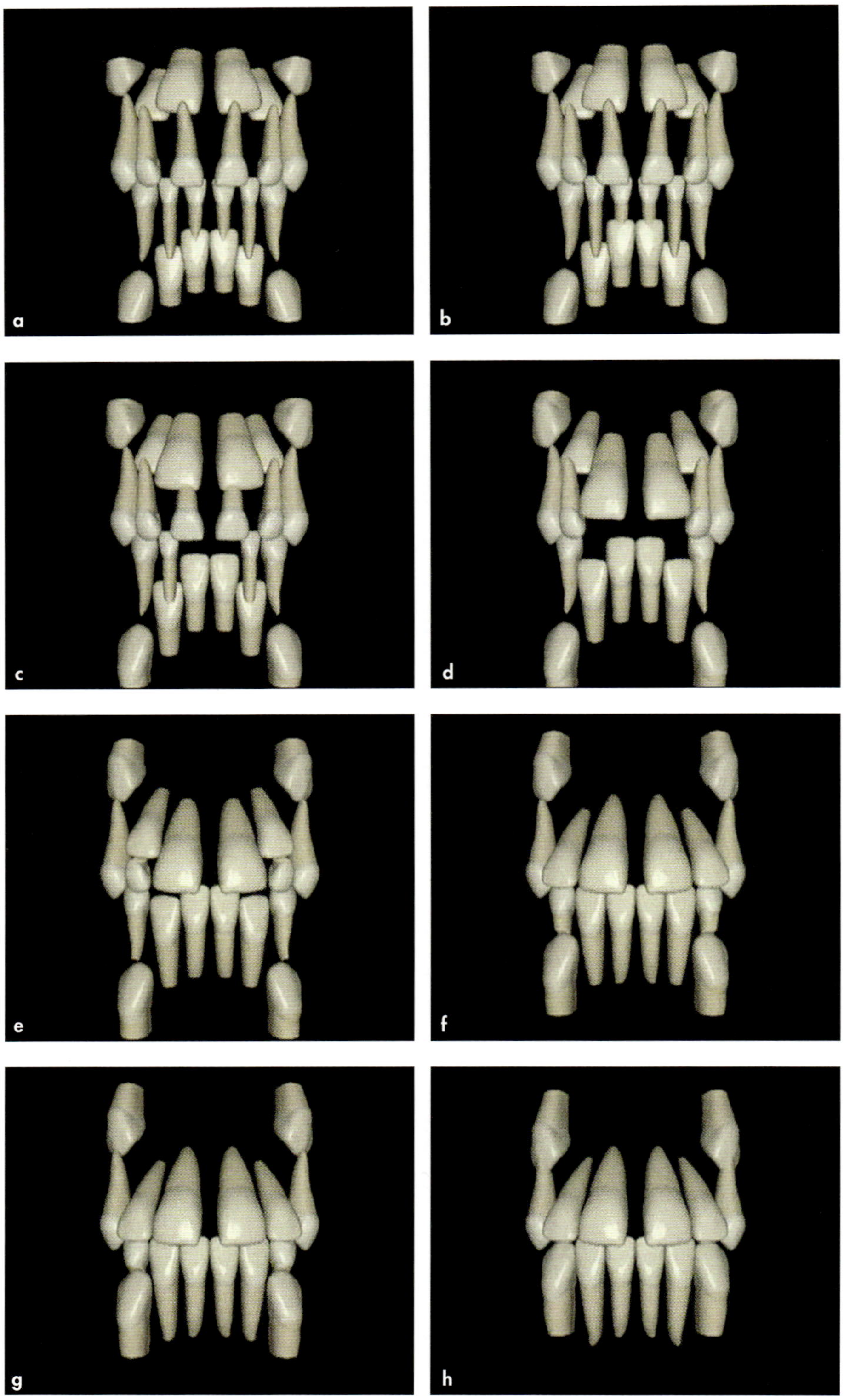

Fig 3-17 Transition of mandibular and maxillary incisors in medium anterior sections of the apical area in both jaws. *(a)* The permanent central incisors are initially the closest to the occlusal plane in the mandible but not in the maxilla. Indeed, the narrowest permanent incisors are formed the closest to the occlusal plane. With this arrangement, the available space within the jaws is used optimally. *(b)* The transition in the mandible precedes the one in the maxilla. *(c)* After the mandibular central permanent incisors have emerged, the adjacent lateral incisors start to erupt, along with the maxillary central permanent incisors. *(d)* They approach the deciduous teeth located distal to them. *(e)* Subsequently, the teeth distal to the mandibular lateral incisors and maxillary central permanent incisors migrate distobuccally, which happens in the same period in both jaws. *(f)* The transition of the incisors is completed as the maxillary lateral permanent incisors reach the occlusal level. *(g)* After 1.5 or more years, the mandibular deciduous canines exfoliate, and the permanent ones emerge. *(h)* The maxillary canines are the last of the anterior teeth to be replaced. Until then, the central diastema in the maxilla does not close, and the four maxillary incisors remain distally angulated. In the mandible, where the central permanent incisors can reach contact shortly after emergence, the angulation of the incisors changes only slightly after emergence of the permanent canines. See video clip 15. (Printed from Van der Linden et al[5] with permission.)

General Overview of the Transition of the Anterior Teeth and Eruption of the First Permanent Molars

To conclude this chapter, the transition of the anterior teeth in both jaws is shown from the front (see Fig 3-17) and the eruption and position of the first permanent molars are shown from various view points (Fig 3-18).

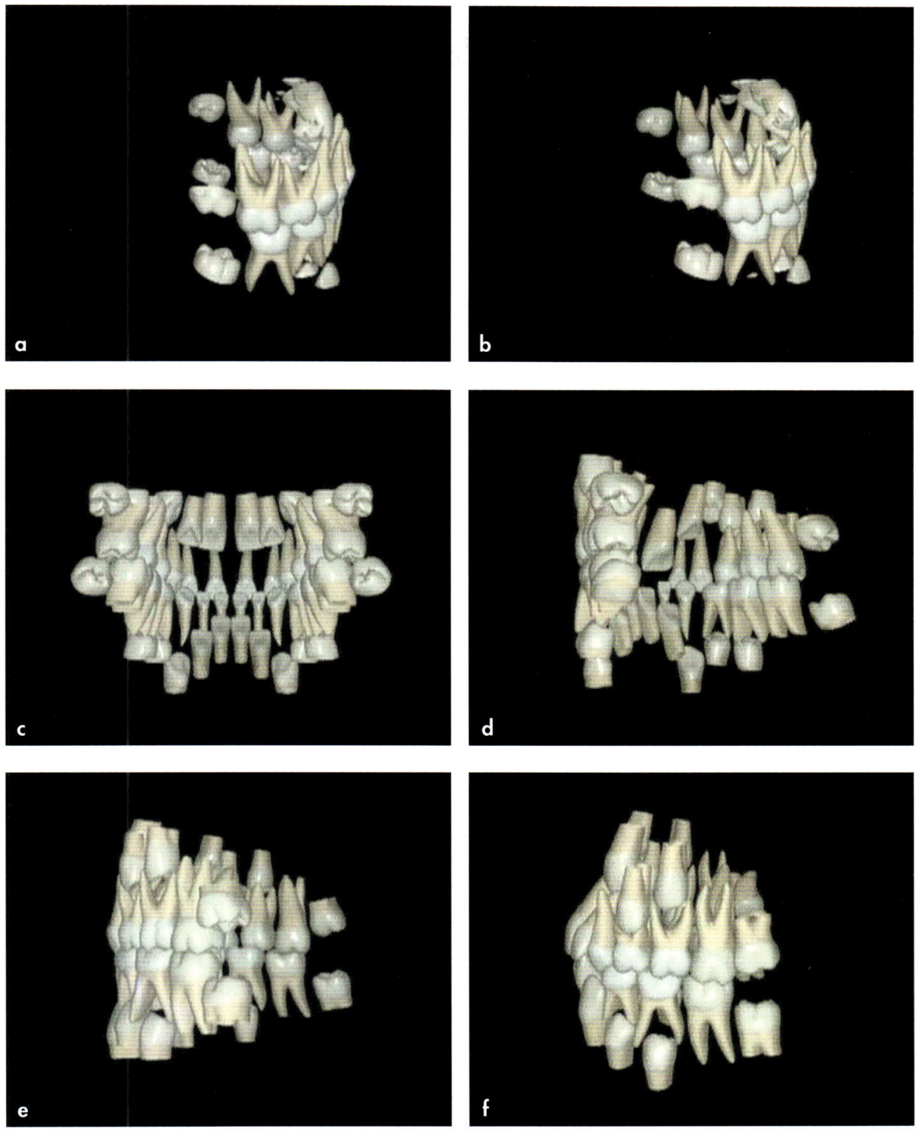

FIG 3-18 Eruption and position of first permanent molars. (a) Prior to emergence, there is sufficient room for the first permanent molars in both jaws. *(b)* With eruption, they become more upright. *(c and d)* After reaching occlusal contact, they are guided by the cone-funnel mechanism. *(e)* With narrow mandibular second deciduous molars, they can immediately reach maximal intercuspation. *(f)* Their angulation does not alter prior to the emergence of the second permanent molars.

References

1. Farsi NMA, Salama FS. Characteristics of primary dentition occlusion in a group of Saudi children. Int J Paediatr Dent 1996;6:253–259.
2. Moorrees CFA, Chadha JM. Crown diameters of corresponding tooth groups in the deciduous and permanent dentition. J Dent Res 1962;41:466–470.
3. Feasby WH. A radiographic study of dental eruption. Am J Orthod 1981;80:545–560.
4. Smith RJ, Rapp R. A cephalometric study of the developmental relationship between primary and permanent maxillary central incisor teeth. J Dent Child 1980;47:36–41.
5. Van der Linden FPGM, Radlanski RJ, McNamara JA Jr. Dynamics of Orthodontics: Normal Development of the Dentition [DVD 3A]. Berlin: Quintessence, 2000.
6. Broadbent BH. The face of the normal child. Angle Orthod 1937;7:183–208.
7. Broadbent BH. Ontogenic development of occlusion. Angle Orthod 1941;11:223–241.
8. Bakker PJMR, Wassenberg HJW, Van der Linden FPGM. Change in the upper incisors [in German]. Inf Orthod Kieferorthop 1979;11:239–270.
9. Jacobsson SO. Diastema mediale. En longitudinell undersökning. Odontol Tidskr 1965;73:127–148.
10. Baume LJ. Physiological tooth migration and its significance for the development of occlusion. I. The biogenetic course of the deciduous dentition. J Dent Res 1950;29:123–132.

11. Baume LJ. Physiological tooth migration and its significance for the development of occlusion. II. The biogenesis of the accessional dentition. J Dent Res 1950;29:331–337.
12. Moorrees CFA. The Dentition of the Growing Child: A Longitudinal Study of Dental Development Between 3 and 18 Years of Age. Cambridge, MA: Harvard University, 1959.
13. Moorrees CFA. Normal variation in dental development determined with reference to tooth eruption status. J Dent Res 1965;44:161–173.
14. Moyers RE, Van der Linden FPGM, Riolo ML, McNamara JA Jr. Standards of Human Occlusal Development, monograph 5, Craniofacial Growth Series. Ann Arbor: University of Michigan, 1976.
15. Yang J, Shinji H. Study on developmental changes of dental arch from pre-dental period to mixed dentition. Part 1. Changes of dental arch widths. Pediatr Dent J 2001;11:67–84.
16. Giles NB, Knott VB, Meredith HV. Increase in intraoral height of selected permanent teeth during the quadrennium following gingival emergence. Angle Orthod 1963;33:195–206.
17. Van der Linden FPGM. Orthodontic Concepts and Strategies. Chicago: Quintessence, 2004.
18. Bakker PJMR, Wassenberg HJW, Van der Linden FPGM. Exchange of the lower incisors [in German]. Inf Orthod Kieferorthop 1979;11:144–168.
19. Bakker PJMR, Wassenberg HJW, Van der Linden FPGM. Changes in the incisal area in relationship to the change of the lower lateral incisors [in German]. Inf Orthod Kieferorthop 1979;11:199–212.
20. Van der Linden FPGM, Wassenberg HJW, Bakker PJMR. General aspects of the development of the occlusion [in German]. Inf Orthod Kieferorthop 1979;11:131–143.
21. Berkovitz, BKB. Theories of tooth eruption. In: Poole DFG, Stack MV (eds). The Eruption and Occlusion of Teeth [Proceedings of the 27th Symposium of the Colston Research Society, 3–7 Apr 1975, Bristol, UK]. London: Butterworth, 1976:193–204.
22. Freund G. Canals of dental lamina and their significance for etiology of follicular cysts and tooth retention [in German]. Acta Anat (Basel) 1954;21:141–154.
23. Scott JH, Dixon AD. Anatomy for Students of Dentistry, ed 3. Edinburgh: Churchill Livingstone, 1972.
24. Brash JC. The growth of the alveolar bone and its relation to the movements of the teeth, including eruption. Int J Orthod 1928;14:196–223, 283–293,398–405,487–504.
25. Moorrees CFA, Fanning EA, Grön AM, Lebret L. The timing of orthodontic treatment in relation to tooth formation. Trans Eur Orthod Soc 1962: 87–101.
26. Nolla O. Development of the permanent teeth. J Dent Child 1960;27:254–266.
27. Angle EH. Classification of malocclusion. Dent Cosmos 1899;41:248–264,350–357.
28. Reichenbach E, Brückl H. Kieferorthopädische Klinik und Therapie. Eine Einführung für den Zahnartz. Zahnärztliche Fortbildung, Heft 7. Leipzig: Barth, 1954:12.

4

Intertransitional Period

Arrangement of the Dentition

During the intertransitional period, the dental arches consist of the permanent incisors, deciduous canines, deciduous molars, and first permanent molars (Fig 4-1). In the maxilla, the incisors are labially inclined. In addition to the central diastema, there are frequently other diastemata in the maxillary anterior region. Initially, there is often some space between the second deciduous molars and the first permanent molars. In the mandible, the incisors are less labially inclined than in the maxilla with fewer diastemata. The incisal edges of the four mandibular incisors are at the same level. In the maxilla, the edges of the central incisors are slightly more occlusal than the lateral ones. The overjet is greater than in the deciduous dentition and also greater than when the permanent dentition is complete and jaw growth concluded.[1] In both jaws, the crowns of the not-yet-emerged permanent canines limit space for the roots of the incisors. The initially lingually positioned mandibular lateral incisors have moved labially and are aligned in the dental arch. Rotations of mandibular incisors are partially or fully corrected through pressure of tongue and lips, provided that space was available.

Effects of Wear

The sharp cusp tips of the deciduous canines have disappeared. Occlusal and approximal surfaces are worn off. Contact points are flattened and mesiodistal crown dimensions are reduced. Except when the first permanent molars are in full intercuspation, the occlusion is less fixed than shortly after the deciduous molars started to occlude and also less than in the later phase when opposing premolars interlock. The slightly anterior movement of the mandibular teeth in relation to the maxillary teeth, associated with the differential anterior growth of the jaws, is not hindered by the occlusion. In modern times, attrition of teeth is limited. However, under primitive living conditions requiring intensive chewing, tooth wear was excessive, particularly when the food contained abrasive material such as sand. Hunter supposed in 1771 that deciduous molars have wider crowns than their successors because otherwise insufficient room would remain in the dental arch for the premolars.[2]

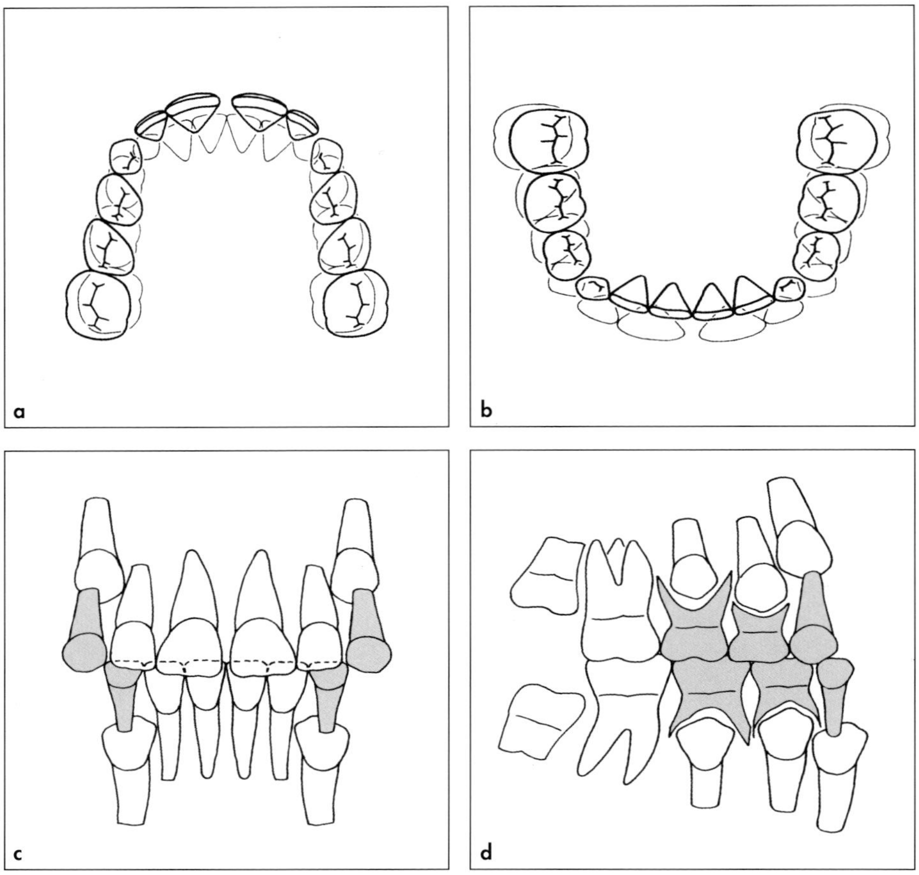

Fig 4-1 The dentition in the intertransitional period. *(a)* The maxillary teeth are arranged in an arch. There is a diastema between the central incisors. These teeth are sometimes in contact with the lateral ones, but in most cases they are not. There are often diastemata distal to the lateral incisors. *(b)* The four maxillary incisors occlude with the six mandibular anterior teeth. The roots of the lateral incisors converge apically, to a greater extent in the maxilla than in the mandible. *(c)* The mandibular teeth are also arranged in an arch. There are few diastemata, except distal to the deciduous canines, in which the maxillary deciduous canines fit. *(d)* There is less room for the permanent canines and premolars in the maxilla than in the mandible. The second permanent molars are located posteriorly to the first permanent molars. Their occlusal surfaces are oriented distobuccally in the maxilla and mesiolingually in the mandible.

Changes in Tooth Positions and Root Ends

The mesiodistal angulation of the incisors depends on the position of the permanent canine crowns and their proximity to the roots of the lateral incisors. With the emergence of the permanent canines, space becomes available in the jaw for the distal movement of the roots of the lateral and central incisors. Initially, the incisors diverge—more in the maxilla than in the mandible. After emergence of the permanent canines, the angulation of the maxillary incisors alters more than that of the mandibular incisors.

During the intertransitional period, the root formation of the emerged and not-yet-emerged permanent teeth continues. The space for the elongation is created by vertical growth of the jaws and an increase in height of the alveolar processes.

As mentioned previously, resorption of the roots of the deciduous teeth is preceded by the occlusal movement of their successors. Also, the bone that surrounds the roots of the deciduous molars is broken down. The resorption pattern of the deciduous canines is similar to that of the deciduous incisors.

Characteristic for the intertransitional period is the dominance of the permanent incisors in the face, particularly the maxillary central incisors. Their crown dimensions are intended to fit harmoniously in the larger adult face. In a comparable way, the size of the deciduous incisors is more appropriate to the dimensions of the face of an infant than that of a 6-year-old.

The fact that the permanent incisors are not in the correct position prior to emergence, as deciduous incisors are, is related to the phenomenon that these teeth are formed in a region that is not intended for the temporary housing of their crowns but to provide the space needed for their roots in the future. This explains the typical arrangement of the permanent incisors following their emergence, particularly in the maxilla. This condition, called the "ugly duckling" stage by Broadbent, is temporary and not deviant.[3]

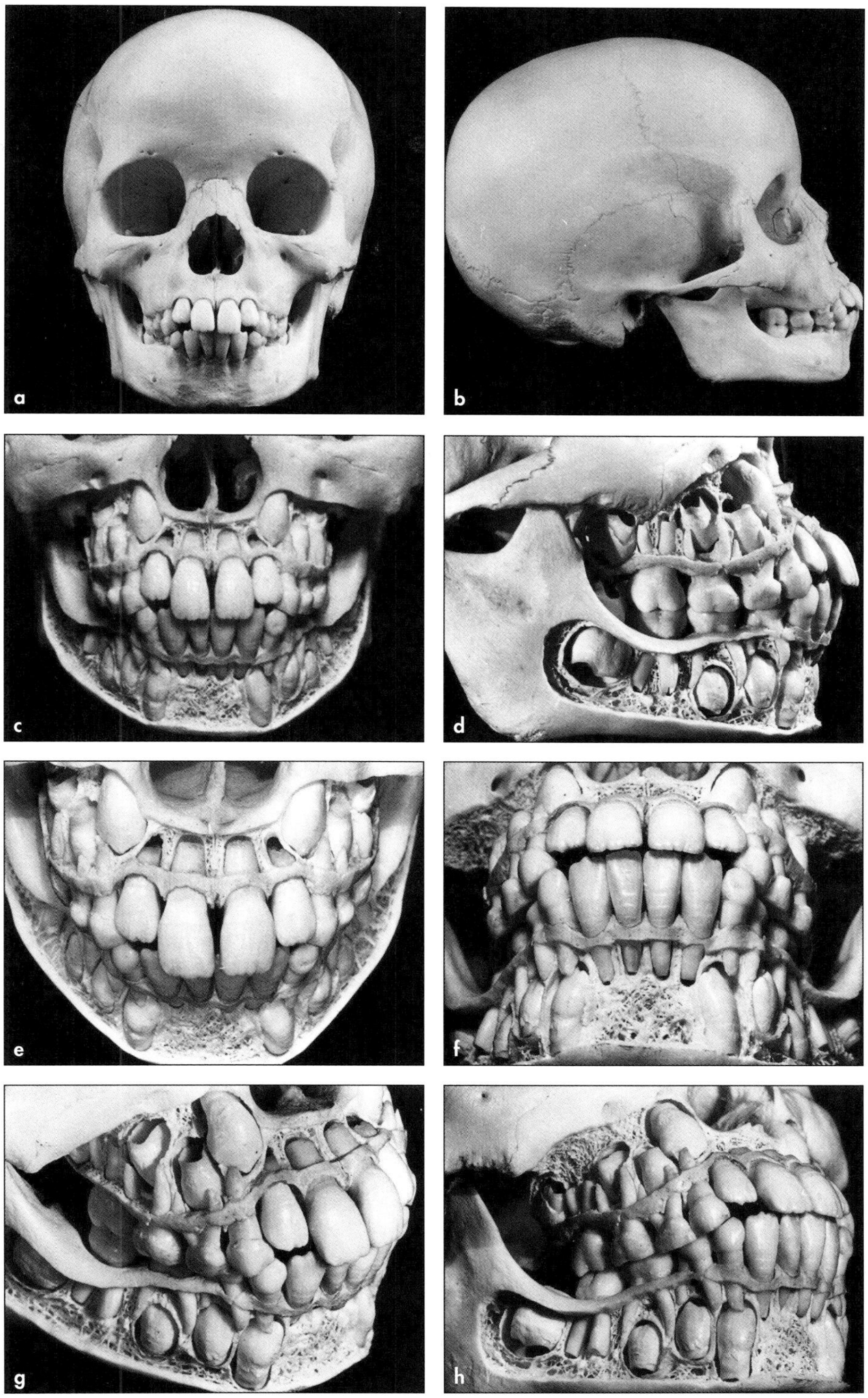

Fig 4-2 Skull at 8 years, at the beginning of the intertransitional period. *(a)* The permanent incisors, particularly the maxillary central ones, are large in comparison with the rest of the skull. *(b)* In this specimen, the incisors in both jaws are more labially inclined than normal. The flush terminal plane of the deciduous dentition hinders optimal intercuspation of the first permanent molars. *(c)* After removal of the buccal alveolar wall it becomes clear that the maxillary permanent canines are located high, adjacent to the piriform aperture. *(d)* In the maxilla, only limited room is available for the developing permanent canines and premolars. There is adequate room for those in the mandible. *(e)* The forming parts of the maxillary central permanent incisors are near the nasal floor. The roots of the lateral permanent incisors are close to the crowns of the permanent canines. Consequently, they are distally angulated. *(f)* There are no diastemata between the mandibular incisors, and their roots converge apically because of the proximity of the permanent canine crowns. *(g)* The maxillary central permanent incisors have completed their eruption, but the lateral incisors have not. *(h)* In the maxilla, the crowns of the permanent canine and first premolar overlap each other vertically. In the mandible, they are situated next to each other and parallel, with sufficient space in between.

Arrangement of Teeth at the Beginning of the Intertransitional Period

A skull at 8 years, representing the beginning stage of the intertransitional period, is shown in Fig 4-2. The buccal alveolar bone is removed, allowing insight into the arrangement of the not-yet-emerged permanent teeth and their relationship with the deciduous teeth. In Fig 4-3, various perspectives of the teeth as they were positioned within the jaws are shown.

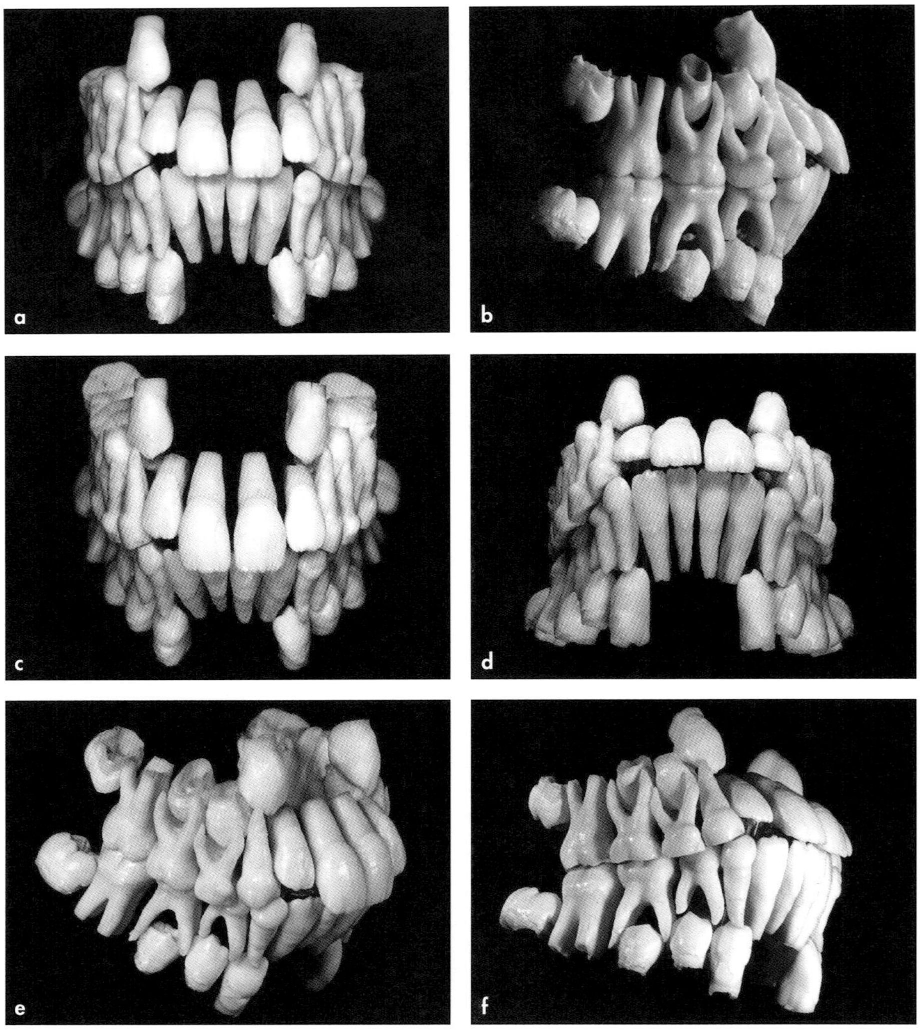

Fig 4-3 The teeth arranged as they were positioned in the jaws. *(a)* The permanent canines are formed at a significant distance from the occlusal plane. *(b)* The crowns of the premolars are situated apical to the roots of their predecessors. There is little difference in the formation stages of the permanent canines and first premolars. In the maxilla, the crown of the second permanent molar is distally angulated and buccally inclined; in the mandible, it is mesially angulated and lingually inclined. The second permanent molars are close to the roots of the first molars. *(c and d)* The dentition is shown frontally from above and from below. *(e and f)* The same perspectives on the three-quarter lateral view.

As mentioned in the previous chapter, there is a large variation in the spatial relationship between the crown of the permanent canine and the root of its predecessor. In addition, the relationship between premolars and their predecessors varies, more in the mesiodistal than in the linguobuccal direction.

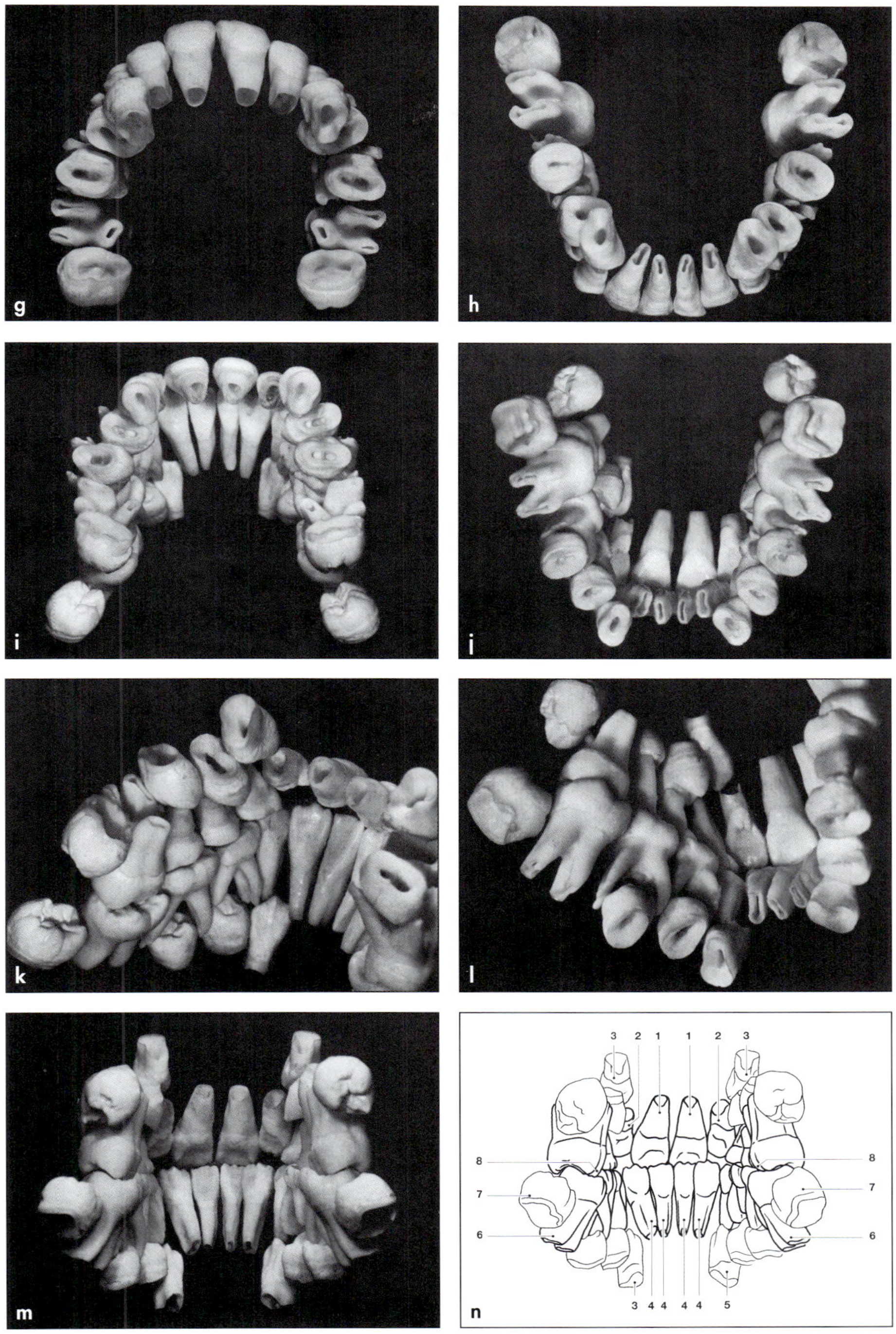

FIG 4-3 *(cont)* *(g and h)* The pictures taken from the apical view show the individual variations in root development of the permanent teeth and the strong resemblance between left and right sides in location, shape, and stage of formation. In both jaws, the forming parts of the permanent canines are more lingually located than those of the premolars. In the maxilla, the arch is the widest at the permanent first molars, in the mandible at the second. *(i to l)* The dentition is shown from additional angles. *(m)* Posterior view. *(n)* A drawing clarifies the elements shown in the posterior view. The roots of the maxillary central permanent incisors (1) converge slightly. The lateral incisors (2) have not completed their eruption. The forming parts of the maxillary permanent canines (3) are located far superiorly. The roots of the mandibular incisors (4) converge. The forming parts of the mandibular permanent canines (5) are the farthest away from the occlusal plane. The mandibular first permanent molars (6) are lingually inclined. The second molars (7) are mesially angulated and lingually inclined. The mesiopalatal cusps of the maxillary first permanent molars (8) occlude in the central fossae of their antagonists.

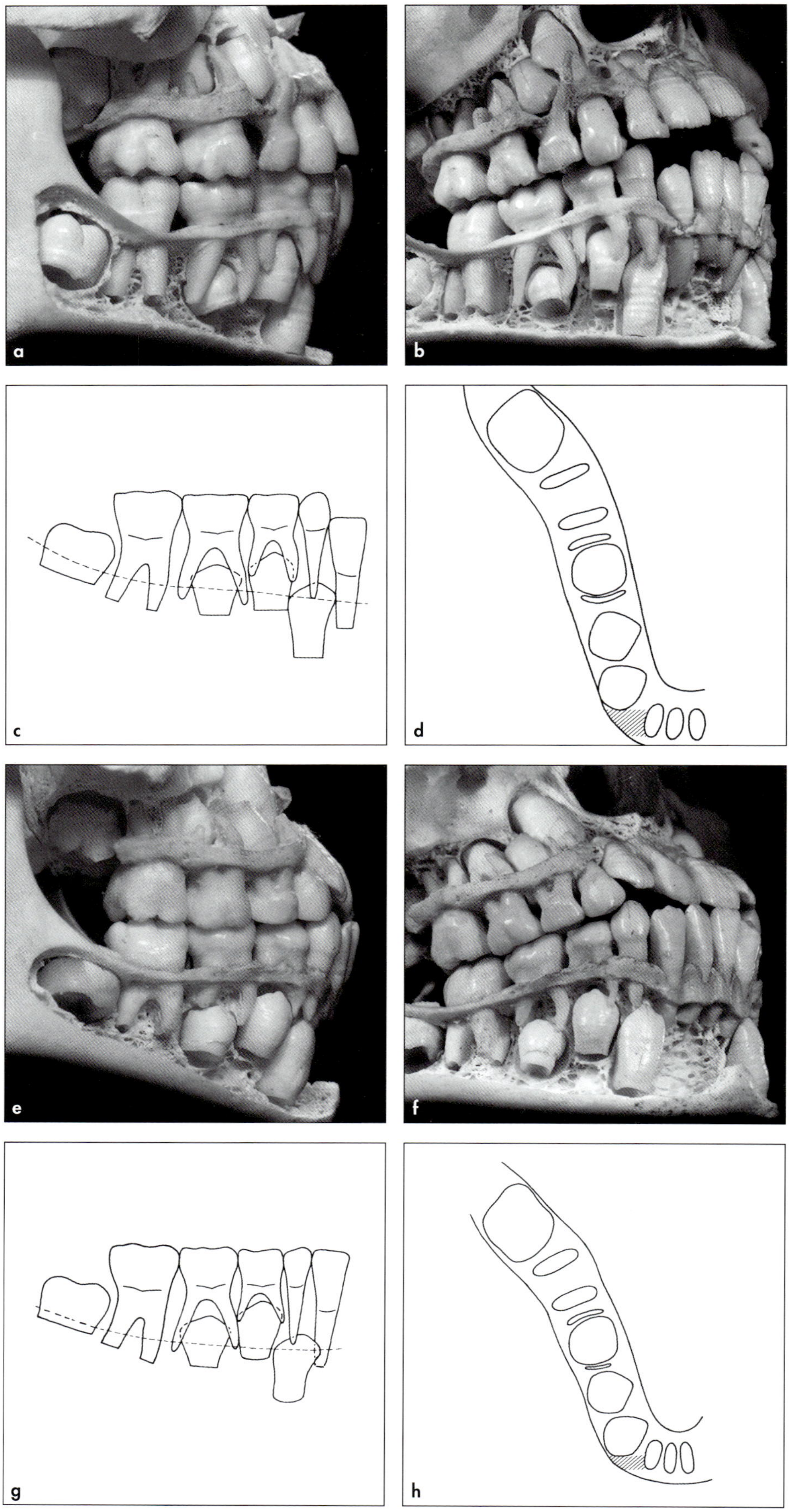

Fig 4-4 Arrangement of the mandibular teeth in the intertransitional period, in relation to the size of the middle section of the apical area. *(a)* The first specimen, with a large middle section, has a large mandibular second deciduous molar crown. Its successor is at a significant distance from the mesial root of the first permanent molar. *(b)* The mandibular permanent canine is slightly mesially angulated and located close to the first premolar. It is situated below the apex of its predecessor and distal to the root of the lateral incisor. There is 3 mm space between the crowns of the premolars. *(c and d)* Drawings based on *a* and *b*, with the *dotted lines* in *c* indicating the sectional plane in *d*. *(c)* The permanent canine does not overlap the root of the lateral incisor. *(d)* There is excess space between the lateral incisor and the first permanent molar for the crowns of the permanent canine and premolars. There is some distance between the canine and lateral incisor *(shading)*. *(e)* In the second specimen, with a medium middle section, the crown of the mandibular second deciduous molar is only slightly wider than that of its successor, which is situated close to the first permanent molar. *(f)* The permanent canine is mesially angulated. There is a 1-mm space between the crowns of the premolars. The first premolar is near the permanent canine, the crown of which overlaps the lateral incisor. *(g)* The cusp tip of the permanent canine crown is situated mesial to the apex of its predecessor. *(h)* The space mesial to the roots of the first permanent molar is just sufficient. The distance between the permanent canine and the lateral incisor *(shading)* is critical.

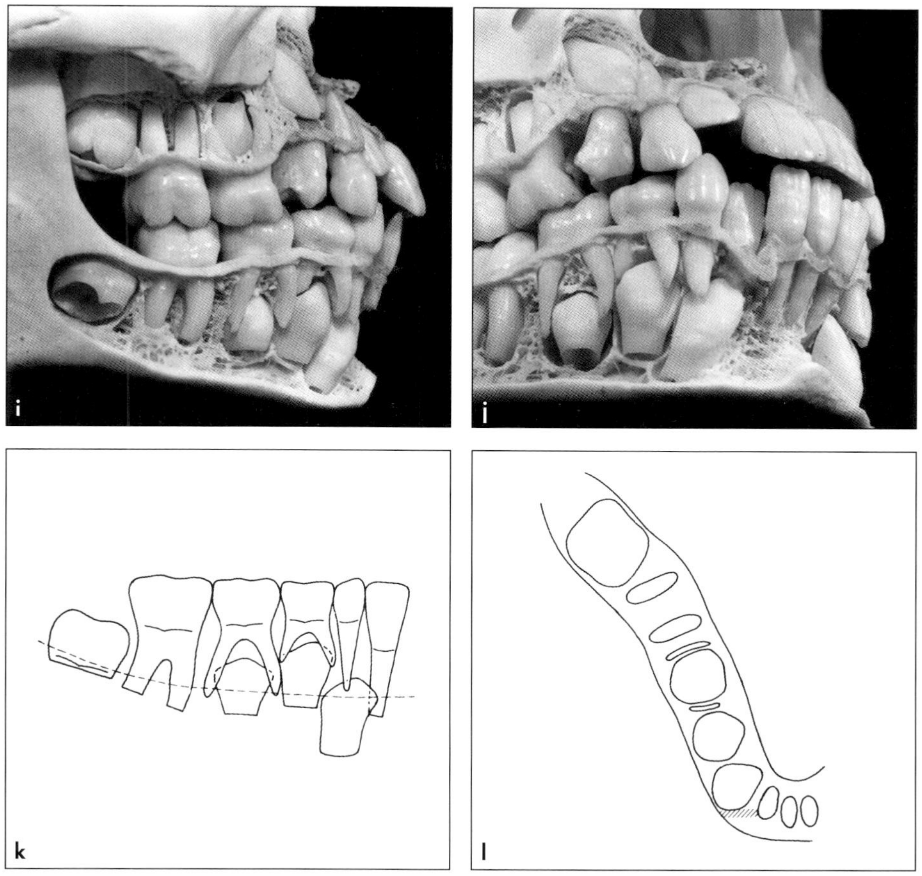

Fig 4-4 *(cont) (i)* In the third specimen, with a small middle section, there is little space between the second premolar and the root of the first permanent molar. *(j)* The canine has a marked mesial position and angulation. The difference in crown width of the corresponding deciduous and permanent teeth is unfavorable. The crowns of the unerupted permanent teeth are close together. The distal aspects of the crown of the permanent canine and of the root of its predecessor are aligned nearly vertically. *(k)* The permanent canine overlaps more than half the root of the lateral incisor, and there is no space for it to move distally. *(l)* The space available in the dental arch is too small for the premolars and permanent canine. The distance between the permanent canine and the lateral incisor is small *(shaded)*, which indicates an unfavorable situation. (Reprinted from Wassenberg et al[4] with permission.)

Variations in the Middle Section of the Apical Area

Like the anterior section of the apical area (see chapters 2 and 3), the middle section of the apical area in the maxilla and mandible may be categorized as large, medium, or small.

Situation in the mandible

In Fig 4-4, the variations in size of the middle section of the apical area in the mandible and the associated arrangement of the permanent teeth are demonstrated on preparations of three skulls. In a large middle section of the apical area, the permanent canine is located in a good position. The differences in mesiodistal crown dimensions among deciduous teeth and their successors are also favorable, and there is enough room for them in the jaw. In a medium middle section, the condition is critical, and in a small one unfavorable.

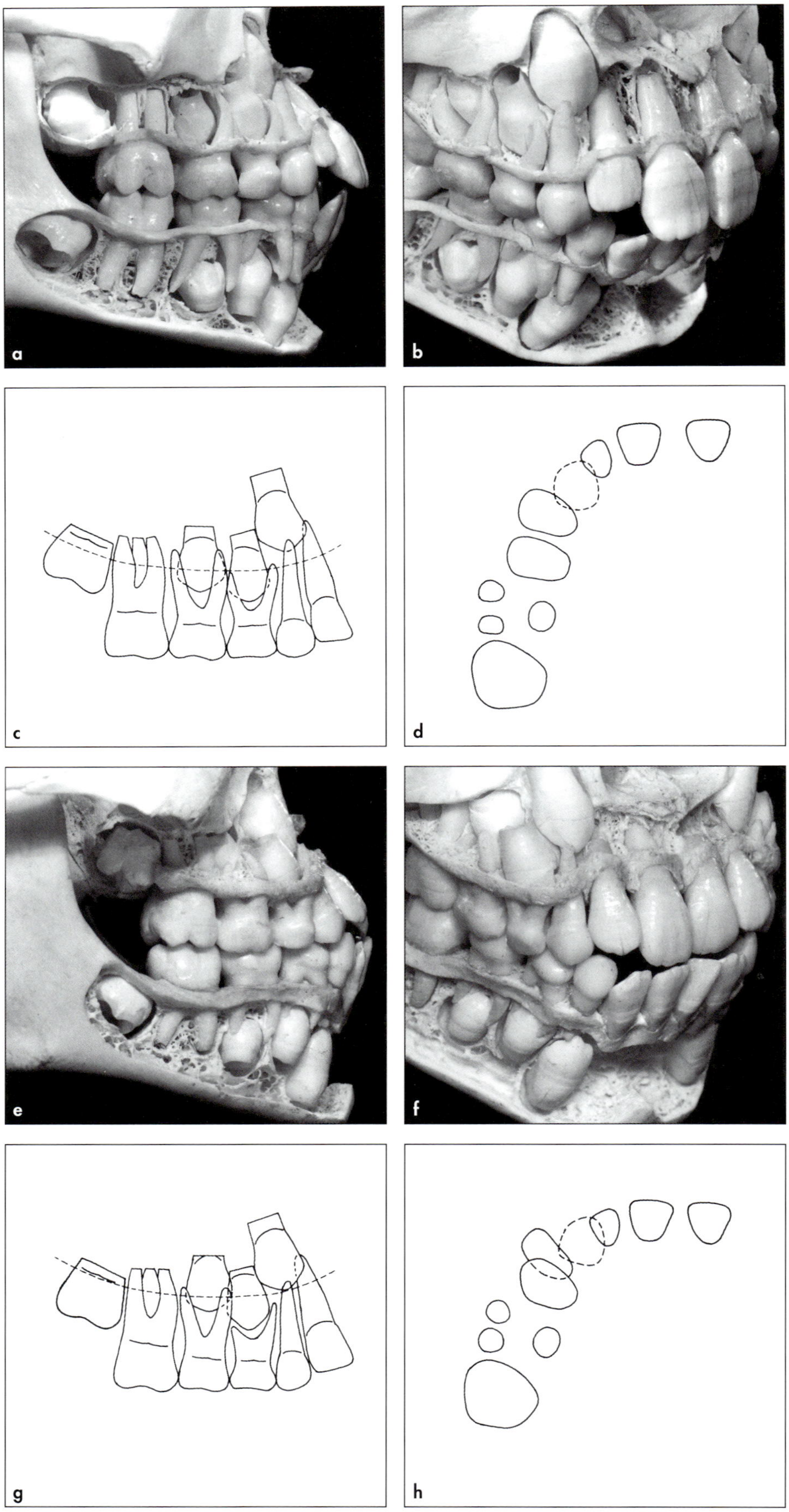

Fig 4-5 Arrangement of the maxillary teeth in the intertransitional period related to the size of the middle section of the apical area. *(a)* The first specimen, with a large middle section, has favorable spatial conditions. The second deciduous molar has a wider crown than its successor. *(b)* The permanent canine is mesially angulated and located more superiorly and palatally than the premolars, which are situated at about the same level. The crown tip of the permanent canine is located palatal and slightly mesial to the apex of its predecessor. The canine is close to the first premolar. *(c and d)* Drawings based on *a* and *b*, with the *dotted lines* in *c* indicating the sectional plane in *d*. *(c)* There is some distance between the root of the first permanent molar and the second premolar crown. The first premolar is slightly mesially angulated. The second premolar is oriented perpendicularly to the occlusal plane. *(d)* The distance between the first premolar and the lateral incisor is relatively large. The canine crown overlaps both adjacent teeth slightly. *(e)* In the second specimen, with a medium middle section, the situation in the maxilla is critical. The premolar crowns are close together. The mesiodistal crown dimensions of the deciduous canine and molars are small in relation to those of their successors. *(f)* The permanent canine is situated palatal and superior to the first premolar and vertically overlaps a large part of it. Both teeth are mesially angulated, particularly the canine. Furthermore, the first premolar is mesiopalatally rotated and extends buccally. *(g)* The crowns of the premolars and canine are in different vertical positions and overlap each other. The distance between the first permanent molar and the lateral incisor is small. *(h)* The distance between the mesial aspect of the first premolar and the distal aspect of the lateral incisor is also small.

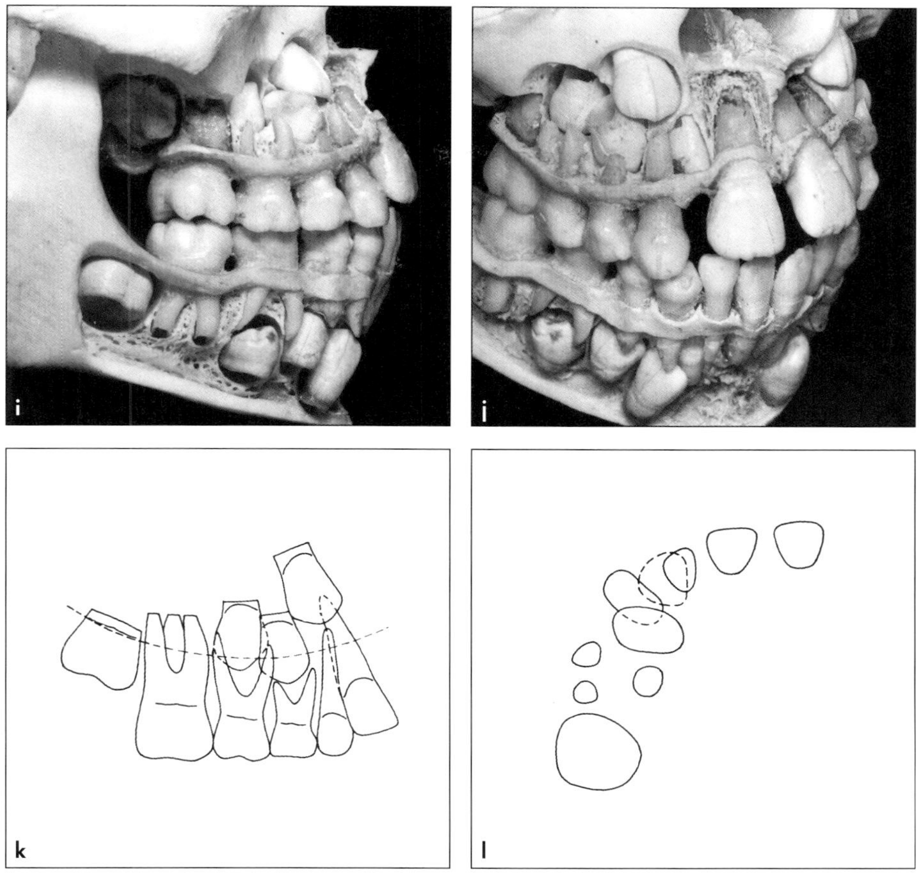

Fig 4-5 *(cont)* *(i)* In the third specimen, with a small middle section, the maxillary lateral deciduous incisor has been lost prematurely, and its successor has not emerged. There is little room between the mesial root of the first permanent molar and the second premolar crown. *(j)* The permanent canine crown is situated far superiorly and considerably mesially angulated. The first premolar is located close to the second premolar and buccal of the canine, which overlaps the first premolar vertically. The canine is distobuccally rotated and overlaps the lateral incisor to a large extent. The first and second premolar crowns are located only partially between the roots of their predecessors. *(k)* The conditions are unfavorable, and after transition, there would have been a marked shortage of space in the dental arch for the three erupting teeth. *(l)* The space between the first premolar and the lateral incisor is very small. (Reprinted from Wassenberg et al[5] with permission.)

Situation in the maxilla

The relationship in size between the middle and the anterior section of the apical area in the maxilla depends on the width and anteroposterior location of the piriform aperture and the associated position of the permanent canines. The middle section exhibits a significant interindividual size variation. These differences are especially evident in the positions of the canine and first premolar. The sagittal and transverse position of these teeth varies more in the maxilla than in the mandible. The variation in size of the middle section of the apical area in the maxilla and the associated arrangement of the permanent teeth is demonstrated on preparations of three skulls in Fig 4-5.

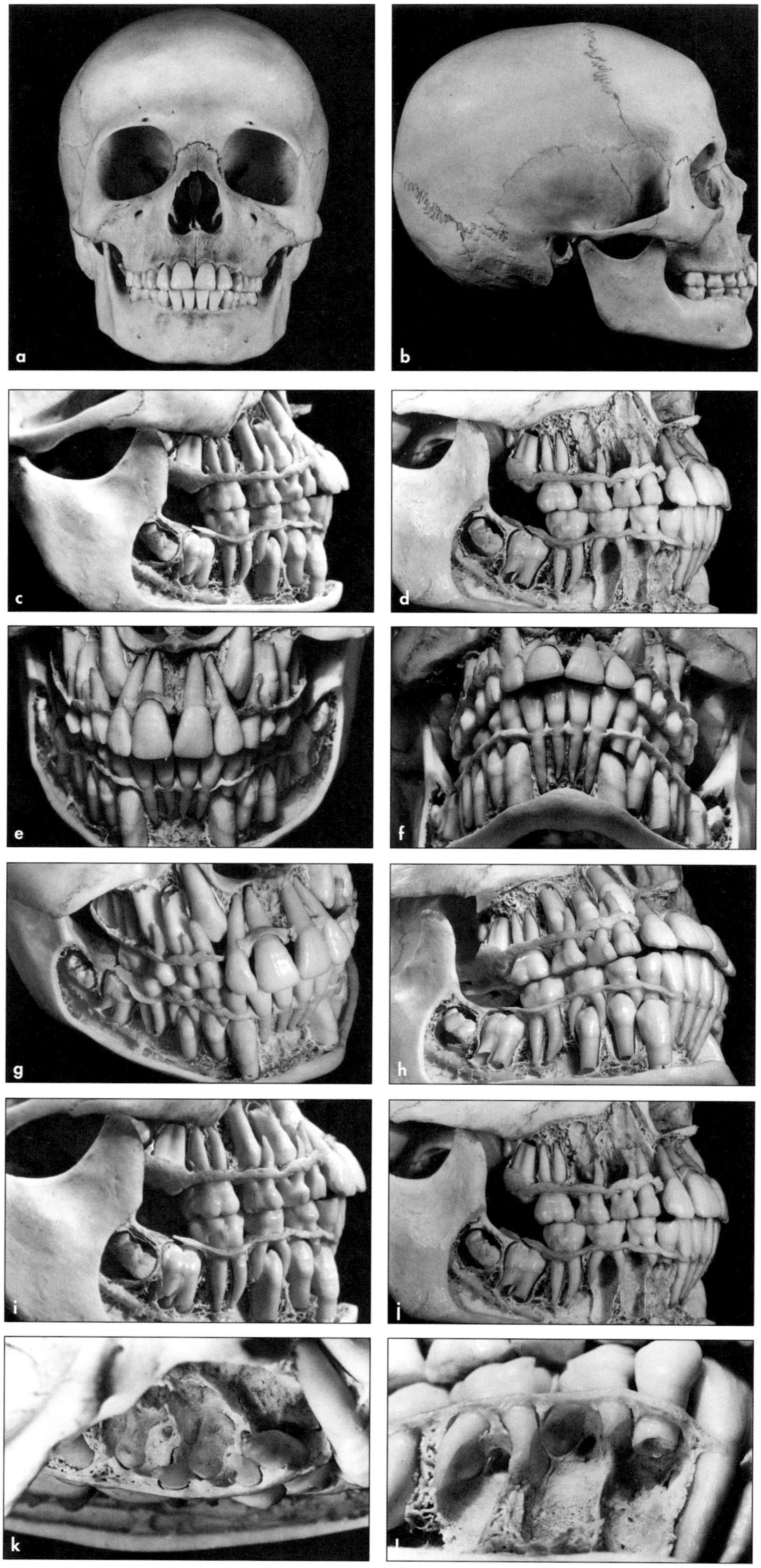

FIG 4-6 Skull at 10 years, the end of the intertransitional period. *(a)* The incisors are labially inclined in both arches, but more so in the maxilla than in the mandible. *(b)* The first permanent molars are in end-to-end occlusion. (c) After removal of the buccal alveolar wall, the lateral view shows the not-yet-emerged canines and premolars. *(d)* With these teeth removed, the contour of the surrounding bone structures reflects their locations. *(e and f)* Frontal views are shown from above and from below. *(g and h)* The same perspectives are shown from a three-quarter lateral view. *(i)* Close-up lateral view with canines and premolars still present in the jaws. *(j)* Same view as *i*, after the removal of the canines and premolars. *(k)* The furcations of the deciduous molars are near the cervical borders, and the roots diverge markedly. This allows the premolars to be close to the crowns of their predecessors, which are maintained for a long period of time because the outer walls of the roots of deciduous molars resorb late. *(l)* The openings of the gubernacular canals are visible in the crypts of the mandibular premolars.

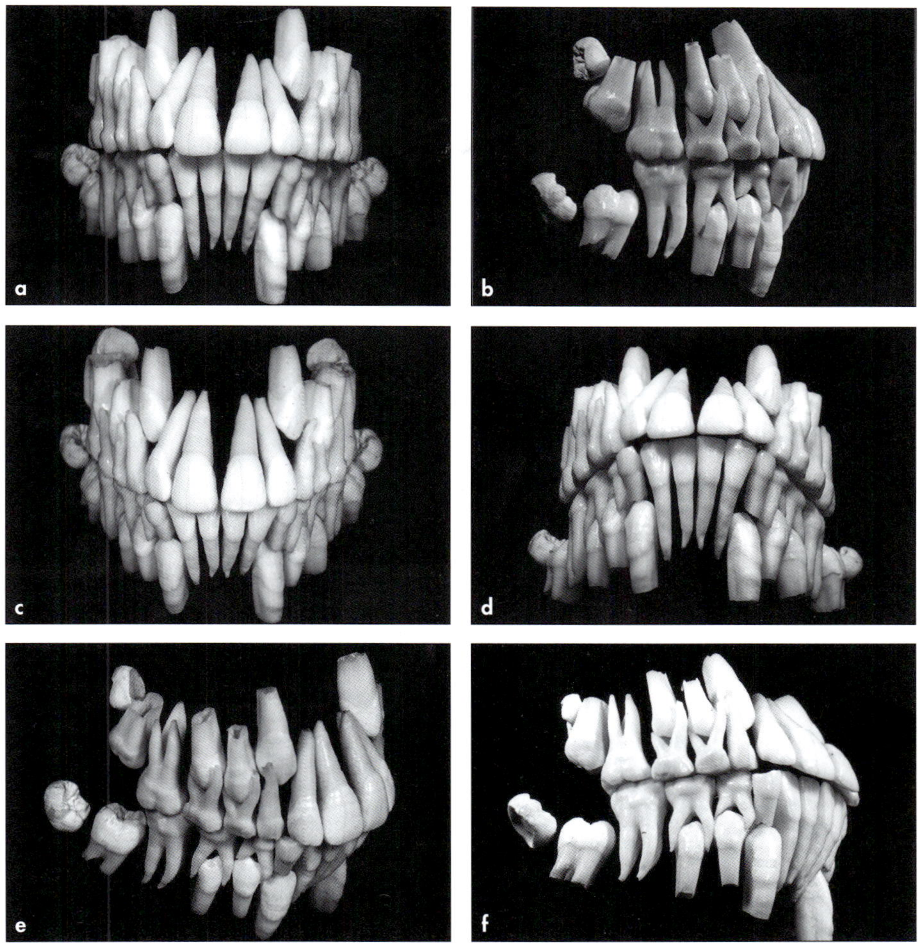

FIG 4-7 The teeth arranged as positioned in the jaws. *(a)* The maxillary right permanent canine is less buccally located than the left canine. Its mesial incisal margin is slightly palatal to the root of the lateral incisor. Also in the mandible, there is a slight asymmetry in the location of the permanent canines and in the resorption pattern of the roots of their predecessors. *(b)* In both jaws, the crowns of the permanent canines and premolars are not far from the occlusal plane. The second and third permanent molars are oriented at the typical angulation and inclination. *(c and d)* Frontal views are shown from above and from below. *(e and f)* The same perspectives are shown from a three-quarter lateral view.

Arrangement of Teeth Late in the Intertransitional Period

Figures 4-6 and 4-7 show a skull at 10 years in the late phase of the intertransitional period. For its presentation, the same approach is used as for the skull at 8 years (see Figs 4-2 and 4-3). The crucial difference is between the sum of the mesiodistal crown dimensions of the deciduous canine and the two deciduous molars and that of their successors. The correlation between these two sums is not high.[6] Among the corresponding individual teeth, the correlation is moderate for deciduous molars and premolars and low for canines.[7] Hence, a marked difference can exist among the mesiodistal crown dimensions of deciduous canines and molars and their successors, particularly between canines. The differences in crown sizes of corresponding teeth, together with the sequence of emergence, play an important role in the second transitional period.

Concluding Remarks

During the intertransitional period, no or only few changes are seen in the dental arches. However, many changes occur within the jaws. Preparations are made for the second transition. Roots of deciduous teeth and the surrounding bone resorb, including the bone at the cervical margins. The crowns of the third molars start to mineralize, earlier in the maxilla than in the mandible. At about the same time, furcations are formed in the adjacent second permanent molars. The roots of the teeth still to emerge elongate.

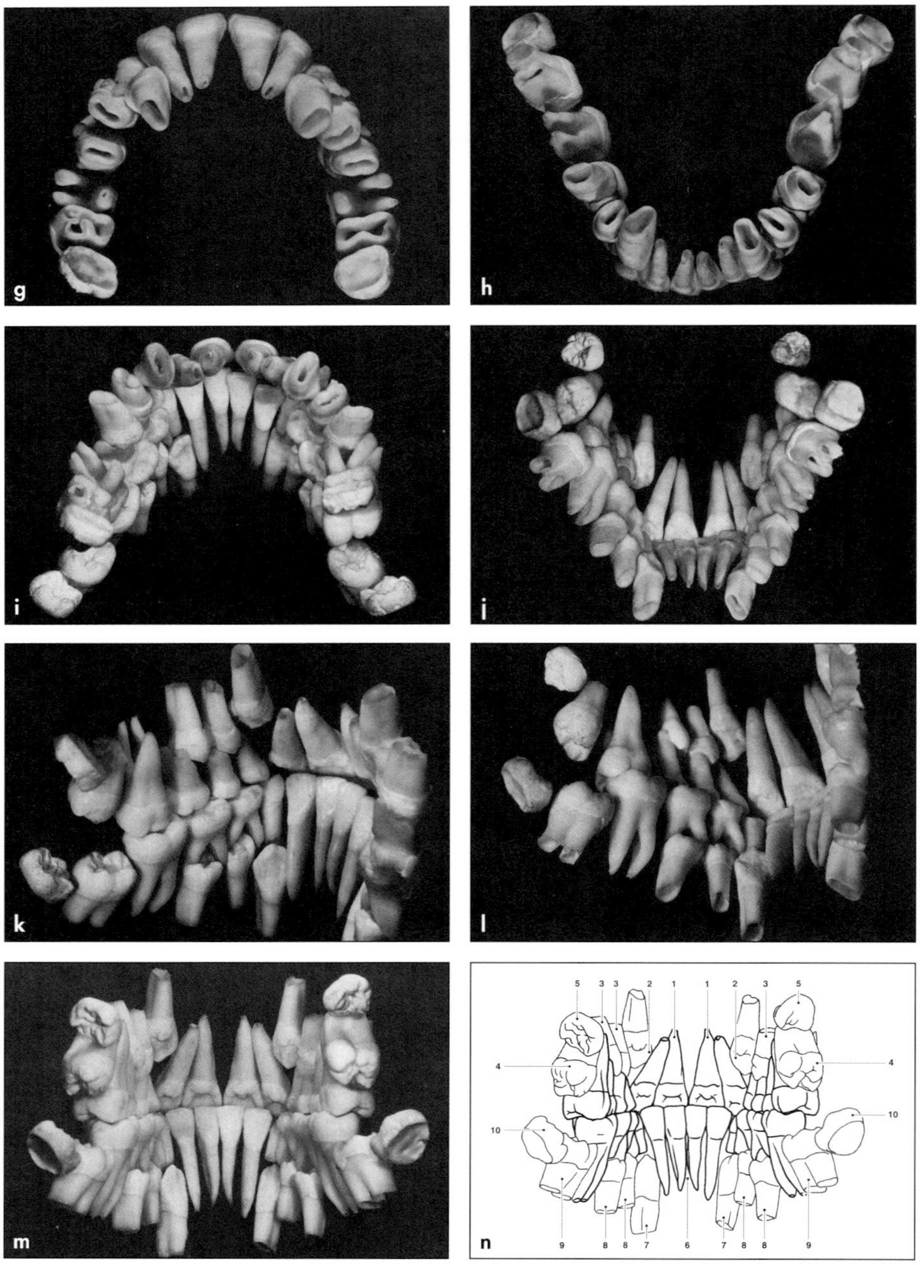

Fig 4-7 *(cont) (g and h)* The apical view shows the differences in root formation stages and the symmetry in root arrangement of the teeth with the exception of the maxillary and mandibular canines. *(i to l)* The dentition is shown from various lingual views. *(m)* Posterior view. *(n)* A drawing clarifies the elements shown in the posterior view. The maxillary central incisors (1) are oriented almost perpendicular to the occlusal plane. The mesial incisal margin of the maxillary permanent canine (2) is located slightly palatal to the root of the lateral incisor on the right side and buccal to it on the left side. The maxillary premolars (3) are located directly above their predecessors. The maxillary second permanent molars (4) are distally angulated and buccally inclined. The crowns of the maxillary third molars (5) are partly formed. The roots of the mandibular incisors (6) converge. The mandibular permanent canines (7) are slightly buccally inclined. The mandibular premolars (8) are located directly below their predecessors. The roots of the mandibular second permanent molars (9) are partly formed. Their crowns are mesially angulated and lingually inclined. The mandibular third molar crowns (10) are partly formed, mesially angulated, and lingually inclined.

References

1. Thilander B. Dentoalveolar development in subjects with normal occlusion. A longitudinal study between the ages of 5 and 31 years. Eur J Orthod 2009;31:109–120.
2. Hunter J. The Natural History of the Human Teeth: Explaining Their Structure, Use, Formation, Growth, and Diseases. London: J. Johnson, 1771.
3. Broadbent BH. Ontogenic development of occlusion. Angle Orthod 1941;11:223–241.
4. Wassenberg HJW, Bakker PJMR, Van der Linden FPGM. Exchange of the lower lateral teeth [in German]. Inf Orthod Kieferorthop 1979;11:169–198.
5. Wassenberg HJW, Bakker PJMR, Van der Linden FPGM. Change in the upper lateral teeth [in German]. Inf Orthod Kieferorthop 1979;11:271–304.
6. Moorrees CFA, Chadha JM. Crown diameters of corresponding tooth groups in the deciduous and permanent dentition. J Dent Res 1962;41:466–470.
7. Moorrees CFA, Reed RB. Correlations among crown diameters of human teeth. Arch Oral Biol 1964;9:685–697.

5

The Second Transitional Period: Transition of Canines and Deciduous Molars/Premolars and Emergence of Second Permanent Molars

Emergence Sequence

The second transitional period lasts 1 to 1.5 years. At about 10 years of age, 2 years after the emergence of the maxillary lateral permanent incisors, the first tooth, usually a mandibular deciduous canine, is shed. In contrast to the predictable emergence sequence of the permanent incisors, a large variation exists in the sequence of emergence of permanent canines and premolars. The spatial conditions in the anterior region allow only one eruption sequence for incisors. There is more space for the not-yet-emerged permanent teeth in the buccal region, and they can be arranged with space in between. However, the maxillary permanent canine is often situated close to and above the first premolar, in which case the premolar emerges first. The distal corner of the canine lies next to the first premolar at the junction of its crown and root. The maxillary first premolar has a corresponding concavity at its mesial side and two roots. The second premolar does not have such a concavity and has only one root; otherwise, the crowns of the premolars are alike in shape and size.

The most common sequence of emergence in the mandible is: canine, first premolar, second premolar; in the maxilla: first premolar, second premolar, canine[1] (Fig 5-1). In both jaws, the first two mentioned teeth quite often emerge at the same time or shortly after each other. In the mandible, all possible variations in sequence of emergence can occur. In the maxilla, the first premolar generally precedes the canine. For the frequency of various sequences of emergence[3–6] and also for times of emergence[7,8] and other statistical data, see chapter 17.

There is a large variation in the age at which permanent teeth emerge. There is a range of 3 years for the incisors and 6 years for the canines and premolars. Sequences and times of emergence can differ between the left and right side. Furthermore, the transition in the mandible precedes that in the maxilla. Generally, the second permanent molars erupt when all deciduous teeth, with the exception of the mandibular second deciduous molar, have been replaced (Fig 5-2).

Leeway Space

Deciduous molars have mesiodistally larger crowns than do their successors. The reverse holds true for canines. Permanent canines are broader than their predecessors, particularly in the maxilla, and more in boys than in girls. The extra space needed for their replacement is usually available because of the presence of diastemata.

Premolars are located between and below (in the mandible) or above (in the maxilla) the roots of the deciduous molars. After emergence, the mandibular premolars are oriented nearly perpendicular to the occlusal plane. The maxillary premolars are slightly buccally inclined, and the first premolar is mesially angulated. The difference in inclination between first premolars and incisors is greater in the maxilla than in the mandible because the maxillary incisors are much more labially inclined than are the mandibular incisors (see chapter 7, Figs 7-3 and 7-4).

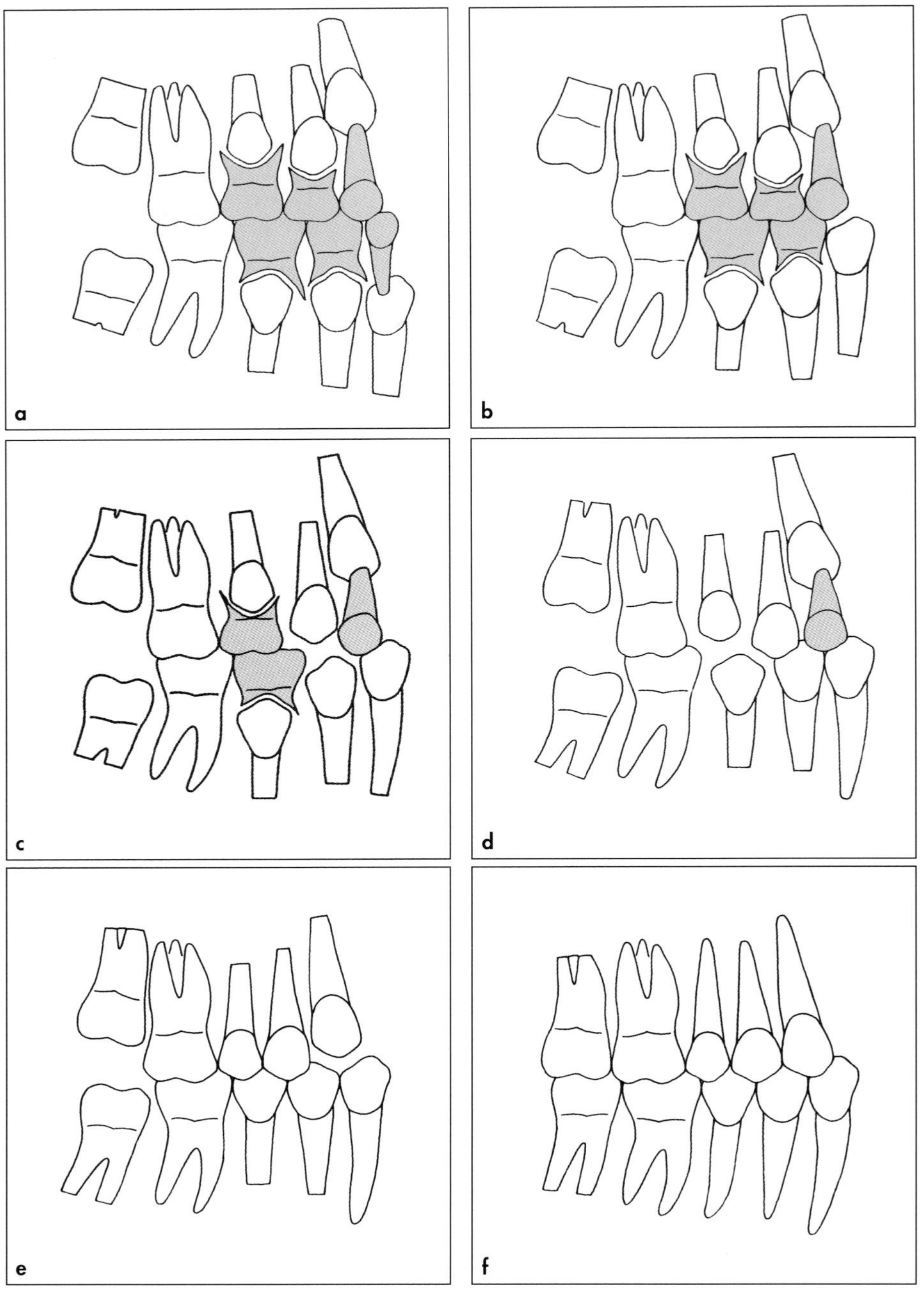

Fig 5-1 Transition in the buccal region and emergence of the second permanent molars. *(a)* In the maxilla, the first premolar is the closest to the occlusal plane; the canine is the farthest away. In the mandible, the permanent canine is also initially farther away from the occlusal plane than the first premolar (see chapter 3, Fig 3-1). In contrast to the situation in the maxilla, there is some space between these two teeth. Usually there is—although not in this drawing—a flush terminal plane of the deciduous dentition.[2] In the maxilla, the canine and first premolar are slightly mesially inclined. *(b)* Some weeks after the loss of the mandibular deciduous canine, its successor emerges with sufficient space in the dental arch and passes the first premolar while erupting. In the maxilla, the erupting first premolar has come free of the canine crown. *(c)* In both jaws, the first premolars emerge with sufficient room. *(d)* Subsequently, the second premolars emerge with excess space in the dental arch. *(e)* In the maxilla, the deciduous canine is the last tooth to be lost, and its successor will erupt a few weeks later. The diastemata, including the central one, provide extra space for the large permanent canine crown. *(f)* After occlusion has been established, the mandibular second permanent molar is mesially angulated and lingually inclined; the maxillary second molar is distally angulated and buccally inclined.

In this context, the term *leeway space*, introduced by Nance in 1947, should be mentioned.[9] Leeway space refers to the difference between the combined widths of the deciduous canine and first and second molars and that of their successors. According to Nance, the average difference for a maxillary quadrant is 1.0 mm and for a mandibular quadrant 1.7 mm (see chapter 17, Fig 17-10). However, there is a large range for these values. The leeway space offers, together with the remaining diastemata, the extra space needed for good alignment of the canines and premolars in the dental arch. With excess space, the first permanent molars can move mesially, especially in the mandible, resulting in improved intercuspation.

Size of the Middle Section of the Apical Area

The sequence of emergence is related to the size of the middle section of the apical area. If it is large, all sequences of emergence can occur (Fig 5-3). However, the mandibular second premolar almost always emerges last in accordance with its late formation. In a medium middle section of the apical area, the three teeth cannot erupt simultaneously, but there is adequate space for the alignment of the teeth (Fig 5-4). In the mandible, the canine emerges first; in the maxilla, it is the first premolar.

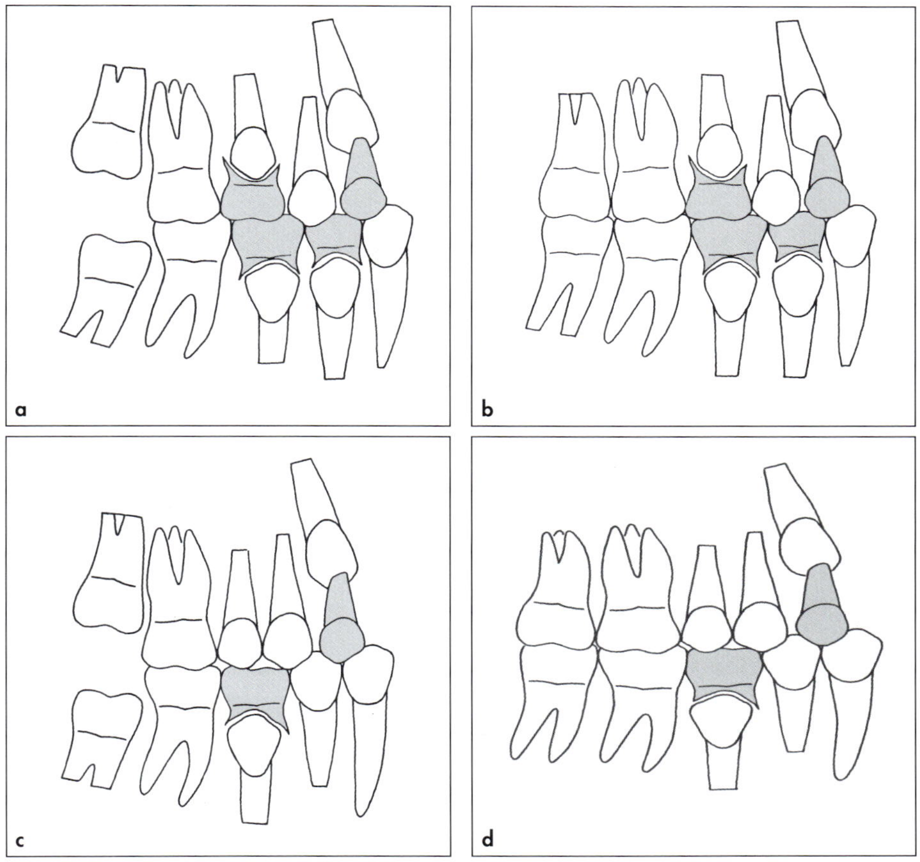

FIG 5-2 Variations in patterns of transition. *(a)* The mandibular permanent canine and the maxillary first premolar have emerged, but the second permanent molars are not yet emerged. The terminal plane of the deciduous dentition has a mesial step. The first permanent molars occlude optimally. *(b)* The second permanent molars have emerged. The terminal plane has a small mesial step. The occlusion of the permanent molars is not optimal. *(c)* Simultaneous emergence of the mandibular permanent canine and first premolar and both maxillary premolars. The second permanent molars have not emerged yet. The wide mandibular second deciduous molar interferes with optimal occlusion of the first permanent molars. *(d)* The second permanent molars occlude prior to the conclusion of the transition. After loss of the mandibular second deciduous molar, the occlusion of the permanent molars can improve.

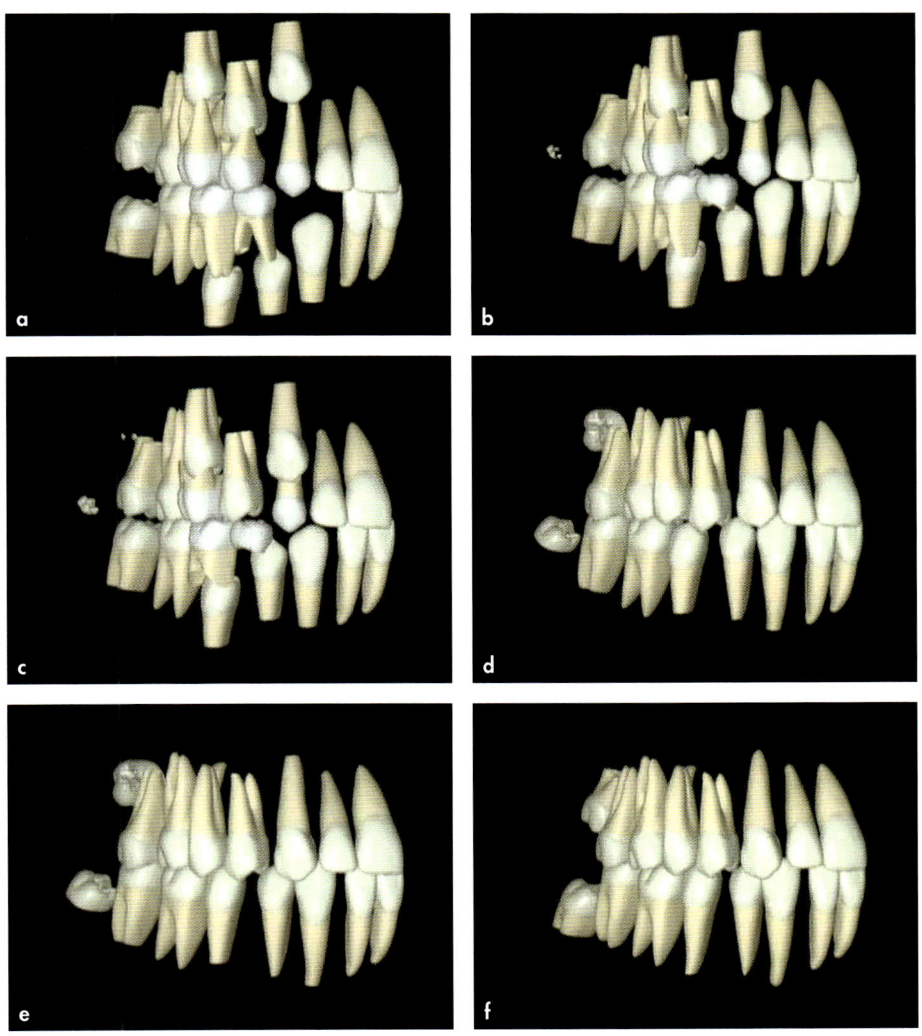

FIG 5-3 Transition in large middle sections of the apical areas. *(a)* In the maxilla and mandible, the canine and premolars can emerge at the same time. *(b)* Usually the mandibular canine comes first, followed by the maxillary first premolar. *(c)* Slightly later the mandibular first premolar emerges. *(d)* After all premolars and canines have emerged, some extra space remains. *(e)* The space gradually disappears. *(f)* In the meantime, the second permanent molars have attained occlusion, and the roots of the maxillary incisors have moved distally. See video clip 16.

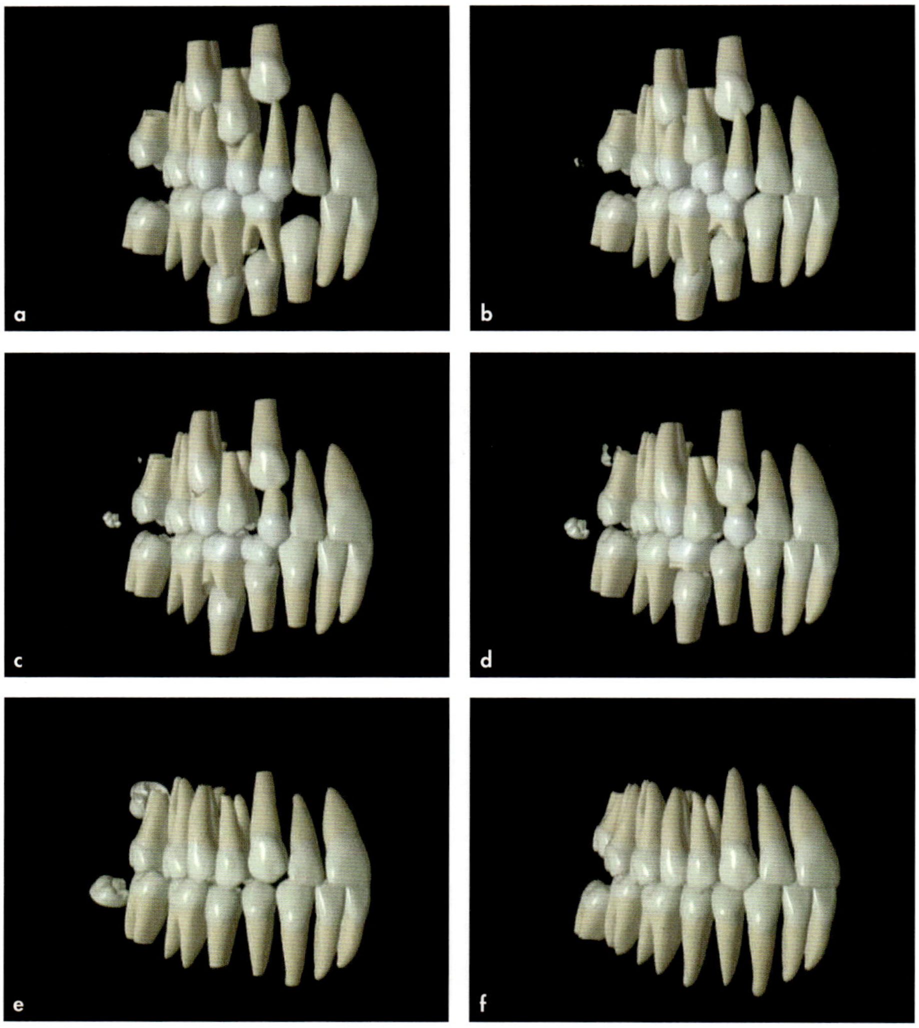

Fig 5-4 Transition in medium middle sections of the apical areas. *(a)* There is enough room in the mandible, where the permanent canine emerges first. *(b)* That is not the case in the maxilla. *(c)* The maxillary first premolar emerges first. *(d)* Subsequently, the mandibular first premolar emerges. In the maxilla, the second premolar often precedes the canine. *(e)* After conclusion of the transition, little space remains in the dental arch. *(f)* Ultimately, there is good dental alignment in the mandible and maxilla. See video clip 17.

In a small middle section of the apical area, the shortage of space especially affects the maxilla (Fig 5-5). The canine ultimately is in a buccal position, outside the dental arch. The same phenomenon can occur in the mandible, with the permanent canine overlapping the lateral incisor.

The relative size of opposing sections of the apical areas quite often differs. For example, a small maxillary anterior section can be combined with a large mandibular anterior section. The same applies to middle sections. In addition, the relative size of the anterior and middle sections may vary within the same jaw. For example, a small maxillary anterior section can be combined with a medium middle section and vice versa.

Emergence of Second Permanent Molars

The emergence of the second permanent molars can occur during or after the conclusion of the transition. The maxillary second molar usually emerges some months to half a year later than the mandibular second molar.

Many factors play a role in the transition in the buccal region and in the emergence of the second permanent molars.[10–17] In Figs 5-6 to 5-9, insight into this topic is provided through the exposure of the dentition in the jaws of four skulls at increasing levels of development.

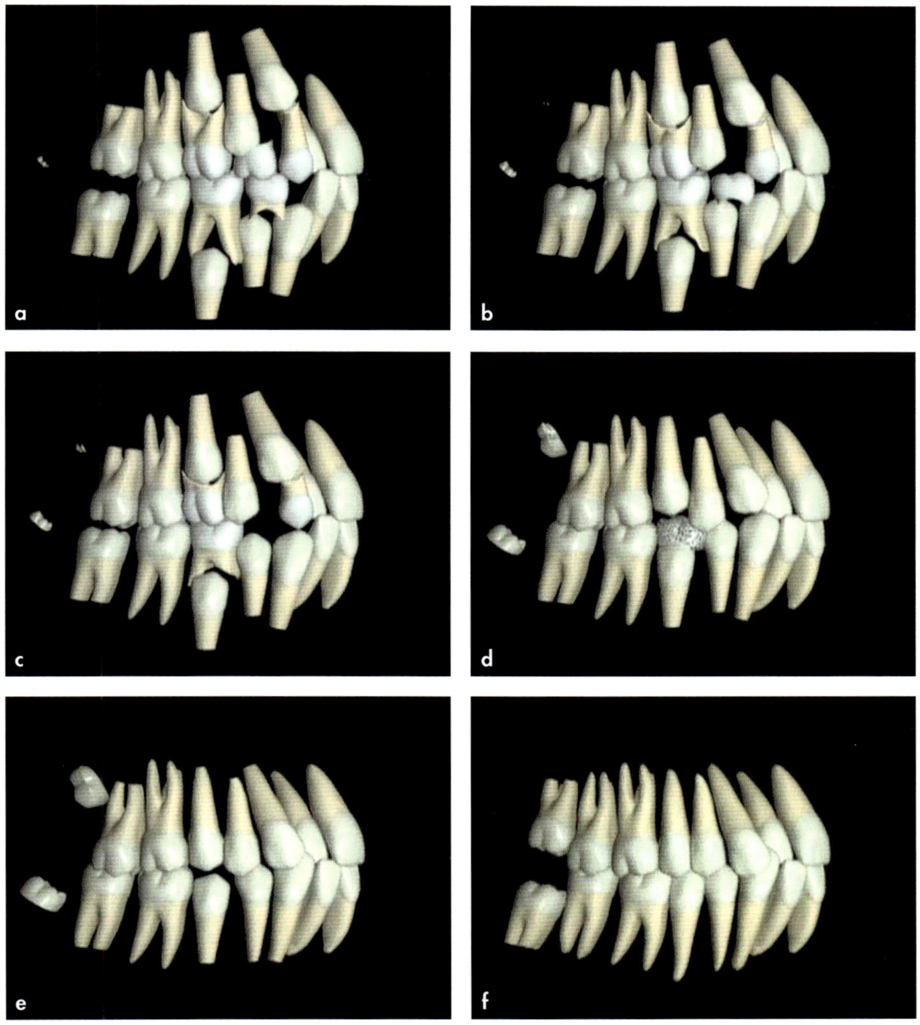

FIG 5-5 Transition in small middle sections of the apical areas. *(a)* The maxillary first premolar can emerge without hindrance. *(b)* The mandibular canine, however, overlaps the lateral incisor labially after emergence. *(c)* In the maxilla, the second premolar emerges well. *(d)* However, the canine ends up in a buccal position outside the dental arch. *(e)* In the mandible, the second premolar also emerges well. *(f)* If the maxillary first premolar moves distally after premature loss of the second deciduous molar, the canine can erupt well, and the second premolar ends up palatally positioned. If the mandibular second deciduous molar is lost prematurely, and subsequently the space is reduced severely, the second premolar emerges lingually. It can even become impacted if the first permanent molar migrates excessively to the mesial. If the maxillary lateral incisor emerges palatally, it can end up in negative overjet. See video clip 18.

Relationship Between Erupting Permanent Teeth and Their Predecessors

As mentioned before, erupting permanent teeth closely approach their predecessors. Not only their roots resorb but also the surrounding bone, beginning at the cervical margins. A premolar moves into the crown of its predecessor, which becomes positioned like a hat on the premolar crown, the buccal part of which is often visible. Hence, there is no time interval between the loss of a deciduous molar and the emergence of its successor, as is the case for incisors and canines. Indeed, the gubernacular canals of premolars end in the alveolar sockets, not at the alveolar process to the lingual of their predecessors, as do those of incisors and canines.

Seen from the occlusal, the cusp tip of an erupting permanent canine is situated lingual to the buccal side of the root of its predecessor. Its buccal surface is more buccally located and can be seen and palpated at the gingiva as a bulge. This is more exaggerated in the maxilla than in the mandible.

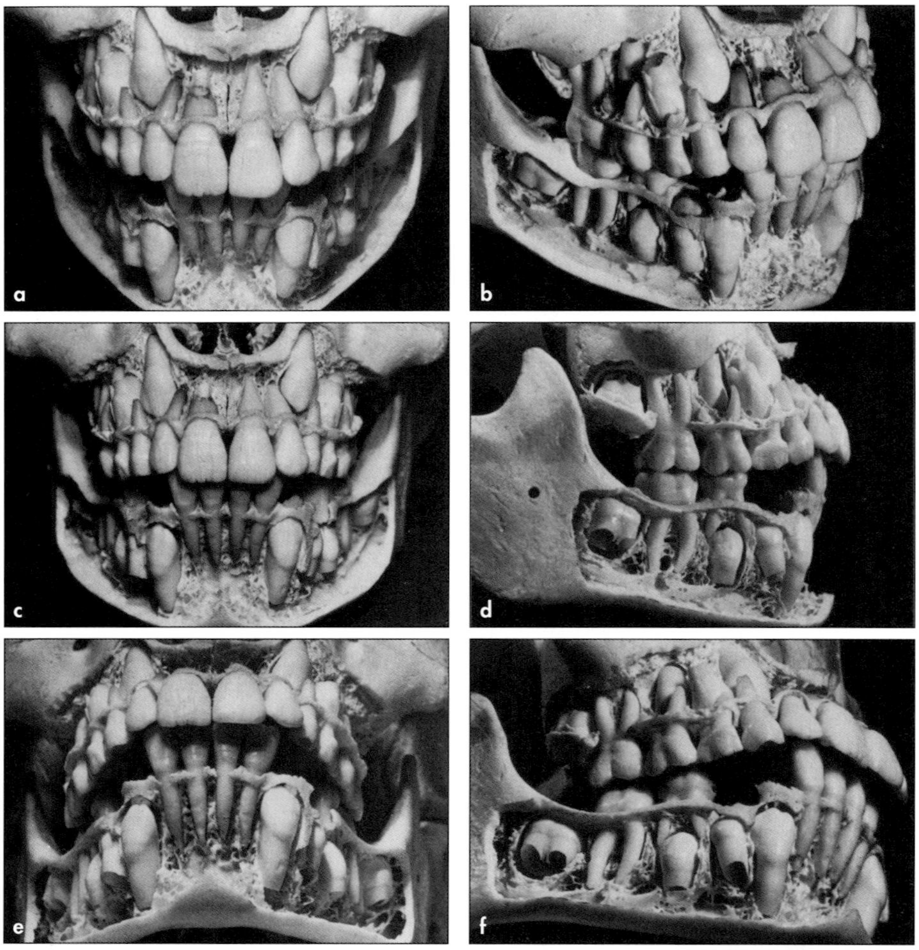

FIG 5-6 Exposed dentition in a skull at 10 years. *(a and b)* In this specimen, the maxillary permanent canine crowns are close to the roots of the lateral incisors. *(c and d)* In both arches, the root formation of the canines is ahead of that of the premolars. *(e and f)* Before the mandibular canines can emerge, remnants of alveolar bone occlusal to them must be resorbed. This is not necessary, however, for the emergence of the premolars.

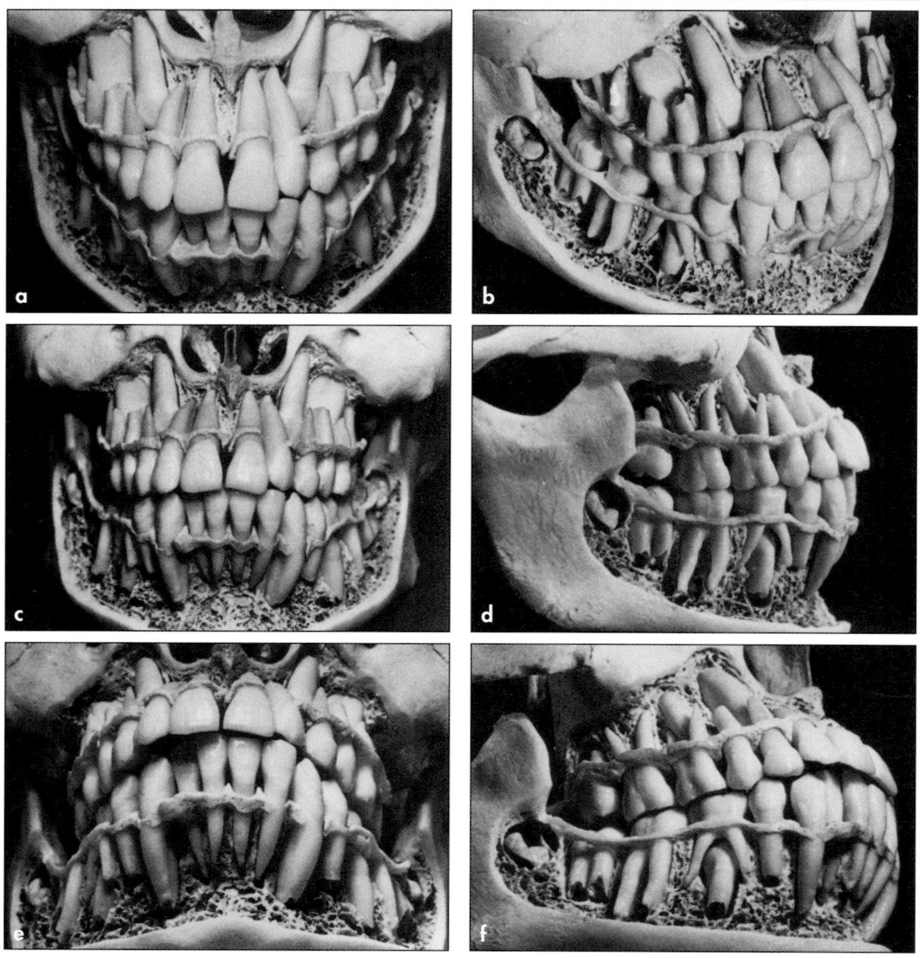

FIG 5-7 Exposed dentition in a skull at 10.5 years. *(a and b)* In this specimen, the maxillary first premolars and the mandibular canines and first premolars have already emerged. *(c and d)* The maxillary permanent canines are located palatal to the deciduous canines, the roots of which are resorbed only slightly. *(e)* The mandibular incisors converge apically. *(f)* The apices of the second deciduous molars also show little resorption, although their successors have already begun to erupt.

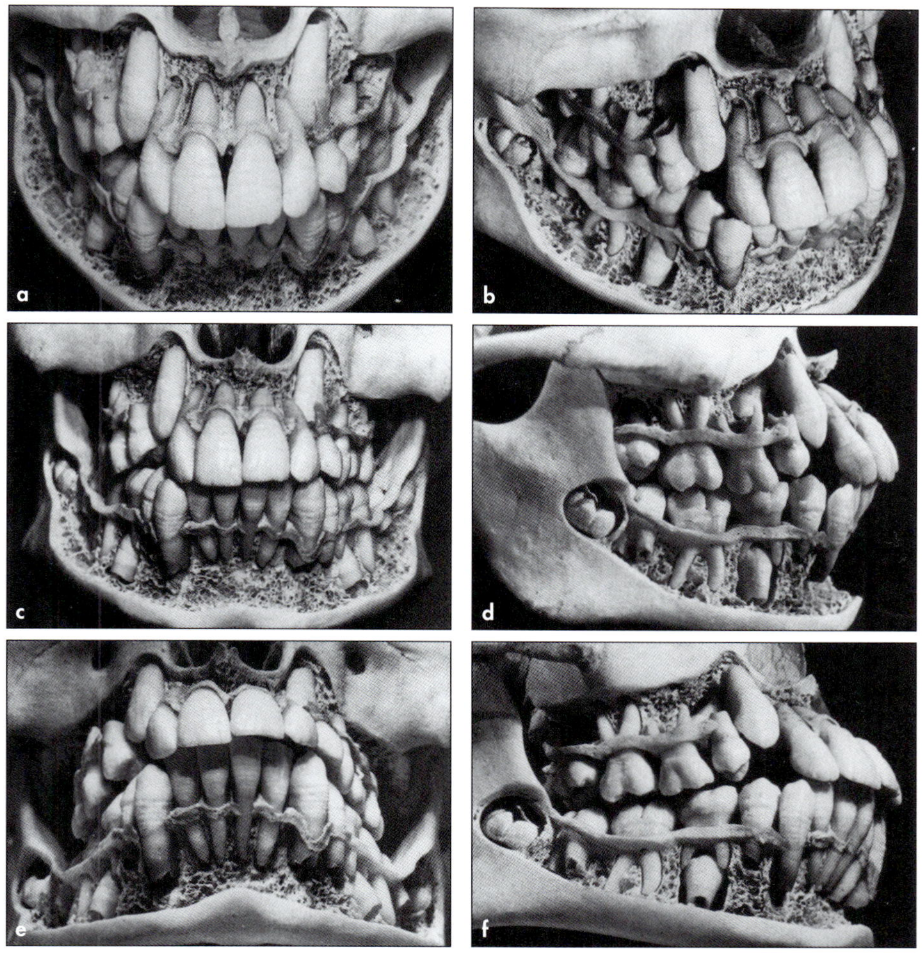

FIG 5-8 Exposed dentition in a skull at 11 years. *(a and b)* In this specimen, the maxillary left permanent canine is more palatally located than the right canine. *(c and d)* The maxillary right first premolar is almost fully emerged, although its root is only halfway formed. Indeed, in this specimen, the roots of all completely formed teeth are short in comparison with the crown heights. *(e and f)* There is no central diastema in the maxilla, which is unusual when the permanent canines have descended halfway.

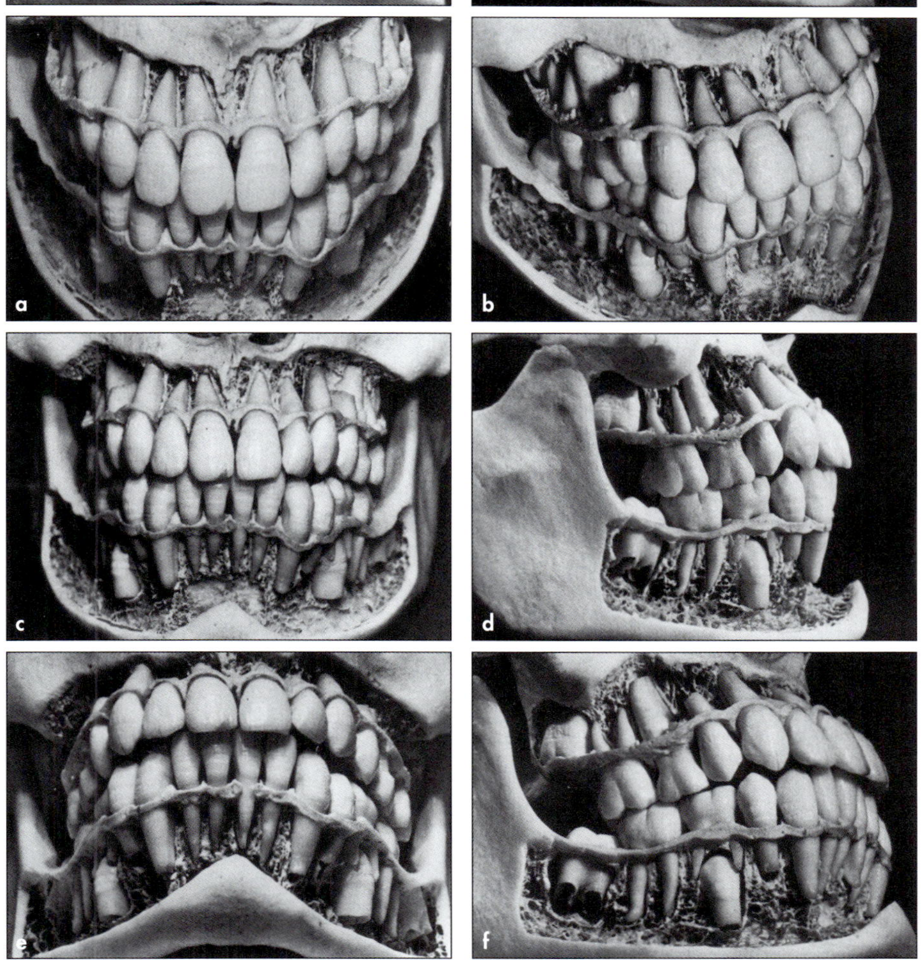

FIG 5-9 Exposed dentition in a skull at 11.5 years. *(a and b)* In this specimen, the maxillary canines have emerged, and the incisors are mesially angulated. There is no central diastema. *(c and d)* The canines and first premolars are not yet occluding. *(e and f)* The roots of the first permanent molars are completely formed. The distobuccally oriented maxillary right second molar crown is positioned close to the apices of the first molar. The mandibular right second molar is oriented linguomesially.

Correlations in Timing of Emergence of Permanent Teeth

The times of emergence of the permanent molars are more closely related to those of the deciduous teeth than of the other permanent teeth. Indeed, the permanent molars are in that respect more synchronous with the deciduous teeth than with the other permanent teeth. Furthermore, the mode of formation of the permanent molars is similar to that of the deciduous molars, and the shape of the crowns of the first permanent molars corresponds strongly with that of the second deciduous molars in both the maxilla and the mandible.[18]

It generally holds true that early emergence of deciduous teeth coincides with an early transition and vice versa. However, the correlation between these two is less than the one between the times of emergence of deciduous teeth and permanent molars, as mentioned above.[18] The emergence time of second permanent molars depends partly on the available space. Space restrictions are correlated with slower eruption and later emergence of all teeth.

The correlations among skeletal age, dental age, and sexual maturity age are limited.[19-21] However, skeletal age is more related to chronologic age than dental age. That also applies for sexual maturity age. Overall, girls are more advanced than boys in development of the dentition.[22] In the second transitional period, the difference is 6 months.[7] However, boys enter puberty 2 years later than girls. Consequently, girls usually experience the adolescent growth spurt during the second transitional period, while boys undergo the adolescent growth spurt after the transition is concluded.

References

1. Lo RT, Moyers RE. Studies in the etiology and prevention of malocclusion. I. The sequence of eruption of the permanent dentition. Am J Orthod 1953;39:460–467.
2. Farsi NMA, Salama FS. Characteristics of primary dentition occlusion in a group of Saudi children. Int J Paediatr Dent 1996;6:253–259.
3. Knott VB, Meredith MV. Statistics on eruption of the permanent dentition from serial data from North American white children. Angle Orthod 1966;36:68–79.
4. Nanda RS. Eruption of human teeth. Am J Orthod 1960;46:363–378.
5. Savara BS, Steen JC. Timing and sequence of eruption of permanent teeth in a longitudinal sample of children from Oregon. J Am Dent Assoc 1978;97:209–214.
6. Sturdivant JE, Knott VB, Meredith HV. Interrelations from serial data for eruption of the permanent dentition. Angle Orthod 1962;32:1–13.
7. Hurme VO. Ranges of normalcy in the eruption of permanent teeth. J Dent Child 1949;16:11–15.
8. Van der Linden FPGM, Boersma H, Prahl-Andersen B. Development of the dentition. In: Prahl-Andersen B, Kowalski CJ, Heydendael PHJ (eds). A Mixed-Longitudinal Interdisciplinary Study of Growth and Development. New York: Academic Press, 1979:521–536.
9. Nance HN. The limitations of orthodontic treatment. I. Mixed dentition diagnosis and treatment. Am J Orthod 1947;33:177–223.
10. Bakker PJMR, Wassenberg HJW, Van der Linden FPGM. Changes in the incisal area in relationship to the change of the lower lateral incisors [in German]. Inf Orthod Kieferorthop 1979;11:199–214.
11. Van der Linden FPGM. Changes in the position of posterior teeth in relation to ruga points. Am J Orthod 1978;74:142–161.
12. Van der Linden FPGM, Bakker PJMR, Wassenberg HJW. Comments regarding the development of the dentition and the carrying out of orthodontic therapy [in German]. Inf Orthod Kieferorthop 1979;11:319–323.
13. Van der Linden FPGM, Wassenberg HJW, Bakker PJMR. General aspects of the development of the occlusion [in German]. Inf Orthod Kieferorthop 1979;11:131–143.
14. Van der Linden FPGM, Wassenberg HJW, Bakker PJMR. The transition process in retrospect. Inf Orthod Kieferorthop 1979;11:325–330.
15. Wassenberg HJW, Bakker PJMR, Van der Linden FPGM. Exchange of the lower lateral incisors [in German]. Inf Orthod Kieferorthop 1979;11:169–198.
16. Wassenberg HJW, Bakker PJMR, Van der Linden FPGM. Change in the upper lateral teeth [in German]. Inf Orthod Kieferorthop 1979;11:271–304.
17. Wassenberg HJW, Bakker PJMR, Van der Linden FPGM. Variations in the upper incisal region in connection with change in the upper lateral teeth [in German]. Inf Orthod Kieferorthop 1979;11:305–318.
18. Moorrees CFA, Kent RL. Patterns of dental maturation. In: McNamara JA Jr (ed). The Biology of Occlusal Development, monograph 7, Craniofacial Growth Series. Ann Arbor: University of Michigan, 1977:25–41.
19. Filipsson R, Hall K. Correlation between dental maturity, height development and sexual maturation in normal girls. Ann Hum Biol 1976;3:205–210.
20. Marshall WA. Interrelationships of skeletal maturation, sexual development and somatic growth in man. Ann Hum Biol 1974;1:29–40.
21. Prahl-Andersen B, Roede MJ. The measurement of skeletal and dental maturity. In: Prahl-Andersen B, Kowalski CJ, Heydendael PHJ (eds). A Mixed-Longitudinal, Interdisciplinary Study of Growth and Development. New York: Academic Press, 1979:491–519.
22. Demirjian A, Levesque GY. Sexual differences in dental development and prediction of emergence. J Dent Res 1980;59:1110–1122.

6

Changes in the Molar Region

The region where the permanent molars are formed and emerge increases gradually in size. The posterior growth of the alveolar process is limited to 1 to 2 mm a year.[1,2] The mineralization of the third molars starts 6 years after the second molars. There is also a 6-year period between times of emergence of the three permanent molars.

Available Space for Molar Development and Orientation of Tooth Buds

There is a large difference between the maxilla and mandible regarding the space available for the development of the molars and in the orientation of the forming molars.

The mandibular ramus provides space for the second and third molars to begin their formation. Initially they are located superior to the level of the occlusal plane and partially overlap each other. Through vertical growth of the mandibular body and the alveolar process, they attain an inferior position in relation to the other mandibular teeth. Furthermore, the roots of the forming mandibular second and third molars are positioned posterior to their crowns. This mesial angulation gradually decreases (Fig 6-1).

In the maxilla, the second and third molars are formed in the limited region of the maxillary tuberosity. They cannot be arranged horizontally as forming deciduous molars are. Rather, they are stacked in a posterosuperior direction and overlap each other vertically. They are formed at a distal angulation, and their roots are close together[2] (Fig 6-2).

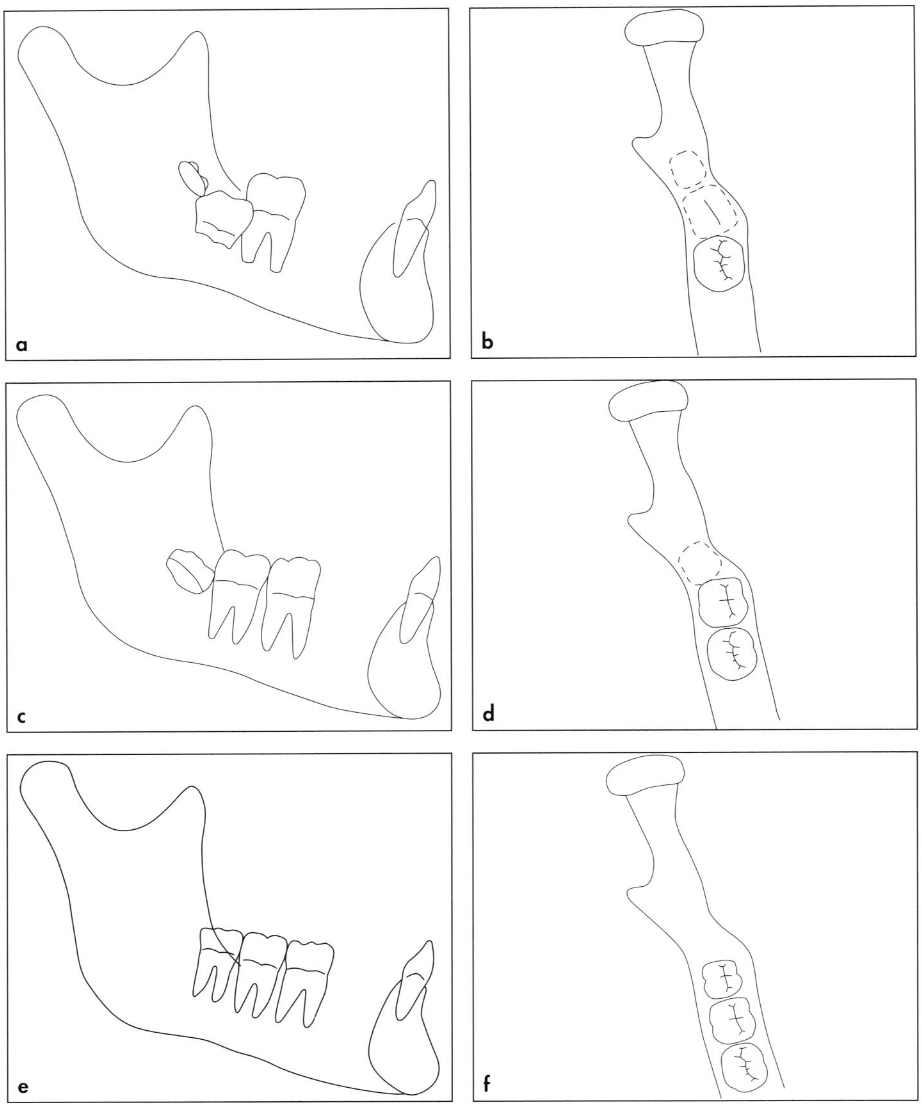

Fig 6-1 Relationship between mandibular growth and development of permanent molars. The mandibular second and third molars are formed in the part of the jaw where the corpus intersects with the ramus. *(a and b)* At 6 years of age, when the first permanent molar has reached the occlusal plane, the forming second molar is located at the slight lateral bend of the mandible. The second molar is then mesially angulated and distobuccally rotated. The third molar starts its formation in the ramus. *(c and d)* By the time the second permanent molar has reached the occlusal plane, its angulation and rotation are reduced. The distal part of the crown has moved to the lingual and is located mesial to the lateral bend of the mandible. *(e and f)* The eruption and change in position of the third molars occurs in a comparable way, 6 years later. In the meantime, the mandible has grown sufficiently to the posterior to house the third molar without distobuccal rotation.

The change in position of the buds of the permanent molars is related to the speed of their formation and the amount of jaw growth. The mandible enlarges about twice as much to the posterior as the maxilla, which is displaced by sutural growth to the anterior in the meantime. Through reconstruction of the bone of their crypts, the buds migrate to the posterior in the mandible and to the anterior in the maxilla.[3–5]

In accordance with the limited space, the maxillary second molars emerge in a distobuccal direction. When they reach occlusion, they are still distally angulated. More space has to be created by growth of the maxillary tuberosity to the posterior before their roots can move distally. After the crowns of the third molars have descended, they can upright and ultimately develop a mesial angulation. Indeed, the position and angulation of the maxillary second and third permanent molars depends on the amount of growth of the maxilla and the presence or absence of third molars.

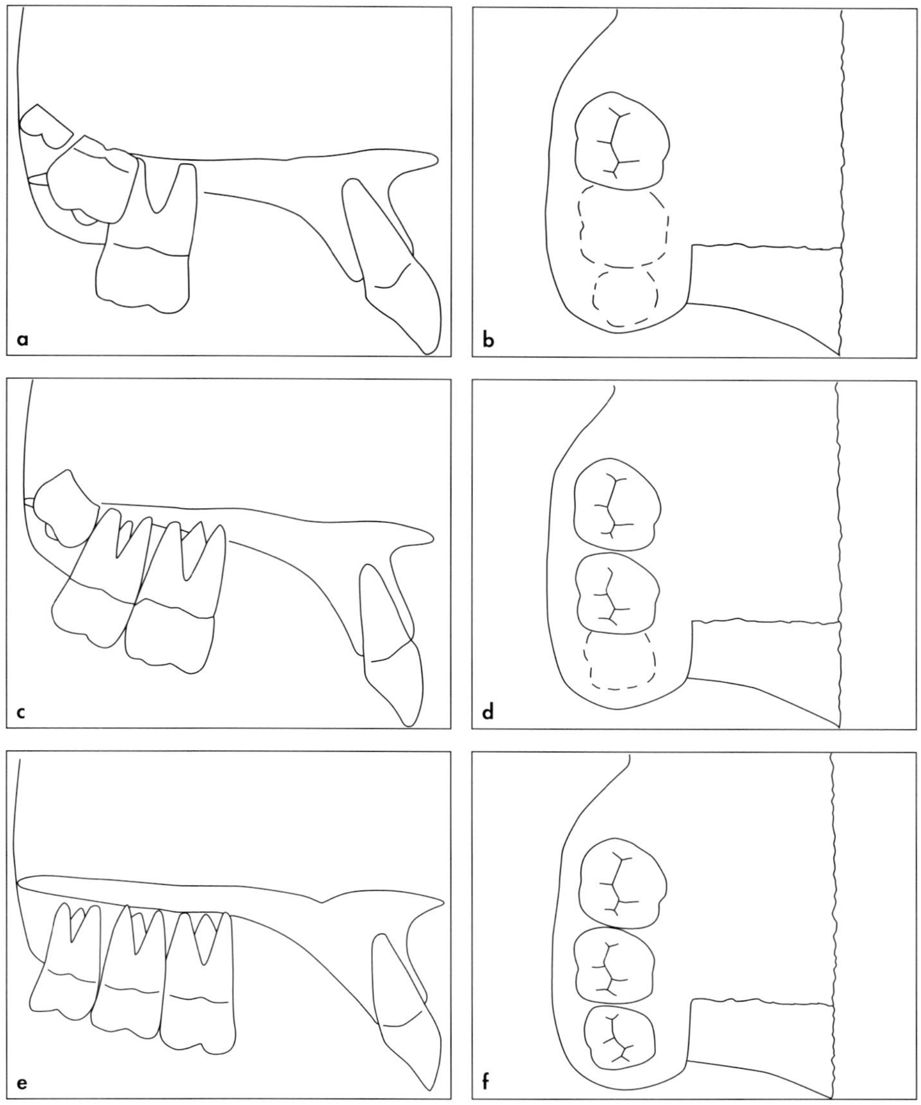

Fig 6-2 Relationship between maxillary growth and development of permanent molars. *(a and b)* The formation of the second and third molars precedes the growth of the jaws. In contrast to that in the mandible, the region in the maxilla where the second and third molars are formed is limited in size. There is sufficient space for the first permanent molars that mesiodistally, emerge perpendicular to the occlusal plane. The crown of the second molar is located at the most apical aspect of the roots of the first molar and is distally angulated, which minimizes the amount of space it occupies. The third molar is formed in a superior location in the tuberosity. *(c and d)* The second molar has emerged in a distobuccal direction. Its angulation has already changed slightly. The third molar is positioned close to the most apical part of the roots of the second molar and blocks their distal movement. *(e and f)* When the third molar has descended, space becomes available for the distal movement of the roots of the second molar. Finally, the maxillary third molar becomes mesially angulated.

It often occurs that the growth of the jaws to the posterior is insufficient for adequate emergence of third molars. Mandibular molars can remain impacted without necessarily causing any problems. However, if they are partially emerged and only the mesio-occlusal aspect of the crown is visible, an infection can develop between the unexposed portion of the crown and the covering gingiva, leading to a swollen cheek. Surgical intervention is then needed. Maxillary third molars are less frequently impacted. With shortage of space, they emerge distobuccally. Extracting them is a simple procedure.

The change in position of erupting mandibular third molars varies. In addition to spatial conditions, differences in speed of formation between the mesial and distal roots might play a role.[6]

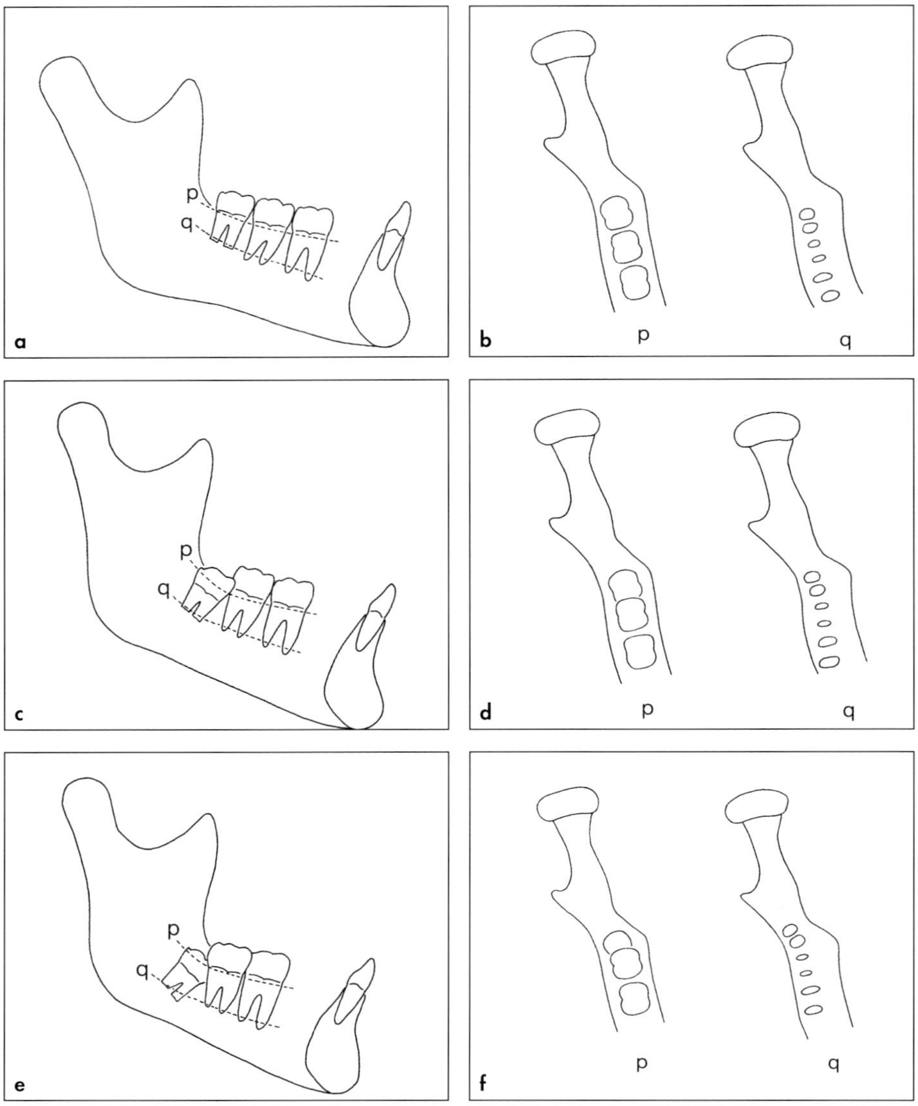

Fig 6-3 Variations in the size of the posterior section of the mandibular apical area in adults. *(a and b)* In a large posterior section, the third molar has adequate space to emerge well. There may even be excess space distally. At the level of the cervical borders, the teeth are positioned at the same height (p). The apices are at equal distances apart (q). *(c and d)* In a medium posterior section, the third molar is tipped mesially and partly emerged. Its crown is distobuccally rotated, and the apex of the distal root is situated in the laterally deviating region of the jaw (q). *(e and f)* In a small posterior section, the third molar is impacted. There is not enough room for it to emerge. Its mesio-occlusal margin is situated close to the cervical border of the second molar. At the level of the cervical margins, there is little room (p). Both apices of the third molar are located in the laterally deviating region of the jaw (q).

Size of the Posterior Section of the Apical Area

The size of the posterior section of the apical area is the decisive parameter in the eruption and emergence of permanent molars. This aspect is illustrated for the mandible in Fig 6-3 and for the maxilla in Fig 6-4.

In both the maxilla and mandible, the size of the posterior sections of the apical areas quite often does not correspond with that of the anterior and middle sections. That also applies, although less frequently, to opposing posterior sections. It is also important to note that the posterior sections are the only areas that continue to increase in size, although the amount of extension varies. The size of the posterior section of the apical area can increase markedly in one individual and only marginally in another. The position and orientation of the molars will vary accordingly.

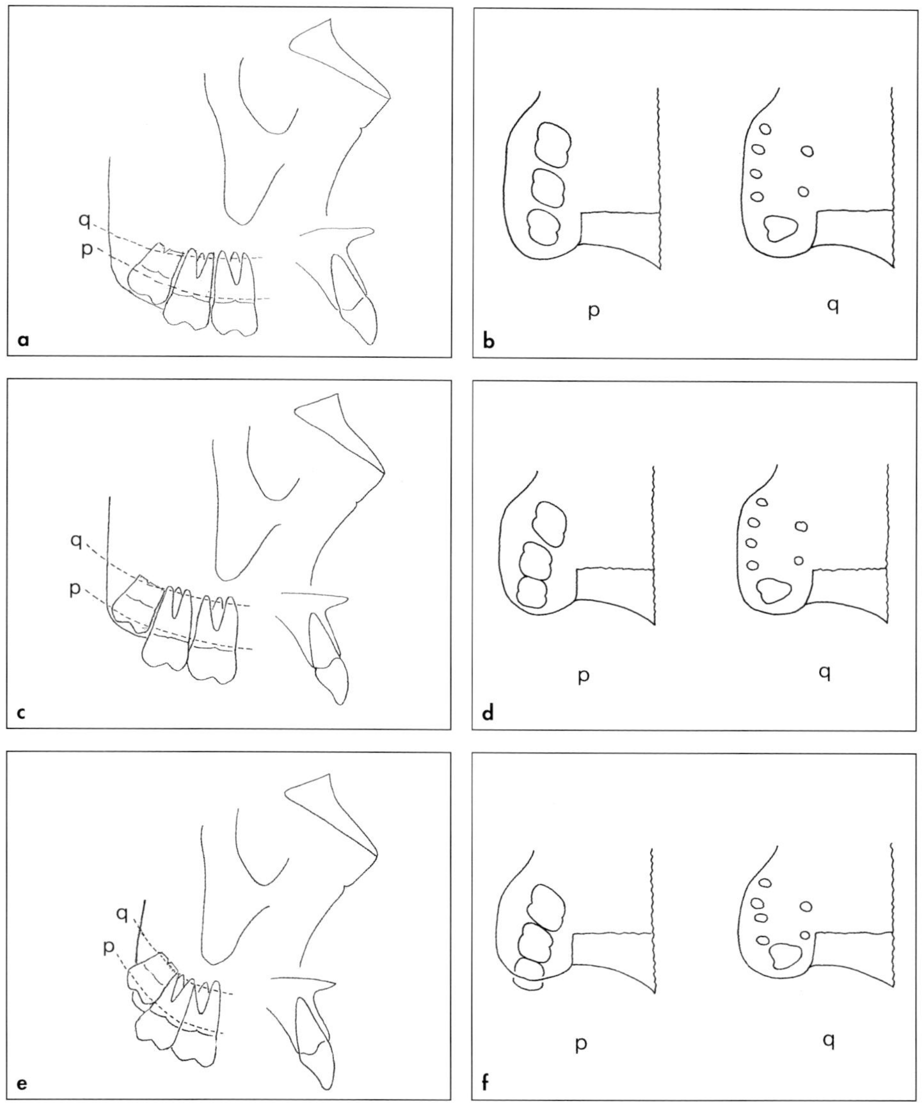

Fig 6-4 Variations in size of the posterior section of the maxillary apical area, shortly before the emergence of the third molar. *(a and b)* In a large posterior section, more than sufficient room is available for the third molar, which has already become somewhat upright prior to emergence. At the level of the cervical margins, there is adequate space (p). At the level of the apices, sufficient room is available for the roots to become separated (q). *(c and d)* In a medium posterior section, the mesio-occlusal margin of the third molar is positioned close to the cervical border of the second molar (p). Adequate room is available for the roots of the second and third molars (q). *(e and f)* In a small posterior section, the crown of the third molar is markedly distally angulated and buccally inclined and can penetrate the distal bony surface of the tuberosity. At the level of the cervical margins, the molars are close together (p). The apices of the second molar and the forming part of the third molar are more mesially and palatally located than they are in favorable spatial conditions (q).

Eruption and Emergence of Molars

Specific aspects of the eruption and emergence of second and third permanent molars can be observed in skeletal material at increasing levels of development (Figs 6-5 and 6-6) and longitudinally collected dental casts and radiographs of growing individuals[7] (Figs 6-7 to 6-9). The changes in the molar region prior to and during the emergence of first, second, and third molars are clarified with virtual illustrations (Figs 6-10 to 6-12).

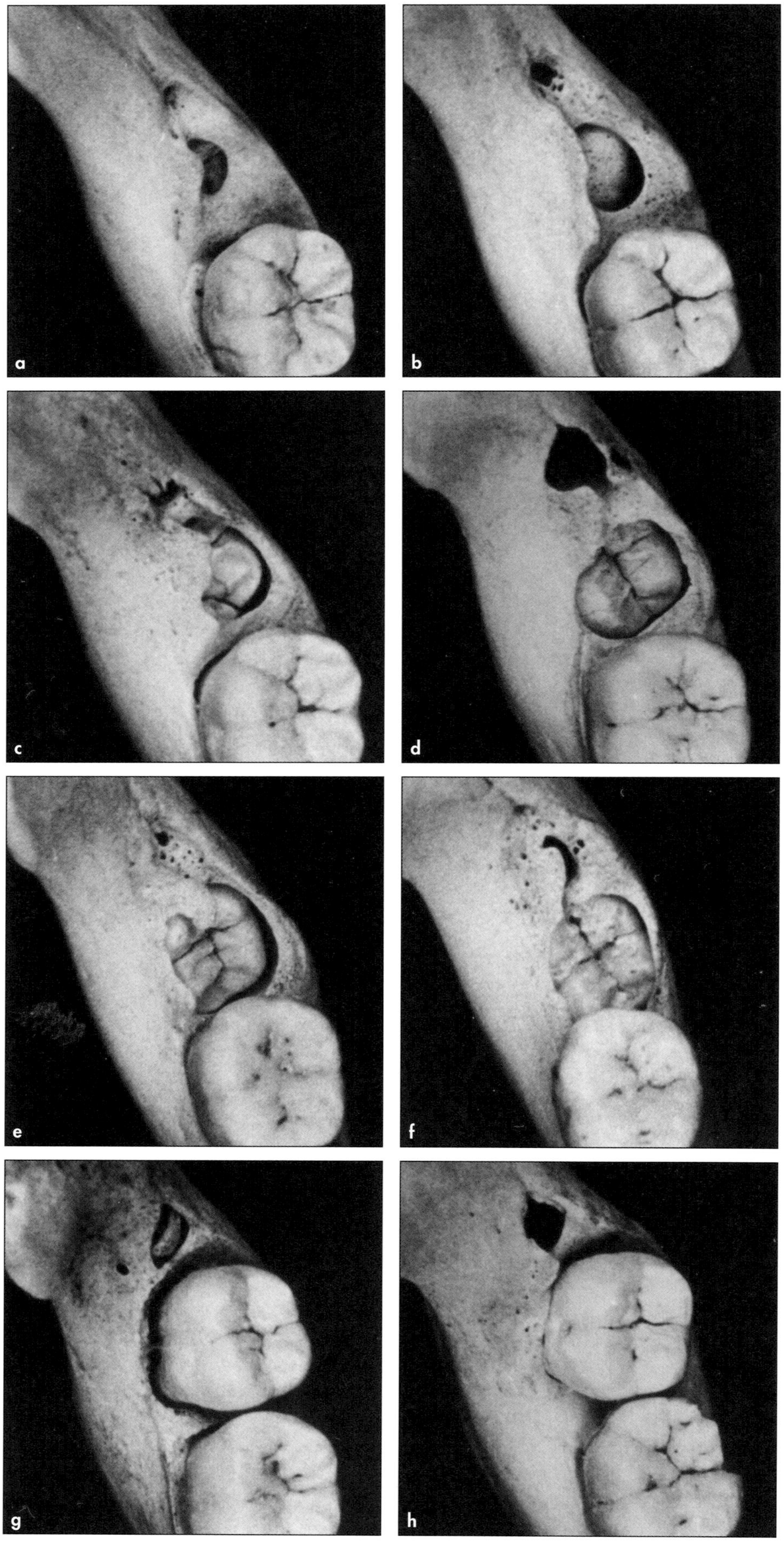

Fig 6-5 Emergence of mandibular second permanent molars, demonstrated in eight right jaw segments. *(a)* Initially, the second molar is located in the part of the jaw posterior to the obtuse lateral bend. *(b to d)* The gubernacular opening enlarges gradually. *(e and f)* Through growth of the mandible to the posterior, the second molar becomes positioned mesial to the obtuse lateral bend. *(g)* Bone resorption creates space for the emergence of the crown. *(h)* As the crown erupts further, new bone is built up at the cervical border.

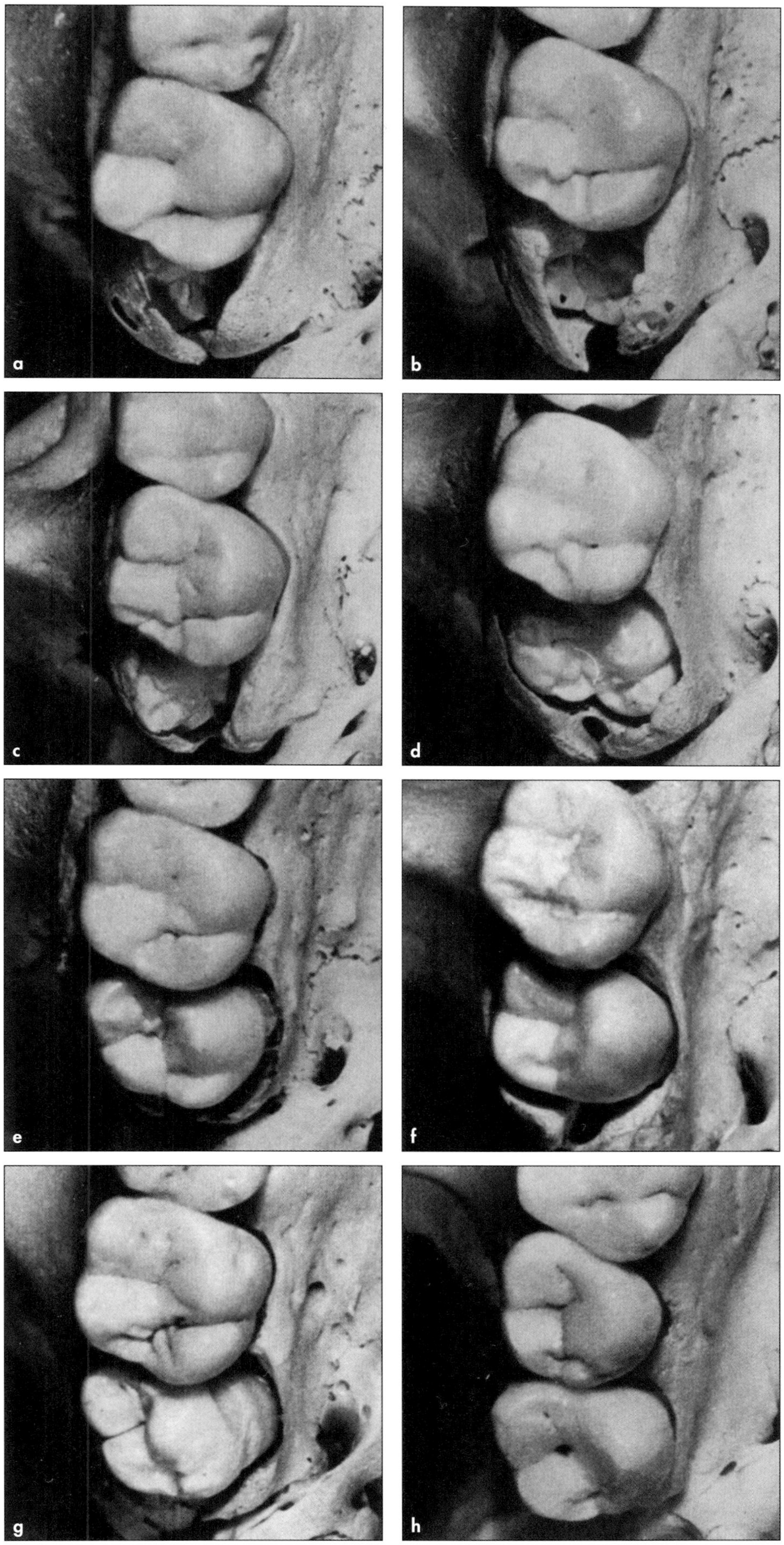

FIG 6-6 Emergence of maxillary second permanent molars, demonstrated in eight right jaw segments. *(a)* Initially, the crown of the second molar is located superiorly in the jaw. The tuberosity needs to extend to the posterior. *(b to d)* The gubernacular opening increases and the tuber enlarges. *(e to g)* Prior to emergence, bone is resorbed widely. *(h)* During the eruption after emergence, the alveolar process is built up, and the cervical border becomes surrounded by bone.

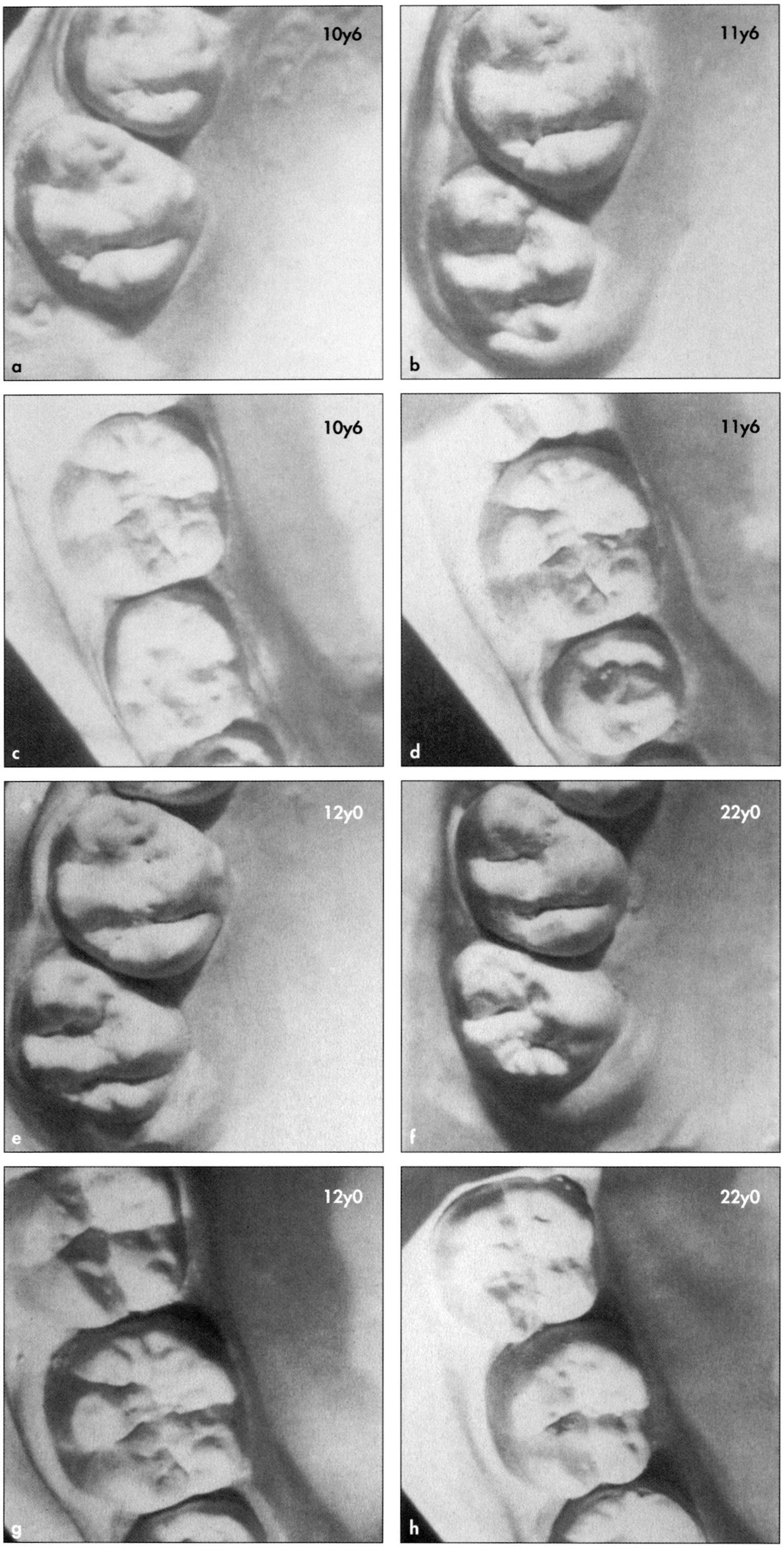

Fig 6-7 Sections of plaster casts collected from one individual. *(a and b)* At 10 years 6 months of age, the second deciduous molars are still present. Shortly before, the mesiobuccal cusp of the maxillary second permanent molar had emerged. *(c and d)* At the age of 11 years 6 months, all second premolars had emerged. The crown of the maxillary second permanent molar has emerged almost completely. However, it has not yet reached the occlusal level. The mesial margin of the mandibular second permanent molar has become visible. That tooth is distobuccally rotated. The distal part of the crown is still located in the laterally deviating part of the mandible. *(e and f)* At the age of 12 years, the slight buccal position of the maxillary second permanent molar has been neutralized. The distobuccal rotation of the fully emerged mandibular second permanent molar has mostly disappeared. *(g and h)* At the age of 22 years, growth to the posterior had resulted in large posterior sections of the apical areas. The third molars could emerge well and attain proper positions in the dental arch. (Reprinted from Schols and Van der Linden[7] with permission.)

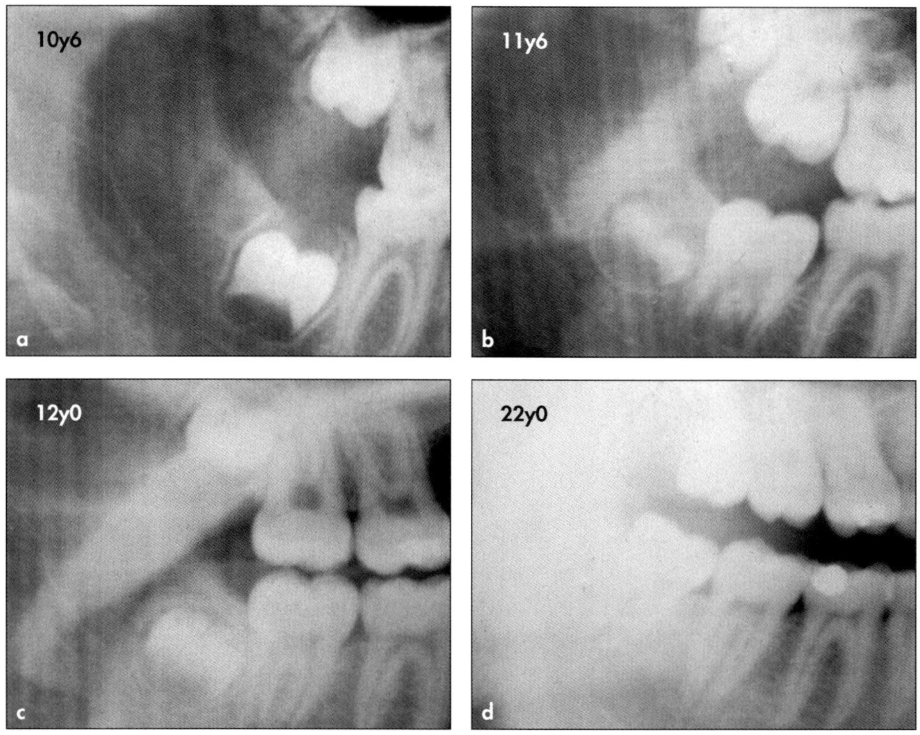

Fig 6-8 Corresponding sections of panoramic radiographs of the person whose casts are shown in Fig 6-7. *(a)* At the age of 10 years 6 months, the crown of the maxillary second molar is positioned close to the roots of the first molar and distally angulated. There is some space between the mandibular first molar and the mesially angulated second molar. *(b)* At 11 years 6 months, the second molars have penetrated the occlusal bony surfaces. The distal part of the mandibular second molar is situated in the laterally deviating part of the alveolar process. *(c)* At 12 years, the second molars occlude completely. The third molars have not yet started to erupt. *(d)* At 22 years, all third molars have emerged completely. The maxillary third molar is mesially angulated. (Reprinted from Schols and Van der Linden[7] with permission.)

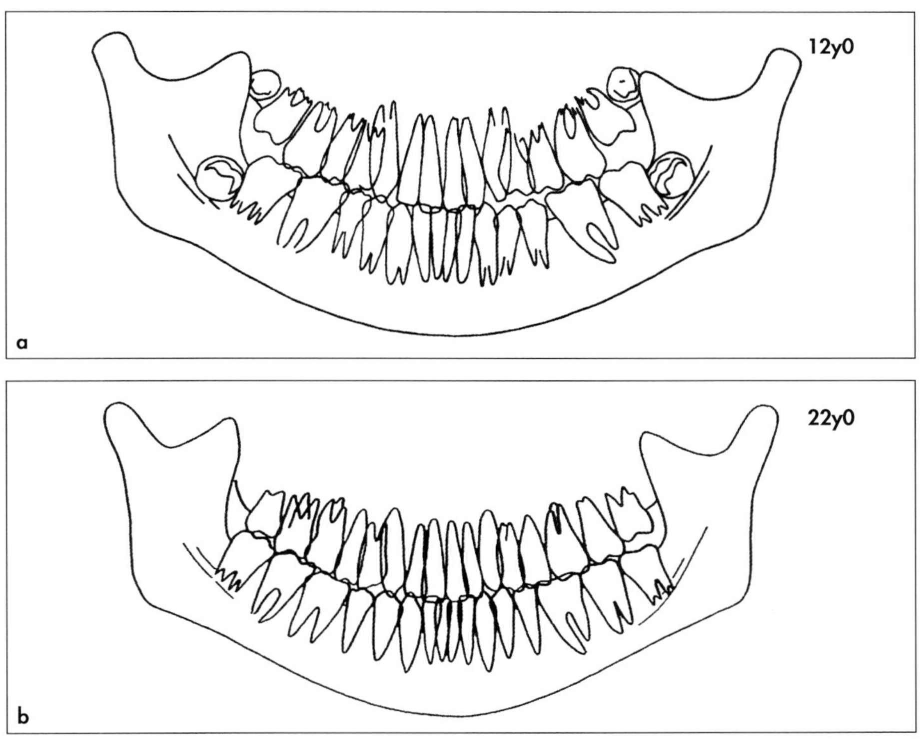

Fig 6-9 Tracings of two of the panoramic radiographs in Fig 6-8. *(a)* At 12 years of age (see Fig 6-8c), the size of the maxillary tuberosities is limited, and the maxillary third molars are positioned superior to the second molars. The mandibular third molars are located in the ramus. *(b)* At 22 years of age (see Fig 6-8d), all molars, except the maxillary left third molar, occlude and are mesially angulated. In the maxilla, the development on the left side is delayed compared with the right side. The maxillary left third molar has to erupt further, and the roots of the first and second molars have not yet moved distally. The final position and angulation of the molars is realized after all of them have reached occlusion. (Reprinted from Schols and Van der Linden[7] with permission.)

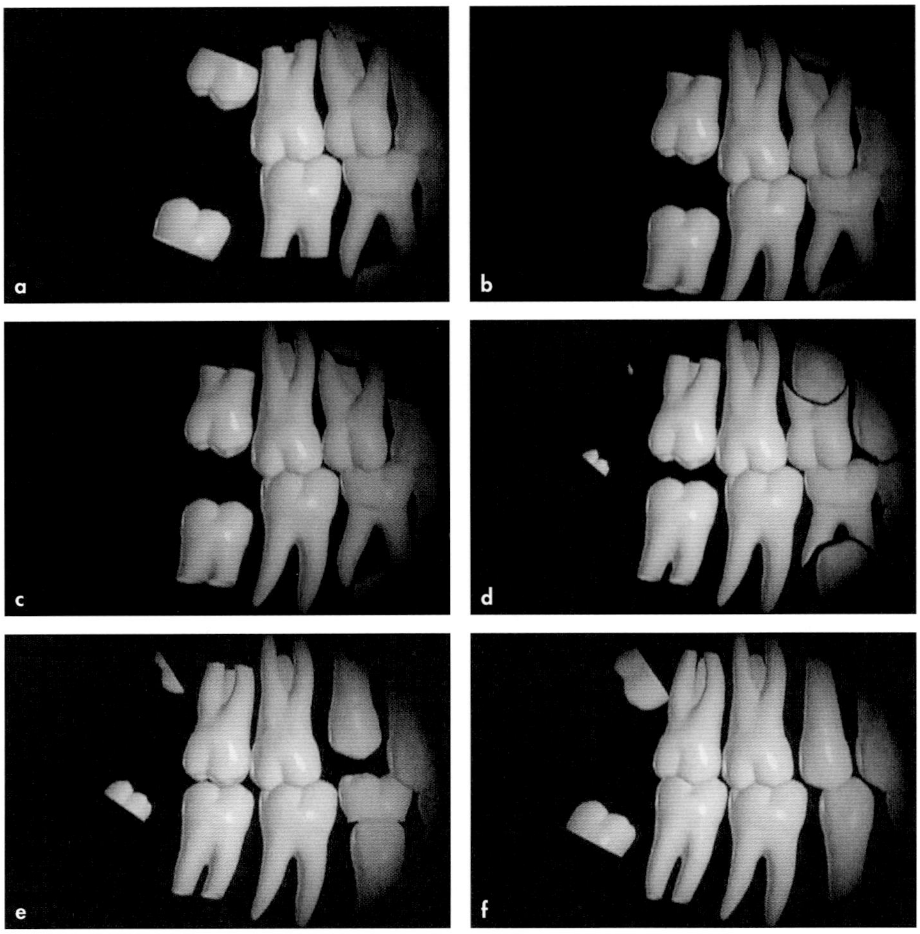

FIG 6-10 Eruption and positioning of second molars. *(a)* Prior to emergence, the mandibular second molar is mesially angulated, and the maxillary second molar is distally angulated. *(b)* The mandibular second molar erupts in a mesial direction, and the maxillary second molar erupts in a distobuccal direction. *(c and d)* With sufficient space, the second molars can erupt and emerge unhindered. *(e and f)* The angulation of the maxillary second molar cannot change as long as the forming third molar is close to its roots. See video clip 19. (Printed from Van der Linden et al[8] with permission.)

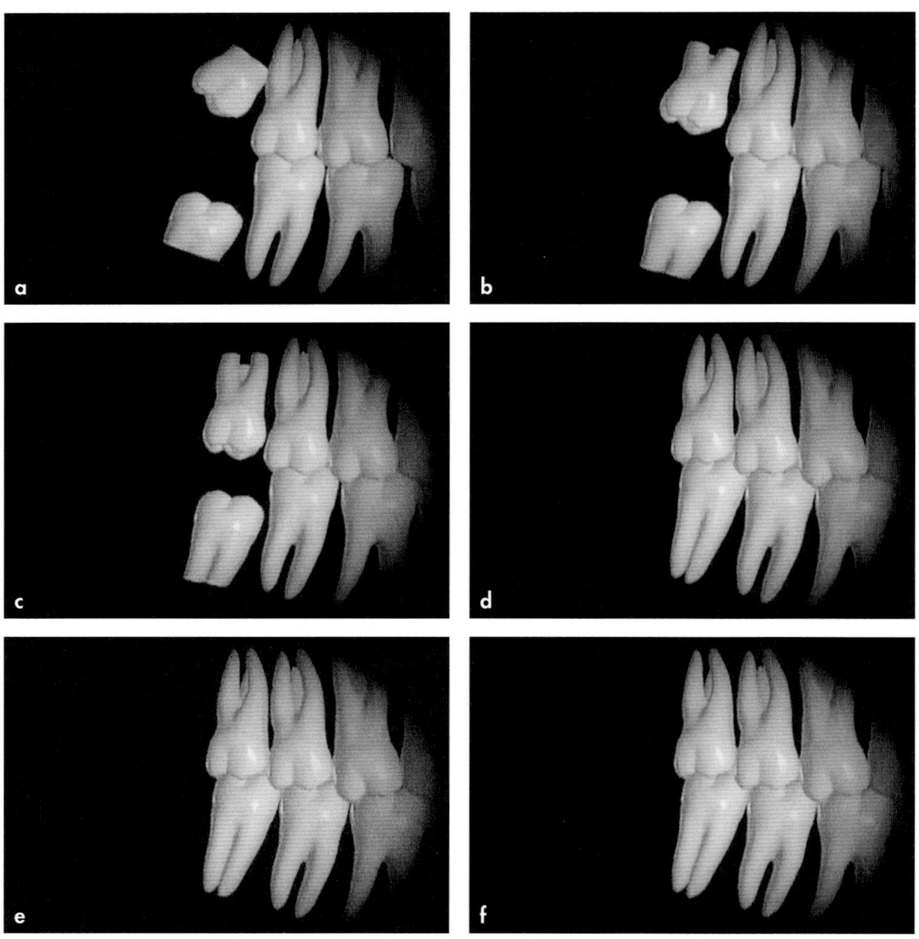

FIG 6-11 Eruption and positioning of third molars. *(a)* The mandibular third molar is mesially angulated, and the maxillary third molar is distally angulated. *(b and c)* With the eruption of the maxillary third molar, space becomes available for the distal movement of the roots of the second molar. *(d to f)* With adequate posterior growth, large posterior sections of the apical area develop. As a result, third molars can emerge unhindered and in good occlusion, and the roots of the maxillary molars can move distally. See video clip 20. (Printed from Van der Linden et al[8] with permission.)

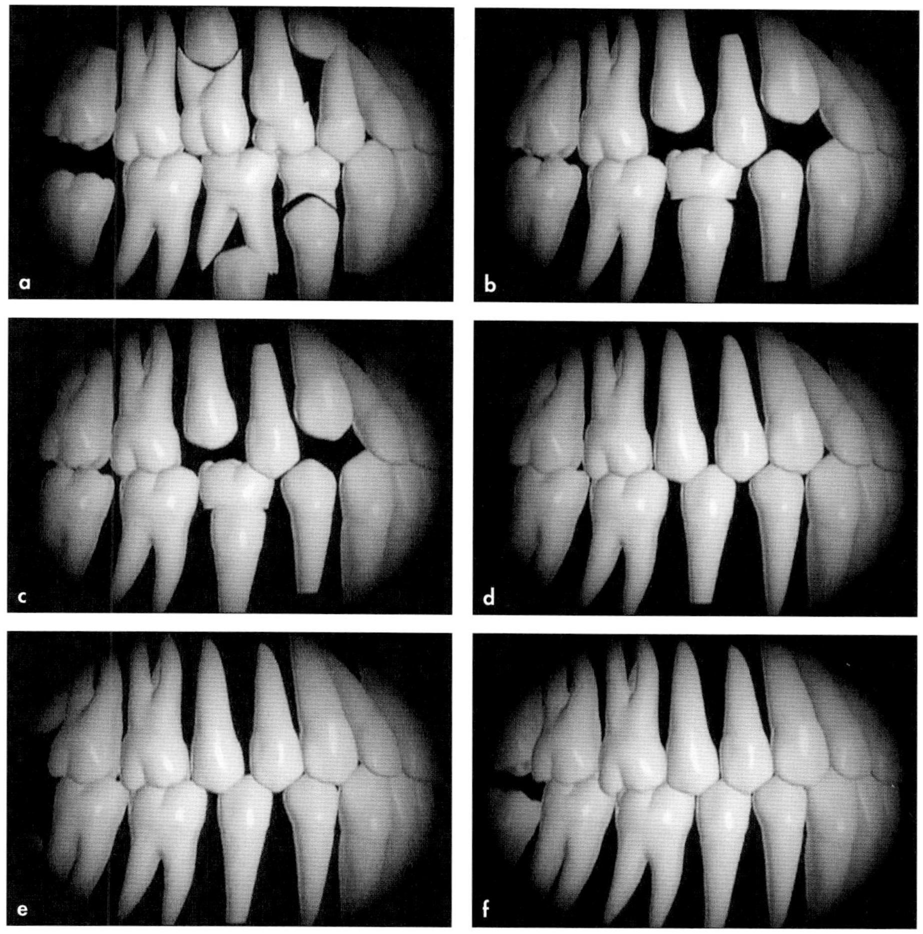

FIG 6-12 Normal development of the molar region. *(a to c)* When the deciduous molars are replaced by their narrower successors, extra space becomes available in the dental arch. *(d to f)* The resulting diastemata are closed by mesial migration of the permanent molars. Subsequently, occlusion of the first permanent molars improves, and their angulation changes. In the maxilla, the mesial angulation increases further if the roots can move distally when the adjacent molar has descended. See video clip 21. (Printed from Van der Linden et al[8] with permission.

Comparison of Anterior and Posterior Eruption

The alteration in angulation of the maxillary second and third molars has some similarity with the alteration in angulation of the maxillary incisors. The latter are also formed in a spatially limited situation. As explained earlier, the roots of the lateral and central incisors cannot move distally prior to the emergence of the permanent canine and until its narrower root is positioned where the bulky crown initially was situated. In addition, the angulation is altered by the mesial migration of the incisor crowns and the closure of the central diastema. A similar phenomenon occurs in the molar region if the extra space that becomes available with the replacement of the deciduous molars is depleted by the mesial migration of the molars. However, there are also clear differences between the posterior and anterior regions. The three molars erupt in intervals of 6 years while the jaws continue to grow posteriorly. In the anterior region, the lateral incisors emerge 1 year after the central incisors, and jaw growth is negligible.

References

1. Chen LL, Xu TM, Jiang JH, Zhang XZ, Lin JX. Longitudinal changes in mandibular arch posterior space in adolescents with normal occlusion. Am J Orthod Dentofac Orthop 2010;137:187–193.
2. Mitani H. Behavior of the maxillary first molar in three planes with emphasis on its role of providing room for the second and third molars during growth. Angle Orthod 1975;45:159–168.
3. Chávez Lomeli ME. Permanent Maxillary Molar Crypts in Man—A Study of Postnatal Development [thesis]. Groningen: University of Groningen, 1987.
4. Duterloo HS. Knochenstruktur und Zahnbewegung. Fortschr Kieferorthop 1980;41:177–185.
5. Jongsma AC. Permanent Molar Crypts in the Human Mandible. A Cross-Sectional Study of Postnatal Development [thesis]. Groningen: University of Groningen, 1985.
6. Richardson ME. Pre-eruptive movements of the mandibular third molar. Angle Orthod 1978;48:187–193.
7. Schols JG, Van der Linden FPGM. Development of posterior apical region [in German]. Inf Orthod Kieferorthop 1988;20:45–55.
8. Van der Linden FPGM, Radlanski RJ, McNamara JA Jr. Dynamics of Orthodontics: Normal Development of the Dentition [DVD 3A]. Berlin: Quintessence, 2000.

7

The Adult Dentition

This chapter deals with the complete permanent dentition. As way of introduction, some aspects of development are mentioned, although most of them have been covered in the previous chapters in another context. Finally, the worn dentition of an elderly individual is shown.

Tooth Positions

After all permanent teeth except the third molars have emerged at 12 or 13 years of age, alterations in tooth positions still take place. The roots of the permanent incisors, particularly the maxillary incisors, move distally. After emergence of the third molars, the roots of the maxillary permanent molars spread throughout the available space. If the third molars are absent, this probably occurs earlier. The roots of the second molars move distally, and their angulation alters. Ultimately, all maxillary molars are mesially angulated. The distal margins of the maxillary first molars become positioned more occlusally than the adjacent mesial margins of the second molars.[1] All maxillary teeth except the second premolars are mesially angulated. The maxillary posterior teeth are inclined slightly buccally; the incisors are inclined labially. Mesiodistally, the mandibular premolars are oriented perpendicular to the occlusal plane. The lateral incisors, canines, and molars are mesially angulated. The molars are inclined lingually; the incisors and canines are inclined labially. The premolars are the turning point between the two inclinations (Figs 7-1 to 7-4).

Factors Affecting the Arrangement of the Teeth

In every population, a large diversity exists in the position and occlusion of permanent teeth. The angulation and inclination of teeth vary considerably, even in normal occlusion[2] (see chapter 17, Table 17-30). The same also applies to the shape and relationship of the jaws and to the influence of functional factors. The position of the apices depends on the morphology of the jaws, the spatial conditions within the jaws, and their sagittal and transverse relationships. The position of the crowns and the inclinations are further determined by the occlusion and the pressures exerted by the tongue, lips, and cheeks. In that regard, the dimensions and volume of the soft tissues are of importance, but their position in unstrained conditions is even more essential. Furthermore, the shape and size of the crowns, the tooth-supporting tissues, and the forces generated by the functioning dentition affect the position of the individual teeth. In this context, habits such as thumb sucking, chewing of tobacco and coca leaves, bruxism, and tooth grinding must be considered. In addition, many factors alter slightly with age, including the morphology of the jaws and the craniofacial skeleton and also the tone, texture, and form of the soft tissue. Most of the aspects mentioned above are clarified further in chapter 9.

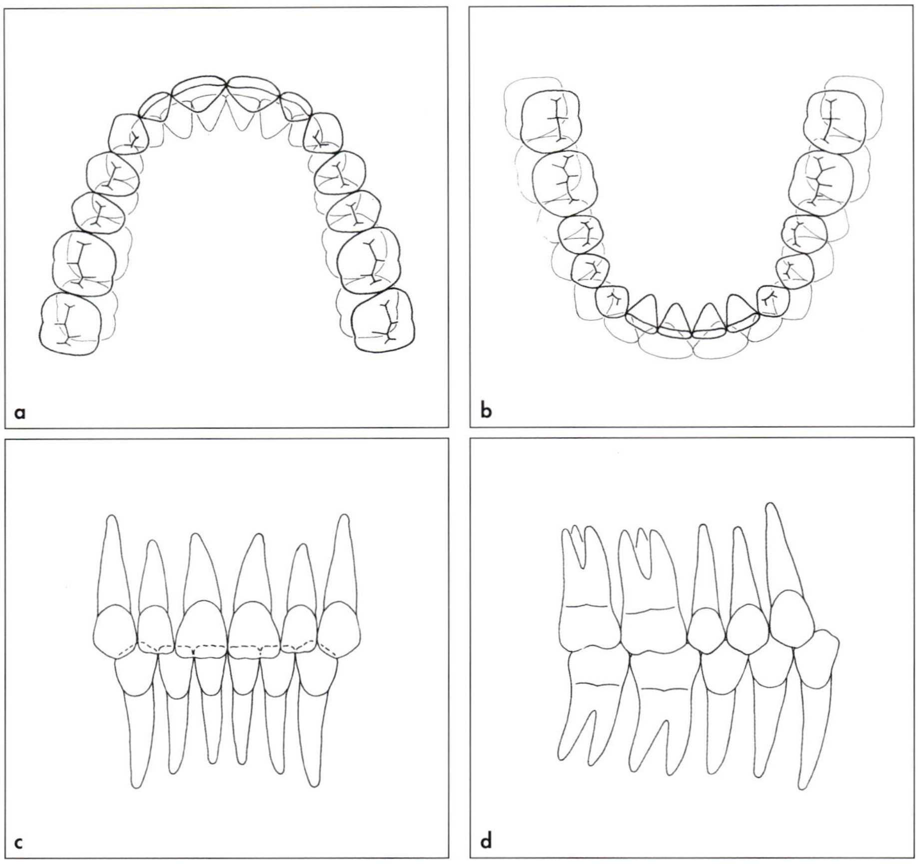

Fig 7-1 Permanent dentition. *(a)* The maxillary teeth are arranged in an arch without diastemata. They occlude slightly outside of the mandibular ones. There is a small overjet. *(b)* The mandibular teeth are in contact with each other and form an arch on which the maxillary teeth fit. All mandibular teeth have occlusal contact with two maxillary teeth, with the exception of the mandibular central incisors. *(c and d)* The roots of the maxillary lateral incisors are directed distally, as are those of the central incisors, although to a slightly lesser degree. The roots of the mandibular lateral incisors are slightly distally angulated. The premolars intercuspate like gears.

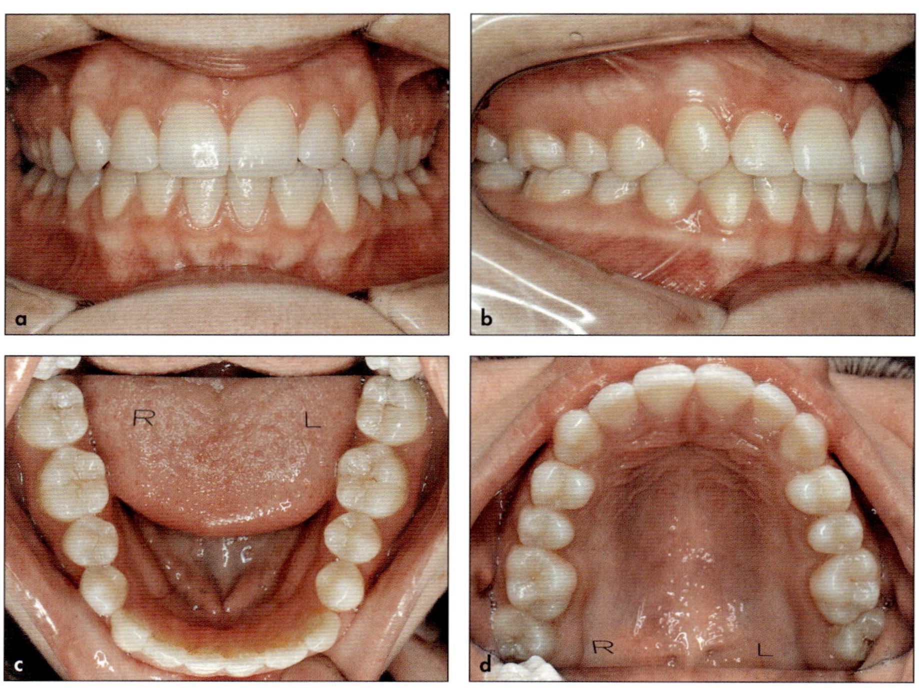

Fig 7-2 Ideal permanent dentition. *(a to d)* In this case, all criteria of an ideal position and occlusion of teeth are met, including the course of the gingival line. The texture and color of the gingiva and the height of the smile line are also optimal. As a result of the availability of sophisticated orthodontic appliances, an ideal arrangement can be reached in many cases.

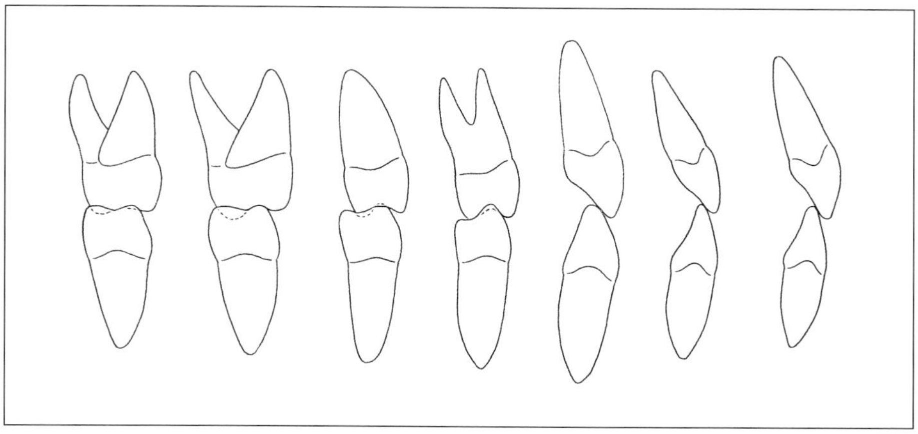

Fig 7-3 Inclination of permanent teeth. The maxillary incisors and canines are more labially inclined than the mandibular incisors and canines. The lateral incisors are more labially inclined than the central incisors, particularly in the maxilla. In the maxilla, the premolars are buccally inclined. In the mandible, their buccolingual orientation is perpendicular to the occlusal plane. The maxillary molars are buccally inclined; the mandibular molars are lingually inclined. Note that the occlusal contacts in this illustration deviate from reality. The distal sides of the teeth are drawn, not cross sections of the points where opposing teeth meet.

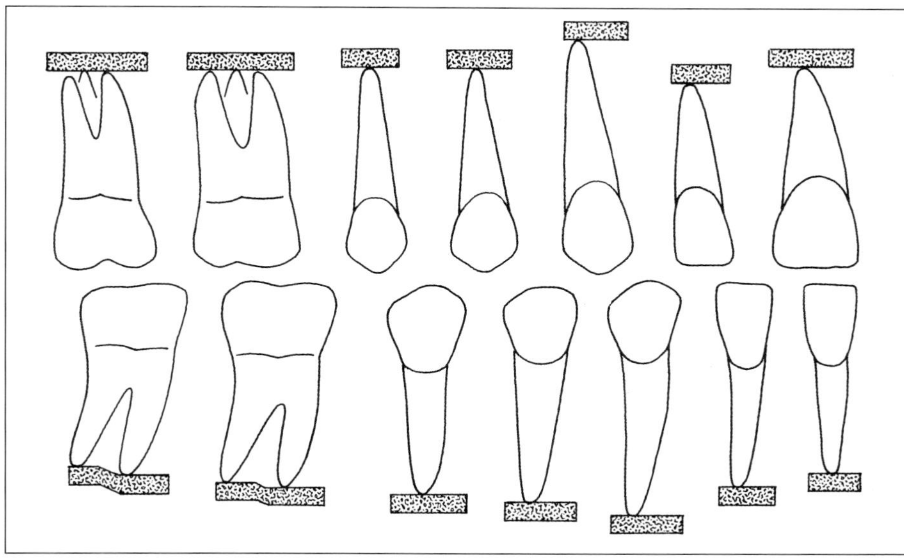

Fig 7-4 Angulation of permanent teeth and the relationship between their length and the level where their formation started *(shaded)*. All teeth are mesially angulated, except both mandibular premolars and the maxillary second premolar. These teeth are oriented perpendicular to the occlusal plane. In both the maxilla and mandible, the canines are formed at the farthest distance from the occlusal plane and ultimately are the longest teeth. In the maxilla, the lateral incisor, which is formed closer than the central incisor to the occlusal plane, is the shortest maxillary incisor. In the mandible, the situation is reversed.

Criteria for an Ideal Dentition

Indeed, the arrangement of the teeth depends on many factors, and an ideal occlusion is quite rare. In most cases, there are some minor shortcomings. A variety of malocclusions, from mild to severe, are found in every population (see chapters 10 to 15). The criteria for an ideal dentition are not limited to specific norms for tooth positions and occlusion, but also include requirements for the course of the gingival line. In the maxilla, the clinical crowns of the lateral incisors should be shorter than those of the central incisors, which in turn should be shorter than the canine crowns. The course of the gingival line corresponds with these differences in clinical crown heights, ie, it is lower at the lateral incisors than at the central incisors and again higher at the canines. In these aspects, symmetry is important.

In the mandibular anterior region, the height of the clinical crowns increases from central incisor to lateral incisor to canine. The course of the gingival line follows accordingly. The incisal edges of the four incisors are at the same level; the canine tips are slightly more superior. In the maxilla, the incisal edges of the central incisors and the canine tips are at the same level. The incisal edges of the lateral incisors are slightly more superior (see Figs 7-1 and 7-2).

As mentioned previously, with the exception of the third molars, the ultimate lengths of the teeth and the position of their apices are related to the locations where their forming parts were situated initially (see Fig 7-4).

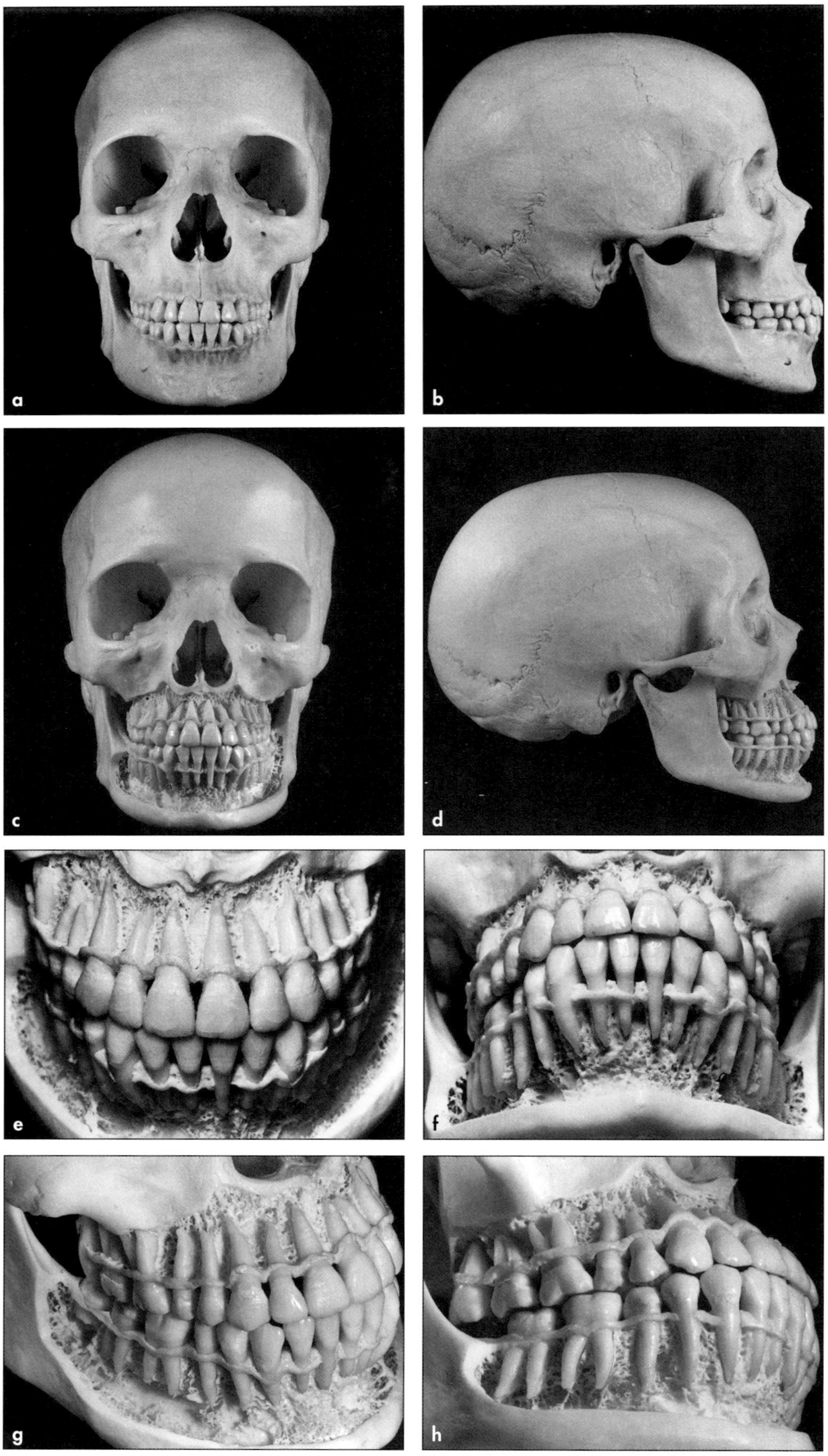

Fig 7-5 Skull of a young adult. *(a)* There is adequate occlusion and position of teeth, although the midlines of the dental arches do not coincide. The mandible is less broad than the neurocranium. The alveolar processes have grown more in a vertical direction than is needed to contain the teeth. *(b)* There is good occlusion in the posterior regions. The third molars are emerged, except the mandibular right one, which is missing. *(c)* The inclination of the anterior teeth is adjusted to the size of the apical areas and the dimensions of the crowns. *(d)* The roots of the maxillary canines are positioned more labially than those of the incisors and premolars. The maxillary and mandibular first and second molars are mesially angulated, as are the maxillary third molars. *(e)* The roots are completely formed and distributed evenly throughout the available space in the anterior region. The alveolar bone at the cervical margins follows the contours of the cemento-enamel junctions. *(f)* The mandible has a heavy cortex; the maxilla has a thin cortex. *(g)* The occlusal surfaces show some attrition; the approximal contacts are slightly worn. *(h)* In the posterior regions, the roots are also evenly distributed throughout the available space.

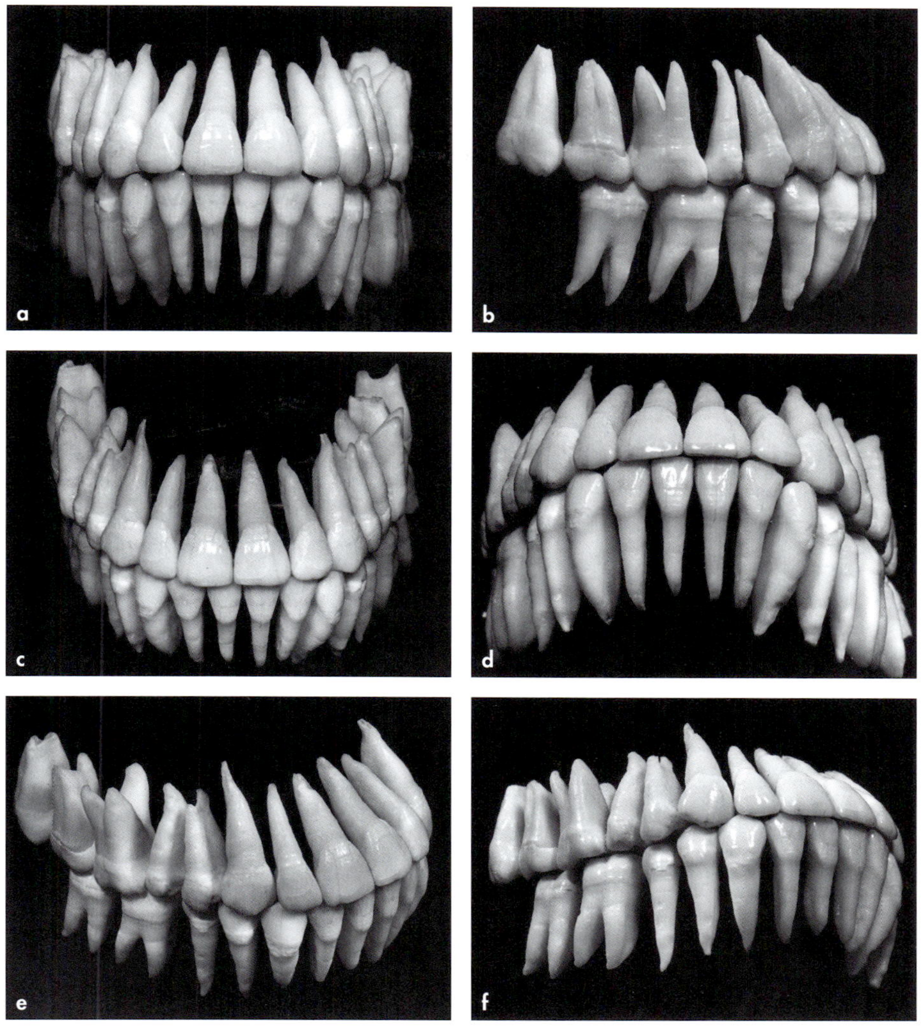

FIG 7-6 Teeth arranged separately as they were positioned in the jaws. *(a and b)* The apices have sharp pointed ends, and some have deviations at their tips. It is assumed that these deviations are caused by alterations in tooth position after emergence, without displacement of the forming parts. *(c and d)* Frontal views are shown from above and from below. *(e and f)* The same perspectives are shown from a three-quarter lateral view.

Comparison of Young Adult and Elderly Dentitions

In Fig 7-5, the skull of a young adult is shown, before and after removal of the vestibular alveolar bone, and in Fig 7-6, the teeth are shown separately, arranged as they were located in the jaws. The same has been done with a skull of an elderly individual (Figs 7-7 and 7-8). In both skulls, there is a noticeable difference in the thickness of the cortex between the two jaws.[5] The cortex is thin in the maxilla. Such fragility is not problematic there because the forces evoked by chewing and biting are transferred to and received by the more superiorly located bones. In that regard, the mandible functions as a solitary unit and has a strong construction. The thick cortex of the mandible serves not only to receive the chewing and biting forces but also is essential in reducing vulnerability to trauma. Furthermore, the mandible serves as the starting point of part of the swallowing musculature, in which the hyoid bone acts as an intermediary.[6,7]

The skull from the elderly individual shows signs of long-lasting, intensive functioning, such as attrition and mesial migration (see Figs 7-7 and 7-8). Today, such severe attrition is rare in the Western hemisphere, where food is processed and contains few grinding substances. However, the dentition does change with aging, particularly when used intensively.

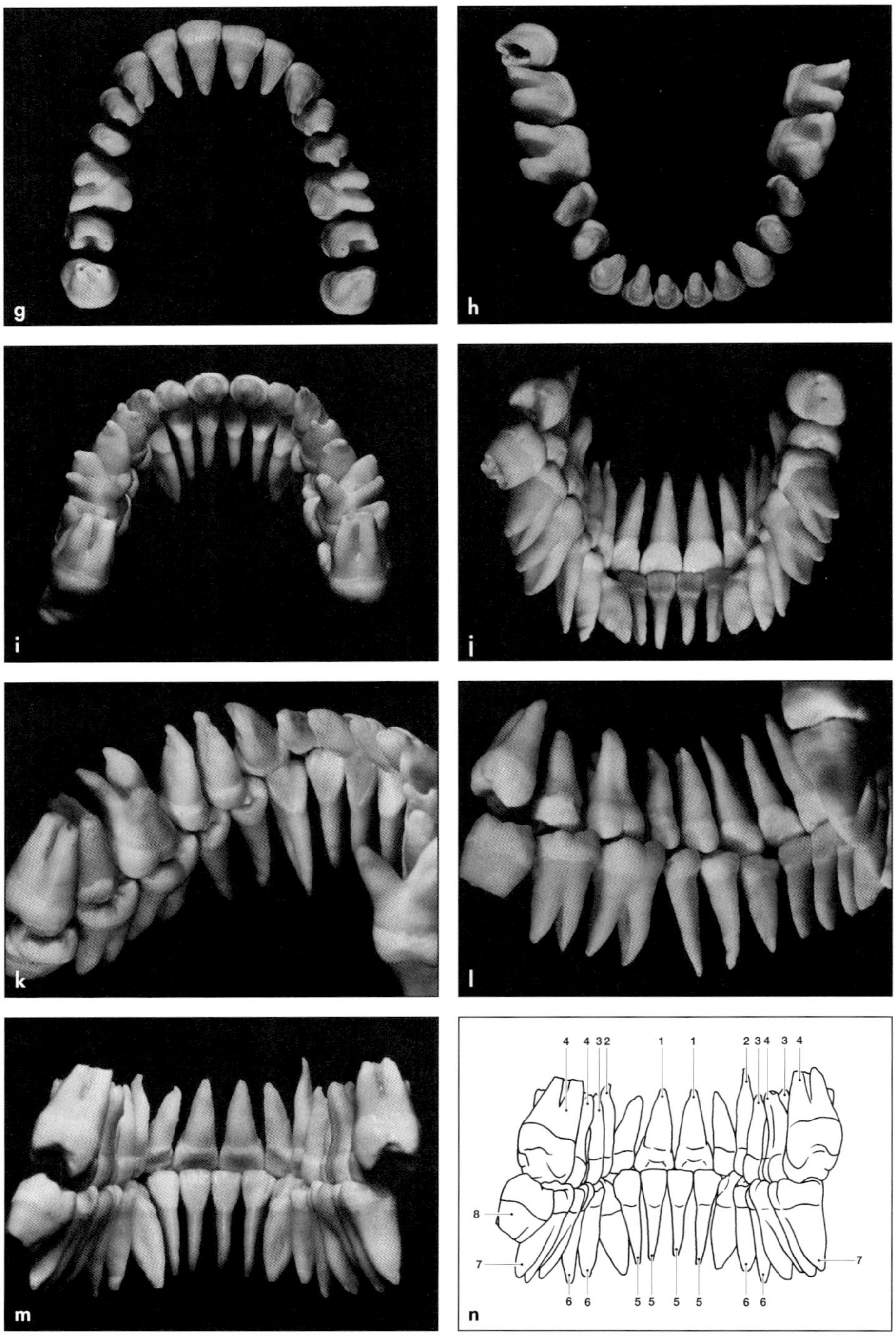

Fig 7-6 *(cont) (g and h)* The apical views show the symmetry in arrangement of the teeth. *(i to l)* The convergence of the maxillary roots and the divergence of the mandibular molar roots are clear. *(m)* Posterior view. *(n)* A drawing clarifies the elements shown in the posterior view. The roots of the maxillary central incisors (1) are positioned quite parallel. The roots of the maxillary canines (2) are longer than those of all other teeth. Of the maxillary premolars (3), the first is slightly mesially angulated, while the second is positioned perpendicular to the occlusal plane. The maxillary molars (4) are buccally inclined—the second more than the first and the third the most. Looking at the roots of the mandibular incisors (5), one can see that those of the central incisors are parallel to each other and shorter than those of the lateral incisors. The mandibular premolars (6) are perpendicular to the occlusal plane. The mandibular molars (7) are progressively more lingually inclined, from the first to the third molar. The roots of the mandibular left third molar (8) are partly formed; the right one is missing.

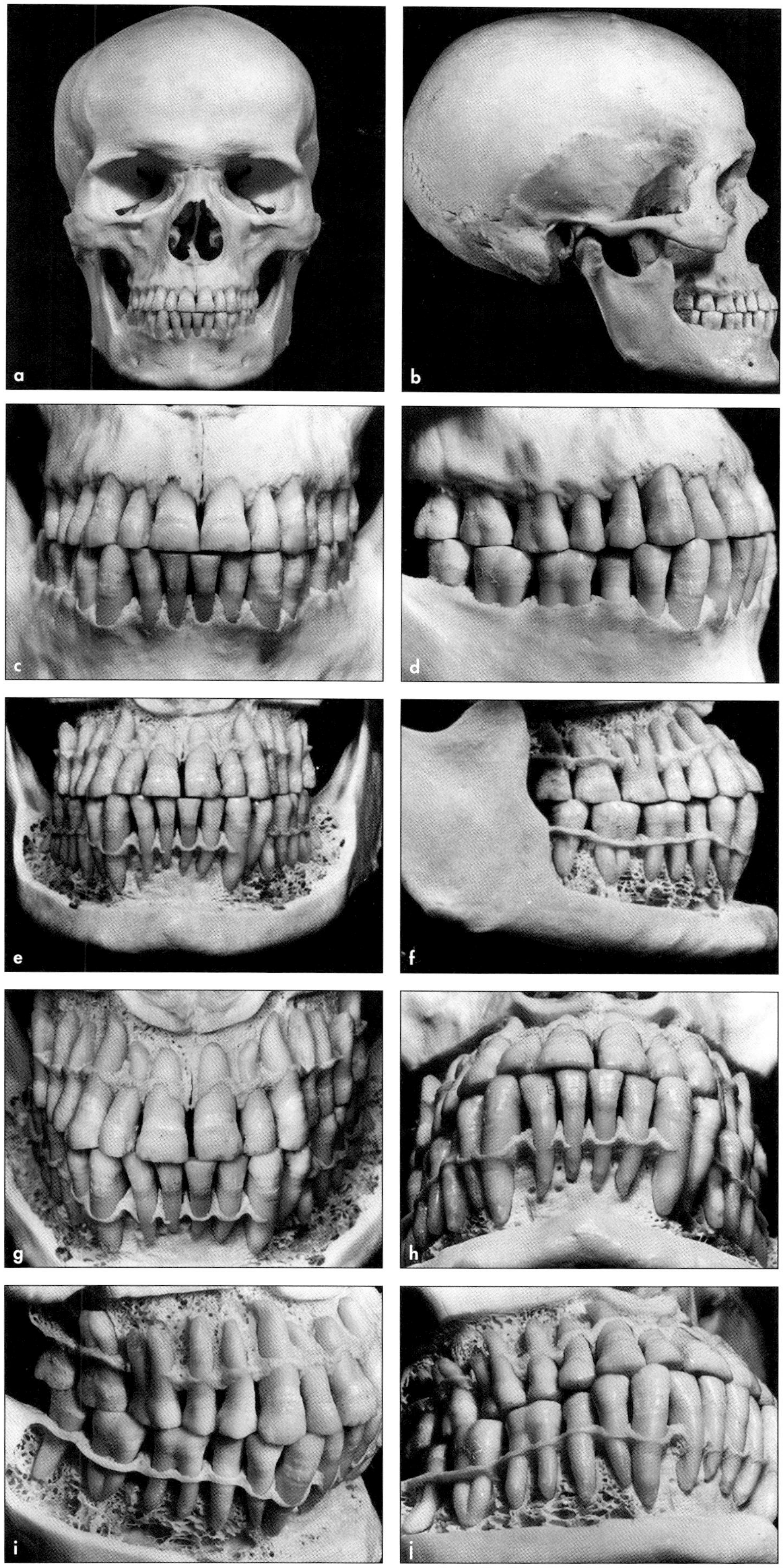

Fig 7-7 Skull of an aged individual. *(a)* This specimen shows marked attrition and breakdown of the cervical alveolar bone. The maxilla is narrow at the roots of the canines, leading to their marked buccal inclination. *(b)* The piriform aperture is posteriorly located; the maxillary incisors are excessively labially inclined. *(c)* The mandibular dentition is located mesially in relation to the maxillary one. Partly due to the attrition of the occlusal surfaces, resulting in loss of their contour, the mandibular posterior teeth are positioned more buccally in relation to the opposing maxillary teeth. *(d)* The pattern of wear, the course and shape of the occlusal plane, and the anterior open bite conform to the description by Murphy.[3,4] The mandibular and maxillary incisors do not overlap. Their incisal edges are in an end-to-end relationship. The cusps of the premolars and molars are worn. Marginal ridges have disappeared. The adjacent occlusal surfaces are at the same level. The interproximal contacts are flat and reach to the occlusal surface. The mesiodistal crown dimensions have decreased. *(e)* The incisor crowns are short. *(f)* The posterior teeth are in a slight mesioclusion. *(g)* The inclination of the maxillary incisors and canines is related to the posteriorly located and narrow piriform aperture. *(h)* Cervical alveolar bone has been lost in the mandibular anterior region. *(i)* The secondary cementum deposition at the apices of the maxillary canines and lateral incisors has not masked the deviations of the root tips. *(j)* The relative buccal position of mandibular molars is combined with occlusal contact without intercuspation.

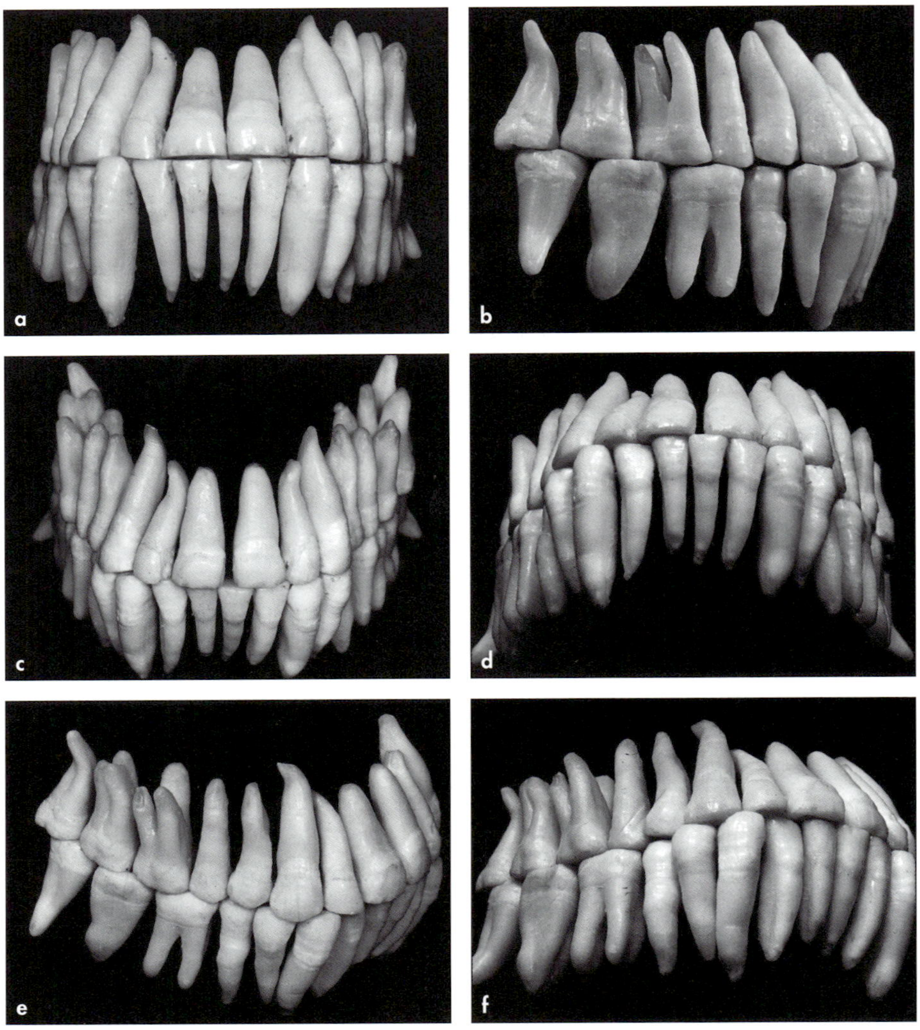

Fig 7-8 *(a)* Teeth arranged separately as they were positioned within the jaws. There is a small midline deviation. *(b)* The crowns of the premolars and molars are rather short. *(c and d)* Frontal views are shown from above and from below. *(e and f)* The same perspectives are shown from a three-quarter lateral view.

Tooth Wear

In normal use, teeth wear at the occlusal and approximal surfaces at a faster rate in the deciduous than the permanent dentition (Figs 7-9 and 7-10).

In the description of tooth wear, three terms are used. Natural wear of the dentition is called *attrition*. This covers the loss of tooth material by repeated physiologic and parafunctional occlusal contact between teeth. Attrition leads to reduction of cusp heights and to flat and smooth occlusal, mesial, and distal surfaces.

The term *abrasion* covers the reduction of tooth material through nonphysiologic mechanical wear. A common form of abrasion is the V-shaped notches found at the buccal aspect of crown-root junctions caused by incorrect and excessive manual tooth brushing. Wear caused by extensive chewing on certain substances, such as tobacco, and biting on pencils and pens is covered by the term *abrasion*, as is the loss of tooth material due to pipe smoking. In addition, abrasion may occur through excessive consumption of carbonated drinks and orange juice or frequent vomiting, which can partially or totally dissolve the enamel on the lingual side of the teeth, resulting in smooth, shiny surfaces.

The third term used in relation to tooth wear is *bruxism*, the diurnal or noctural parafunctional activity that includes clenching, bracing, gnashing, and grinding of teeth.[8] Bruxism is a common cause of excessive tooth wear in modern society.

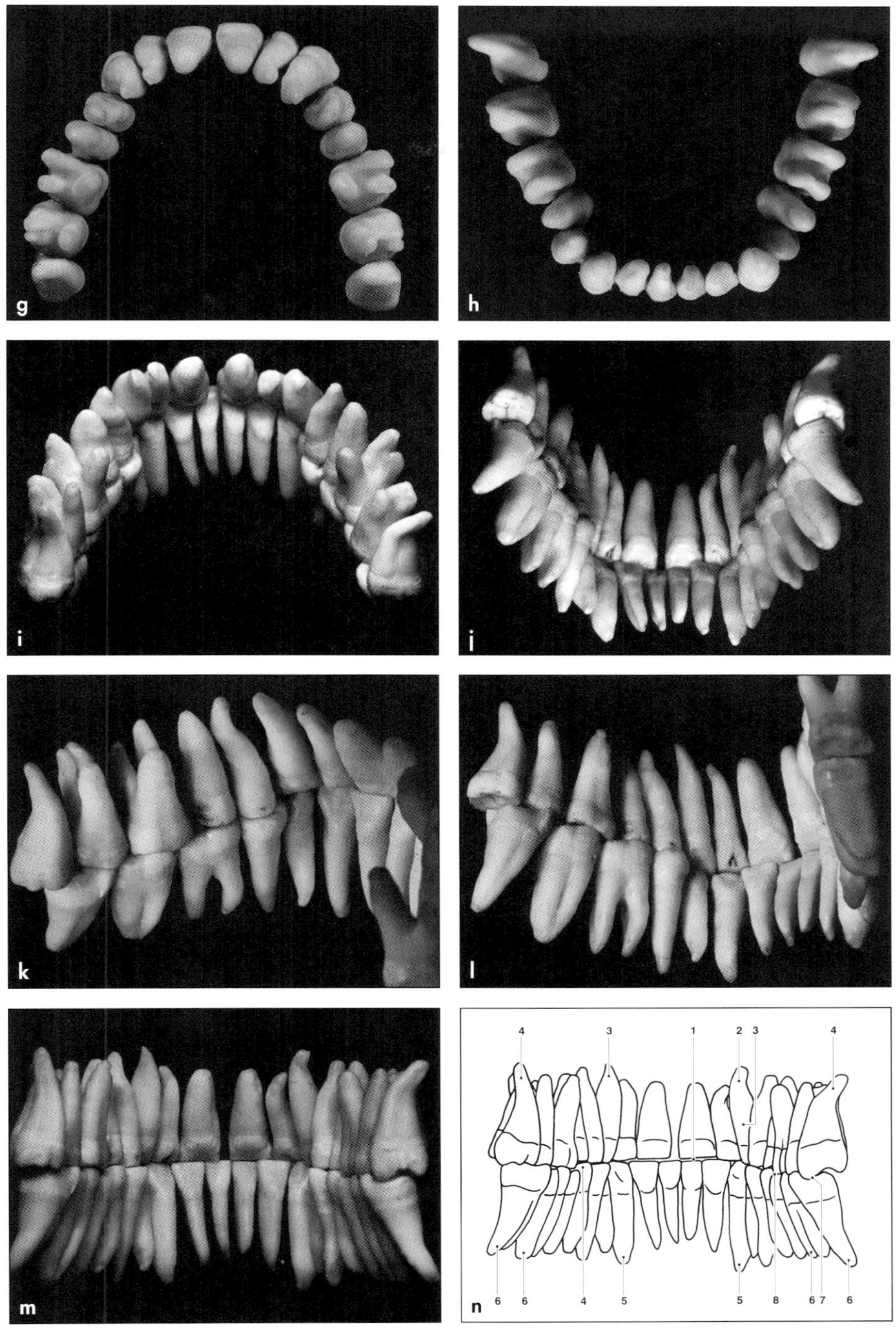

Fig 7-8 *(cont)* *(g and h)* The apical views show the convergence of the maxillary teeth and the divergence of the mandibular posterior teeth. *(i and j)* Secondary cementum deposition has resulted in large, round apices, more so in the maxilla than in the mandible. *(k and l)* In the transverse direction, the molars are just opposite each other. *(m)* Posterior view. *(n)* A drawing clarifies the elements shown in the posterior view. There is a small open bite and an end-to-end relationship of the incisors (1). The apex of the maxillary right canine (2) deviates, as do the apices of some other teeth. The roots of the maxillary canines (3) converge. The maxillary third molars (4) are buccally inclined and have deviating root tips. The mandibular canines (5) are nearly parallel to each other. The mandibular molars (6) are lingually inclined. The right third molars (7) have typical attrition patterns. The transverse occlusal relationship (8) differs from that of an adult without excessive tooth wear.

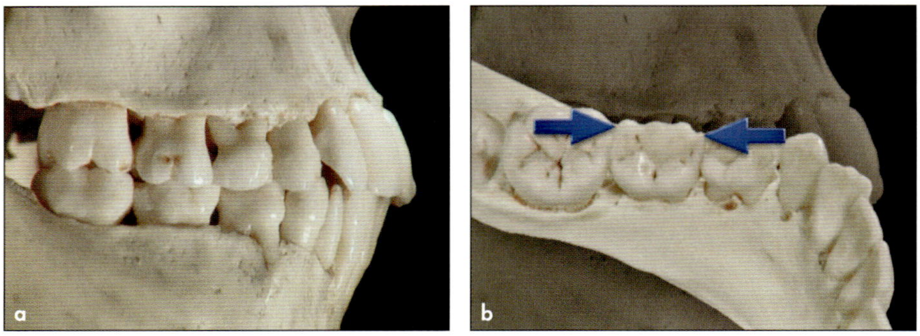

FIG 7-9 Jaws with dentition in the intertransitional stage. *(a and b)* Deciduous teeth are not as hard as permanent teeth and wear more quickly, including approximally.

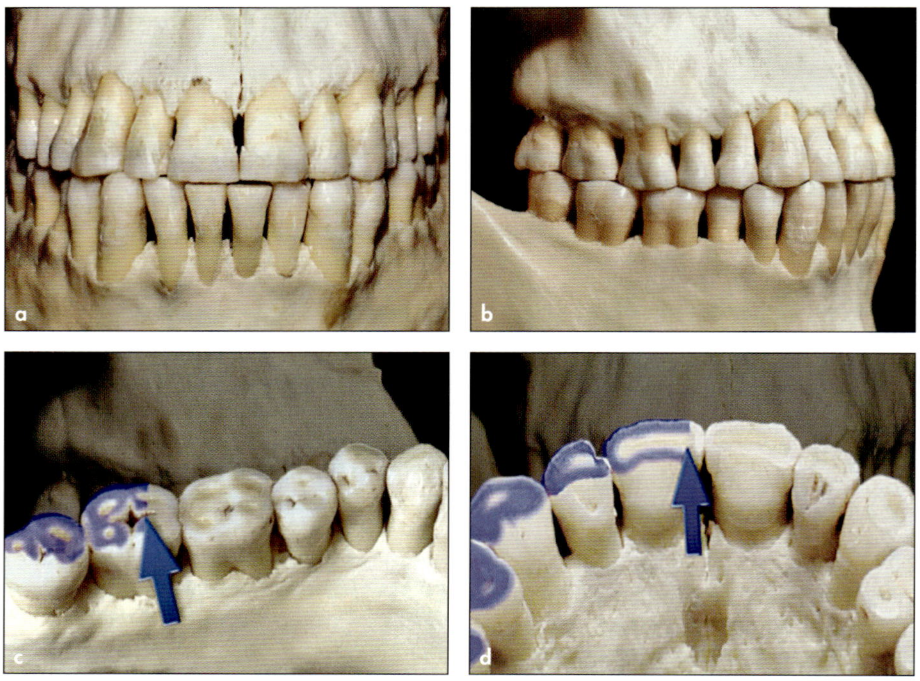

FIG 7-10 Jaws with an intensively used dentition. *(a to d)* In a dentition that has been heavily used for a long time, as was needed in primitive living conditions, much occlusal attrition took place, and the dental arches became shorter through approximal attrition. Contact among the teeth is maintained by mesial migration of the posterior teeth

Concluding Remarks

As indicated above, the ideal occlusion, as defined in dentistry, is not encountered often. An ideal occlusion is a concept created and accepted by dentists and orthodontists that serves as the goal for realizing an optimal esthetic and functional result with orthodontic and esthetic treatment. This goal can often be reached by adequate orthodontic and esthetic treatment in young patients. An ideal occlusion is experienced as youthful, healthy, and attractive. The size, form, and relation of the jaws and the configuration and structure of the face sometimes limit the realization of the ideal goal.

References

1. Stoller AE. The normal position of the maxillary first permanent molar. Am J Orthod 1954;40:259–271.
2. Dempster WT, Adams WJ, Duddles RA. Arrangement in the jaws of the roots of the teeth. J Am Dent Assoc 1963;67:779–797.
3. Murphy TR. A biometric study of the helicoidal occlusal plane of the worn Australian dentition. Arch Oral Biol 1964;9:255–267.
4. Murphy TR. The relationship between attritional facets and the occlusal plane in aboriginal Australians. Arch Oral Biol 1964;9:269–280.
5. Duterloo HS, Atkinson PJ, Woodhead C, Strong M. Bone density changes in the mandibular cortex of the rhesus monkey *Macaca mulatta*. Arch Oral Biol 1974;19:241–248.
6. Brodie AG. Anatomy and physiology of head and neck musculature. Am J Orthod 1950;36:831–844.
7. Houston WJB. Mandibular growth rotations—Their mechanisms and importance. Eur J Orthod 1988;10:369–373.
8. Daskalogiannakis J. Glossary of Orthodontic Terms. Chicago: Quintessence, 2000.

8

General Aspects of the Development of the Dentition

This chapter begins with an overview of the changes in the dental arches and occlusion from birth until adulthood. Subsequently, eruption, emergence, and migration of teeth are clarified. Some aspects presented in previous chapters are discussed again in a broader context.

Changes in Arch Width

The increase in size of the parts of the jaws that contain the teeth prior to emergence and thereafter takes place in sagittal, vertical, and transverse directions. Jaw growth does not occur at a constant rate and differs by region. From birth until 6 months of age, the jaws grow considerably, particularly in the median regions.[1,2] Subsequently, there is only a limited increase in the transverse direction. Consequently, the dental arch width, as measured between left and right deciduous canines and second molars, enlarges only slightly.[3–5] This limited increase in arch width applies not only to the deciduous dentition but also to later stages of development[6,7] (see chapter 17).

The changes in arch width are partially related to the transition. For example, the distance between the deciduous canines increases as part of the process of the replacement of incisors. With the replacement of the canines, the intercanine distance enlarges slightly as the permanent canines become positioned more buccally than their predecessors, more so in the maxilla than in the mandible.

The distances between corresponding left and right deciduous molars and premolars and also between permanent molars increase gradually. This slight increase occurs more in the anterior part of the dental arch than in the posterior part and also more in the maxilla than in the mandible. The increase in jaw height associated with facial growth contributes to the widening of the dental arch. With adequate transverse intercuspation, the mesialization of the mandibular dental arch that accompanies the anterior growth of the jaws leads to an increase in the width of the maxillary dental arch (called the rail mechanism; see video clip 22). The increase in intercanine width, associated with the transition of the incisors, can be considered as superimposed on the overall widening of the dental arches. The changes in the dental arches are illustrated in Figs 8-1 to 8-4.

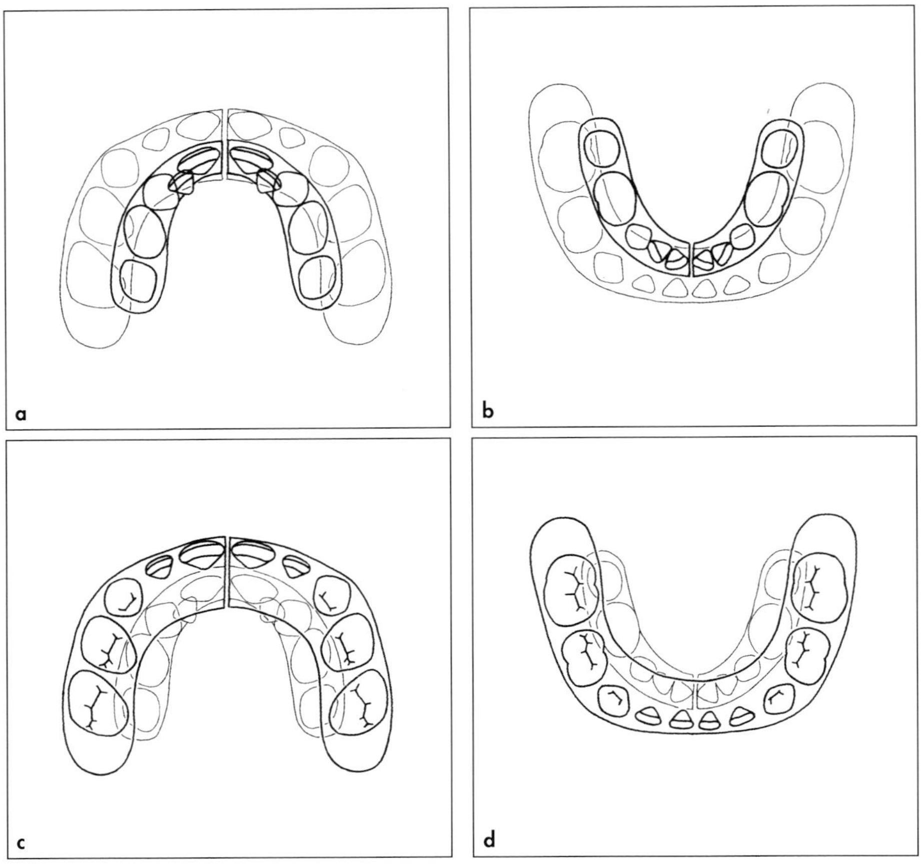

FIG 8-1 Changes in the parts of the jaws that contain the deciduous teeth, from birth (*dark lines, a* and *b*; *light lines, c* and *d*) to complete emergence (*light lines, a* and *b*; *dark lines, c* and *d*). In this period the jaws grow considerably, and space develops for the anterior teeth. The jaws grow posteriorly. The increase in width takes place mainly in the first 6 months after birth, prior to the ossification of the mandibular symphysis. The median suture in the maxilla remains open, allowing further growth in the median plane, a potential that no longer exists in the mandible.

Changes to the Occlusal Plane

The deciduous dentition has a flat occlusal plane. There is no or only a slight overbite. After the transition, the permanent incisors erupt more than their predecessors. This results in an overbite (ie, overlap in height of the maxillary incisors over the mandibular incisors). For an adult dentition, an overlap of one-third of the clinical crown height (ie, the part of the crown that is visible in the mouth) of the mandibular central incisors is considered normal. The overbite is somewhat greater in the intertransitional period, as is the associated overjet.[8–10] In the second transitional period and particularly during adolescence, the labial inclination of mandibular and maxillary incisors decreases, and the overbite and overjet (ie, distance between the anterior side of the incisal margin of the maxillary central incisor and the labial surface of the mandibular central incisor) reduce[11–16] (see video clip 7).

After the permanent incisors are fully erupted, the occlusal plane is no longer flat; the curve of Spee is formed. The curve of Spee is the imaginary curve that is formed by the buccal cusps and incisal edges of the teeth in one arch. In the mandible, this curve is slightly concave, with the incisors more occlusally positioned than the other teeth. In the maxilla, the curve is slightly convex. The curve of Spee arises with the emergence of the mandibular permanent incisors and first molars, increases with the emergence of the second molars, and stabilizes in the permanent dentition.[9]

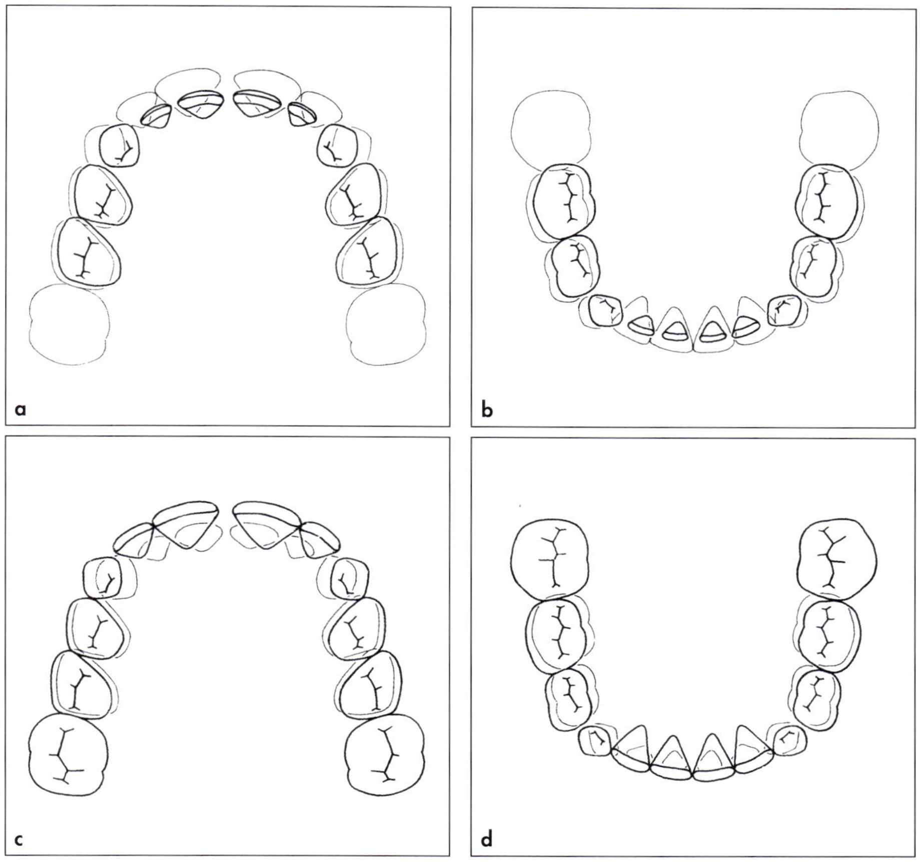

Fig 8-2 Changes in the dental arches from the complete deciduous dentition (*dark lines, a* and *b*; *light lines, c* and *d*) to the intertransitional stage (*light lines, a* and *b*; *dark lines, c* and *d*). The permanent incisors are more anteriorly located than their predecessors. The intercanine distances increase. There is also a small increase in the distances between the corresponding left and right deciduous molars. The first permanent molars are added to the dental arch. The diastemata in the posterior regions decrease, and the distal surfaces of the second deciduous molars move mesially.

Achieving Final Molar Occlusion

The posterior position of the mandible in relation to the maxilla, present in the newborn, disappears largely during the first year of life as the mandible grows more anteriorly than the maxilla. This difference in anterior growth continues in a small measure until adulthood. The mandibular teeth gradually attain a slightly more anterior position in relation to the maxillary ones, which contributes to an improvement of the first molar occlusion. With a flush terminal plane, the largest improvement takes place after the mandibular second deciduous molars are exfoliated and the first permanent molars migrate to the mesial. The third factor involved in attaining the final molar occlusion is the mesial closure of the diastemata in the mandibular dental arch, particularly the diastema between the deciduous canine and the first deciduous molar, in which the maxillary deciduous canine fits.[17]

Alterations over the Life Span

After the permanent dentition is complete, small changes in tooth position, occlusion, and arch width dimensions continue to take place. Initially existing diastemata in the mandibular and maxillary anterior regions reduce or disappear totally.[18] Well-aligned mandibular anterior teeth may become irregular; existing irregularities may worsen.[19–21] In general, the dentition shows slight alterations during the total life span. That is not surprising, as the potential to adapt to alterations in the skeleton and in functional conditions is always present. However, with increasing age, the changes become smaller.[22–24]

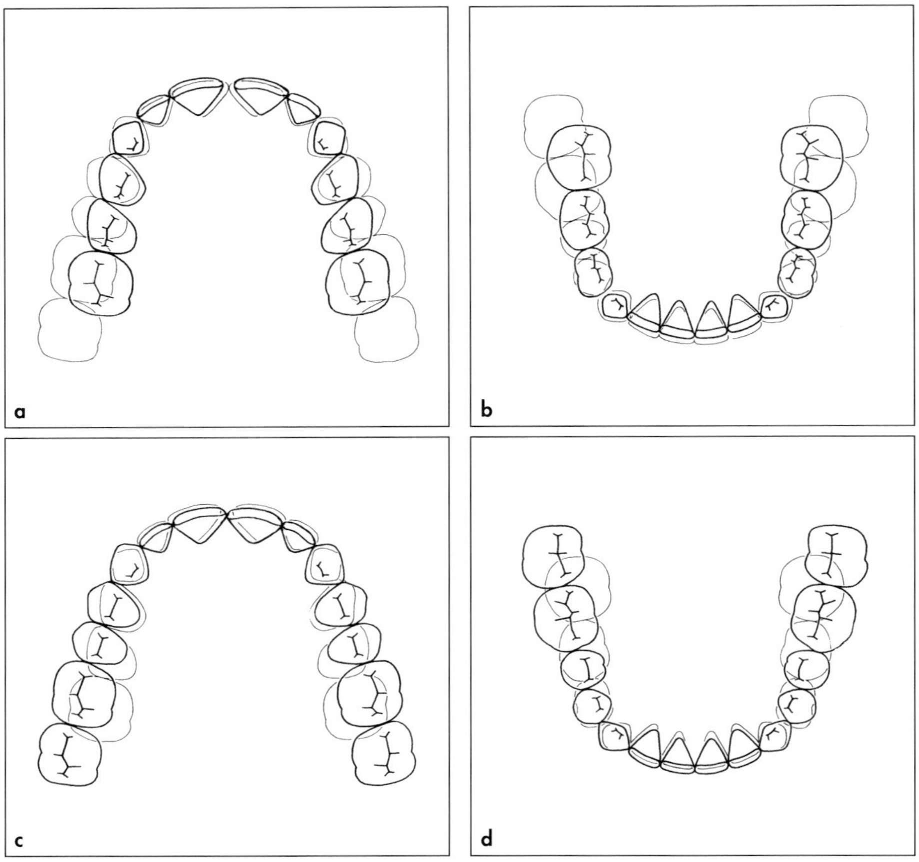

FIG 8-3 Changes in the dental arches from the intertransitional stage (*dark lines, a* and *b*; *light lines, c* and *d*) to the complete permanent dentition (except third molars) (*light lines, a* and *b*; *dark lines, c* and *d*). The permanent canines and premolars attain a more buccal position than their predecessors. The first permanent molars, particularly in the mandible, migrate mesially. This migration is facilitated by the differences in mesiodistal crown dimensions between the premolars and their predecessors and by the closure of diastemata. The second permanent molars are added to the dental arch.

Eruption and Emergence

At a certain developmental stage, forming teeth begin to move occlusally. In that process, a distinction is made between eruption and emergence. Eruption refers to the movement of teeth toward the occlusal plane, from their initial location in the jaws to their functional position in the mouth. The term *emergence* applies to the piercing of the surface and may be distinguished as the penetration of either the alveolar occlusal bone or the gingiva.

The eruption process is divided into two phases: prior to emergence and thereafter. The potential for eruption and displacement of teeth remains throughout an individual's lifetime, as long as the periodontium stays intact. In addition, fully occluding teeth continue to erupt when facial height increases,[25] and eruption occurs to compensate for the attrition of occlusal surfaces in adults.[26] However, when a bony connection develops between the root and the alveolar socket (ie, ankylosis), eruption can no longer occur.

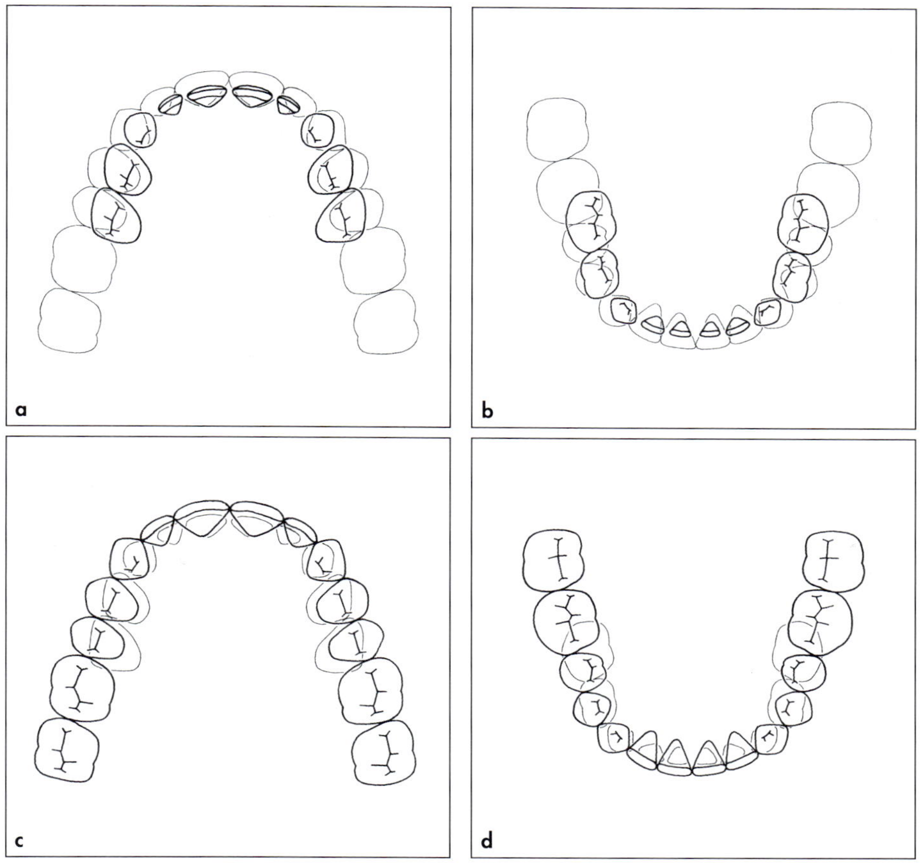

Fig 8-4 Changes from the deciduous dentition (*dark lines, a* and *b*; *light lines, c* and *d*) to the complete permanent dentition (except third molars) (*light lines, a* and *b*; *dark lines, c* and *d*). The anterior parts of the dental arches show only a small increase in size. The widening of the posterior regions is greater in the maxilla than in the mandible. This difference is related to the mesial advancement of the mandibular arch in relation to the maxillary arch (ie, the rail mechanism). The extension with the first and second permanent molars results in lengthening of the dental arches to the posterior.

A tooth germ develops inside a follicle. The increase in length of a developing tooth occurs mainly by dentin deposition in an apical direction. The contribution of enamel deposition in an occlusal direction is limited. The root end, where growth mainly occurs, migrates initially in an apical direction, while the coronal part moves occlusally. Because both displacements occur at about the same speed, the tooth germ itself remains in the same place. At that point, bone resorption occurs at the apical as well as at the occlusal side. When active eruption starts, the tooth bud starts to move occlusally. The rate of apical lengthening of the root stays more or less the same during the whole period of its formation and is slower than the rate at which the tooth bud moves occlusally. Consequently, bone is deposited at the apical side to fill up the otherwise growing open space. Indeed, the start of active eruption coincides with the reversal from bone resorption to bone apposition at the apical side—the first reversal point. When the tooth has reached its functional position, active eruption stops. Because the root is not completed yet, the end of the forming root again moves apically, with corresponding bone resorption—the second reversal point. As the root formation is concluded and facial growth is still going on, the associated passive eruption is accompanied by bone apposition near the apex—the third reversal point.

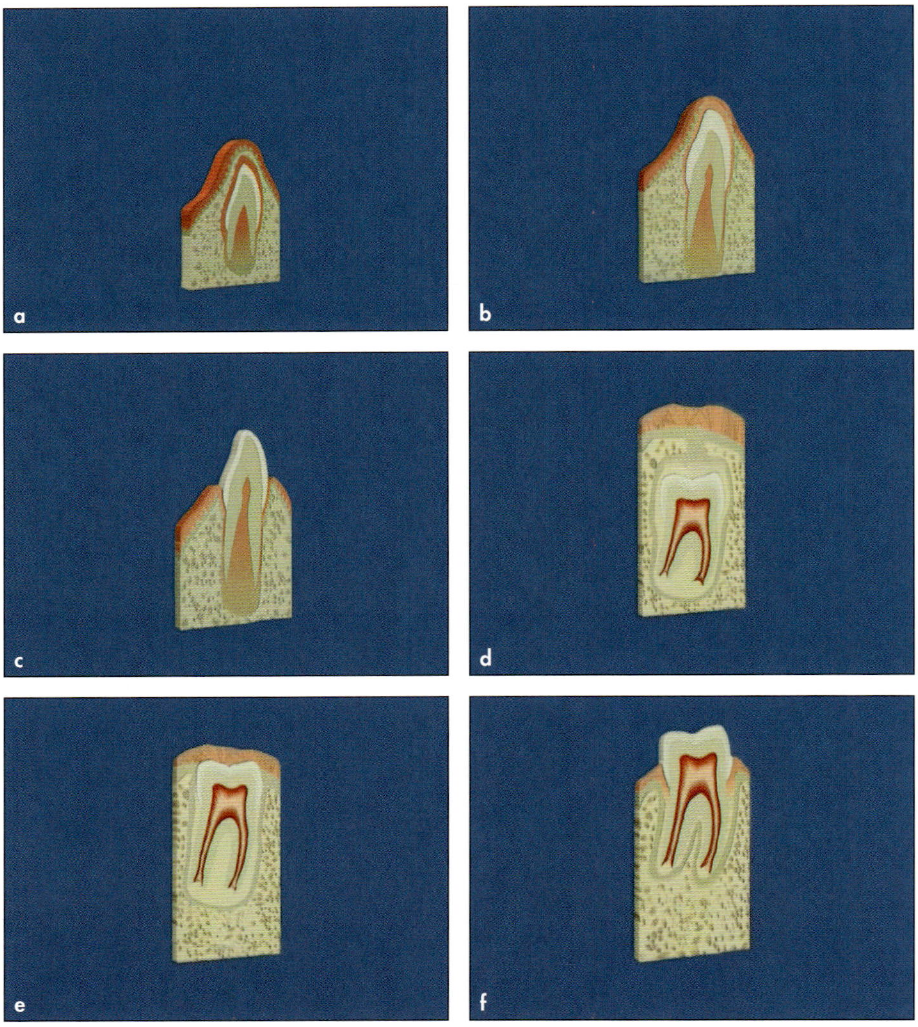

FIG 8-5 Eruption and emergence of a mandibular deciduous incisor *(a to c)* and a permanent molar *(d to f)*. *(a)* During the emergence of a deciduous incisor, the epithelium that covers the tooth bud contacts the oral epithelium. *(b)* The two epithelium layers fuse. *(c)* Together they form the attached gingiva and sulcus. The mesenchyme stays intact the entire time. The same process applies to the emergence of deciduous and permanent molars: *(d)* A permanent molar before emergence. *(e)* The situation after penetration of the occlusal alveolar bone. *(f)* After penetration of the gingiva.

Permanent teeth erupt in the direction in which they are formed.[27] After emergence they become affected by functional factors such as the pressure of the lips, cheeks, and tongue and contact with antagonists, which alter the direction of their eruption. The eruption direction of deciduous molars, premolars, and permanent molars is guided by the cone-funnel mechanism when occlusal contact is reached.

Unlike premolars and molars, incisors and canines are not fixed three-dimensionally by the occlusion. Their eruption is slowed down by the contact established between the antagonists and through the soft tissues on which they rest. In that way, the lower lip contributes to the slowing down and stopping of the eruption of maxillary incisors.

The eruption direction after emergence also depends on the space available in the dental arch. With a shortage of space, an erupting incisor or canine will deviate to the lingual or labial. On the other hand, the situation can improve spontaneously if extra space is created. Extraction of a deciduous canine can provide space for a lateral incisor that otherwise could not emerge within the dental arch. Prior to emergence, it may be evident that the shortage of space is so severe that the permanent canine and two premolars cannot be adequately arranged next to each other in the dental arch. In such an extreme case of space shortage, if the first premolar is removed before or after its emergence, the adjacent teeth can attain a better position prior to emergence. The serial extraction and simultaneous extraction procedures are based on this phenomenon.[28–30]

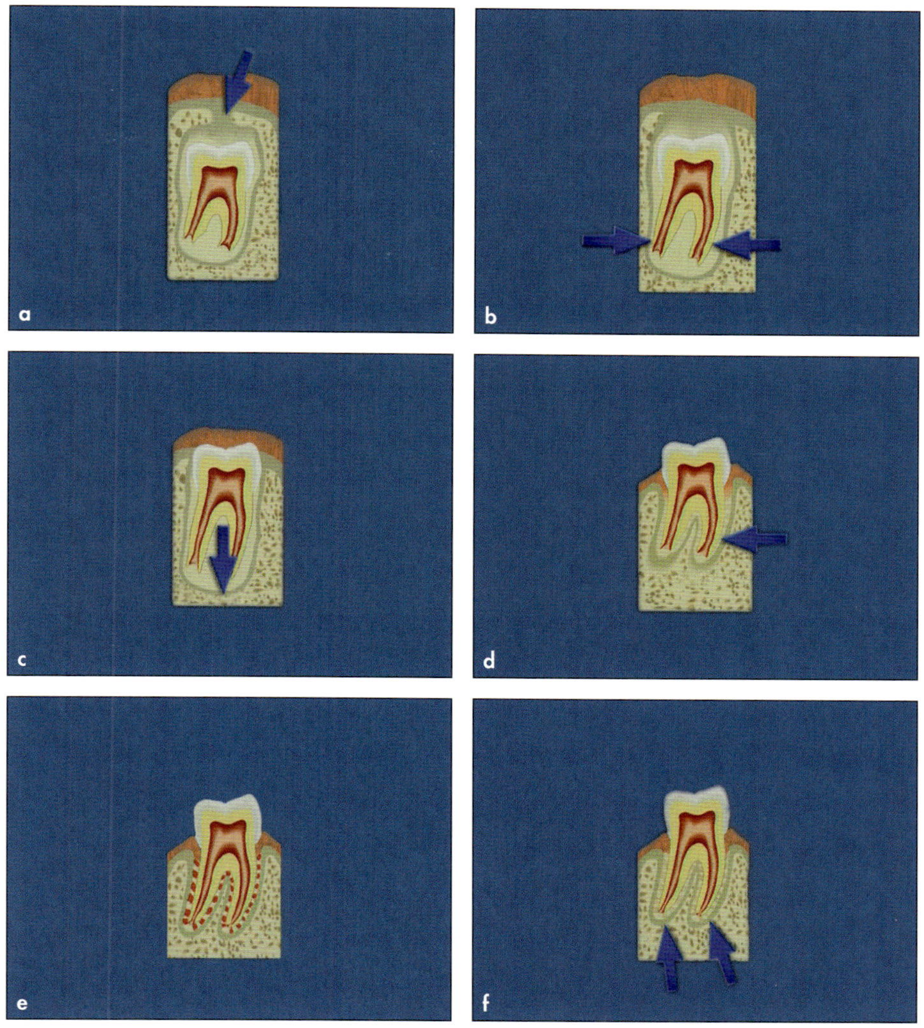

FIG 8-6 Differences in the pre- and postemergence eruption. Prior to emergence, a tooth bud is situated within a follicle. *(a)* Preceding the eruption, bone resorption occurs at the occlusal side. *(b)* In the meantime, the roots elongate. *(c)* Bone deposition takes place below the apices. *(d)* Before emergence, there are no periodontal fibers. Following emergence, they will be formed from the follicle. *(e)* Reconstruction of the fibers of the periodontal ligament and the involved activities are probably the most important factors in the postemergence eruption. *(f)* It is unlikely that apical bone apposition plays a role in the eruption process. Bone resorption will occur apically when the tooth has reached its functional position and while root formation continues.

The eruption process of deciduous teeth differs from that of permanent teeth that replace deciduous teeth. In the newborn, the forming deciduous teeth are only partially covered occlusally by bone. During emergence they become exposed. The same happens in permanent molars, where the overlying occlusal bone has to be resorbed. In this way, permanent molars are more similar to deciduous teeth than to permanent teeth that replace deciduous teeth (Fig 8-5).

The eruption of premolars is preceded by resorption of the roots of corresponding deciduous molars and the bone between and around their roots. Because premolars have smaller crowns than their predecessors, little bone has to be resorbed for their emergence. However, permanent incisors and canines have larger crowns than their predecessors and emerge lingual to them. In comparison with the eruption of premolars, more bone has to be resorbed, which makes the transition process last longer. Hence, there is an interval of several weeks between the loss of deciduous incisors and canines and the emergence of their successors.

The active eruption of permanent teeth starts shortly after the formation of the roots has begun. It is 2 to 3 years before a tooth penetrates the occlusal surface of the alveolar process. At that stage, about two-thirds of the root is formed. About 6 months later, an opening is created in the gingiva, and the tooth emerges without the occurrence of bleeding because the epithelium that covers the tooth bud occlusally fuses with the oral epithelium without disturbing the integrity of the mesenchyme. At that stage, about three-quarters of the root is formed.[31–33]

After emergence, the eruption initially proceeds quickly. An erupting maxillary central permanent incisor will have 50% of its crown exposed after 4 months and 80% after 8 months.[34–36] The eruption process prior to emergence differs from that which occurs after (Fig 8-6), as is explained in more detail later in this chapter.

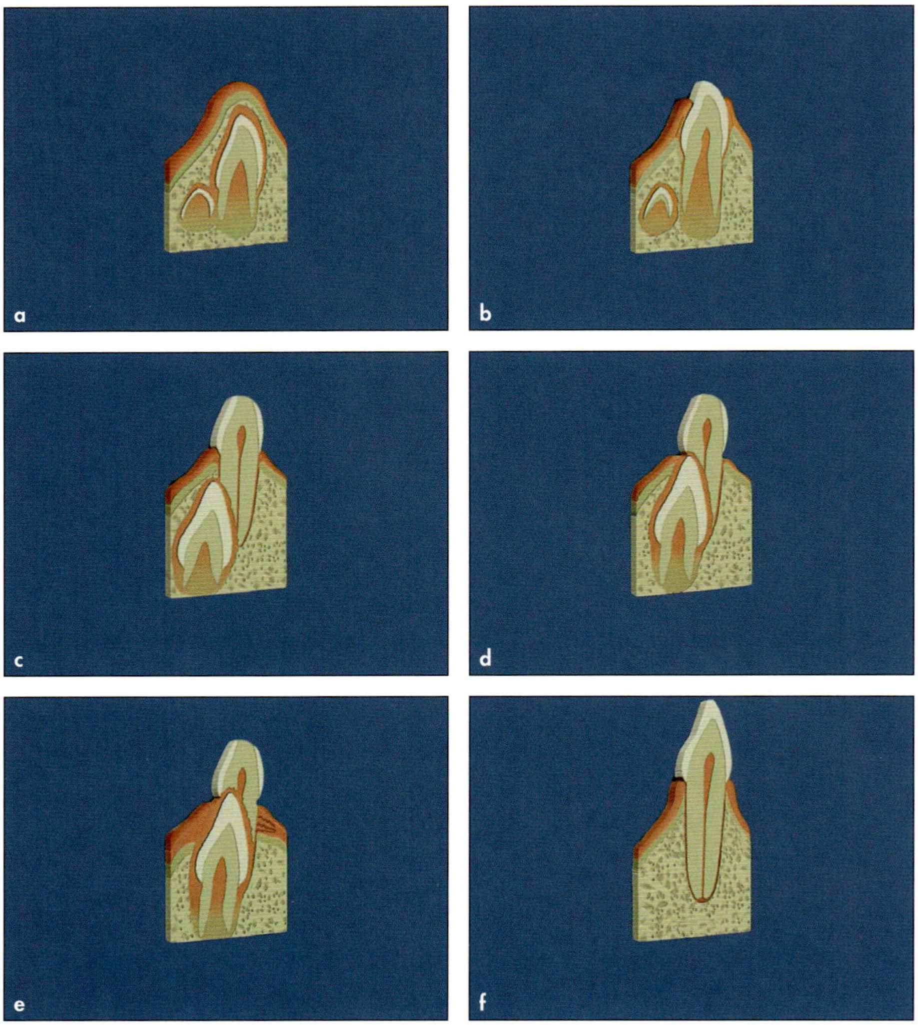

Fig 8-7 Eruption, emergence, and replacement of incisors. *(a)* The formation of a permanent incisor starts before its predecessor begins to erupt. *(b)* The formation of a deciduous and permanent tooth is accompanied by bone resorption. *(c)* When a permanent incisor erupts, bone as well as the root of its predecessor are resorbed. *(d and e)* Gradually, the permanent incisor erupts farther, and its predecessor resorbs more. *(f)* The emerging and erupting incisor builds up its own alveolar process.

The eruption of teeth that replace deciduous teeth is accompanied by resorption of the cementum and dentin of their predecessors and of the surrounding alveolar bone[37] (Fig 8-7). Enamel is not resorbed. A deciduous crown, together with a small remaining part of the root, exfoliates after a stage of high mobility. This happens because in the last phase there is no longer a fibrous connection between the remaining part of the root and the alveolar bone. Indeed, the alveolar bone that surrounded the deciduous tooth cervically has been resorbed. The root is then only fixed by fibers that run from the remaining part of the root into the gingiva.[38,39] If that connection is very small and not completely circumferential, the crown can be moved by the tongue or a digit over a large distance. A loose tooth ready to be shed is not a pleasure for the average child. In addition, deciduous molars extrude above the occlusal plane and therefore will make contact first when the child occludes.

Deciduous incisors are smaller than their successors. The defect in the gingiva caused by the loss of the deciduous crown is repaired, and a new opening is created for the emergence of the successor (Fig 8-8).

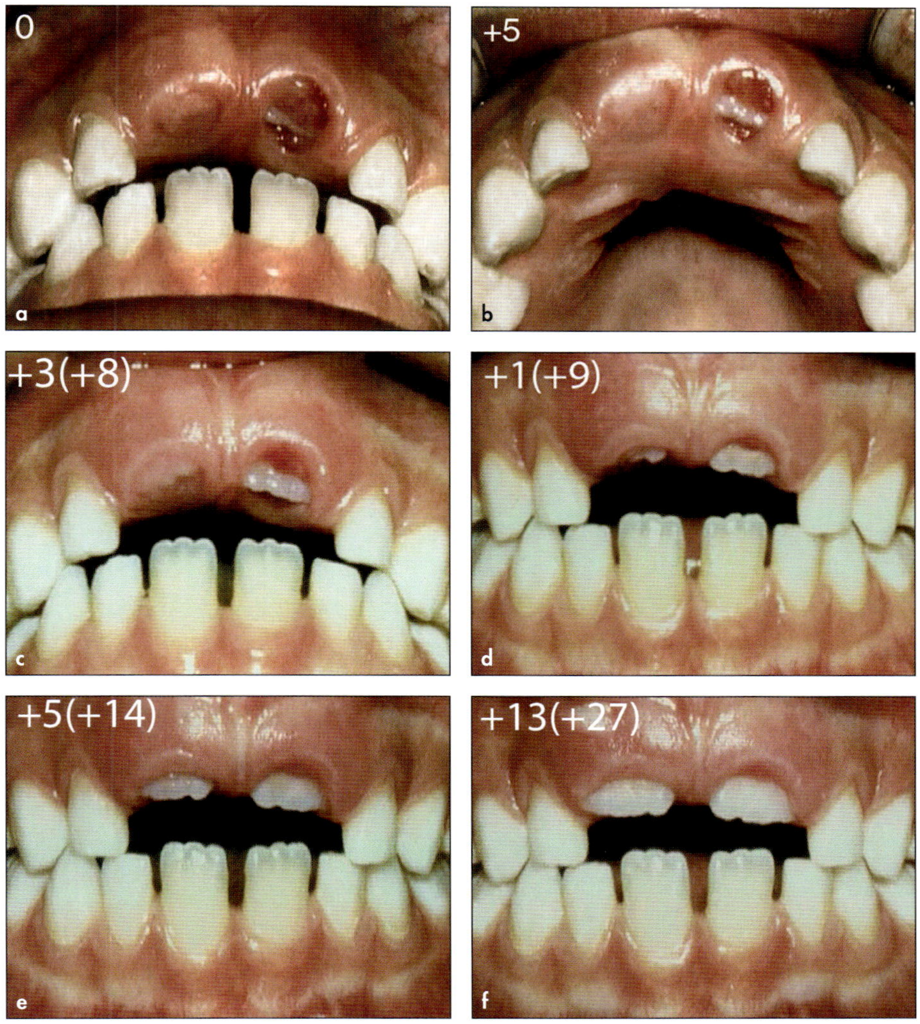

FIG 8-8 Emerging and erupting maxillary central permanent incisors. The first number in the images indicates the number of days that has passed since the preceding photograph; the number in parentheses is the number of days that has passed since the first photograph. The series covers a total of 27 days. *(a and b)* After the deciduous tooth has been shed, the gingiva closes over the remaining opening, as shown here on the right side. On the left side, the emerging crown causes reconstruction of the gingiva, resulting in an opening. *(c)* This opening becomes larger, freeing the complete incisal edge. On the right side, the incisal edge appears through the thinning gingiva. *(d to f)* The continued eruption is accompanied by retraction of the gingiva. (Courtesy of Dr H. S. Duterloo.)

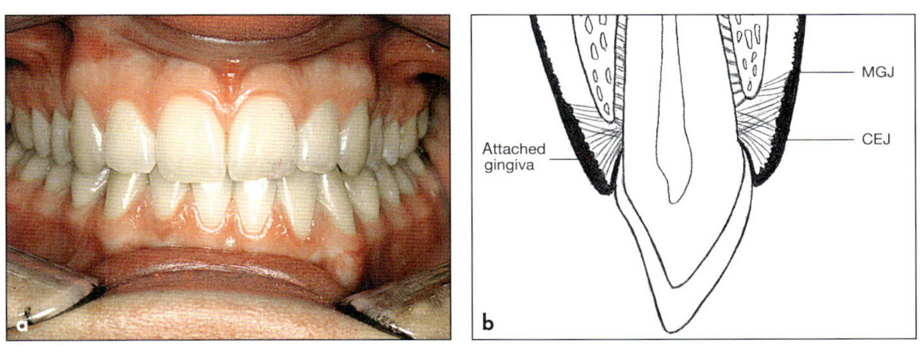

FIG 8-9 Attached gingiva. *(a)* The gingiva is rigidly connected with the alveolar bone over a zone of 2 to 4 mm. *(b)* The mucogingival junction (MGJ) is the point at which the attached gingiva converts to the movable oral mucosa. CEJ, cementoenamel junction.

Every tooth has at its labial/buccal and lingual aspect a zone where the gingiva and the alveolar bone are rigidly connected: the attached gingiva (Fig 8-9). It runs at the buccal side from the bottom of the sulcus to the mucogingival junction, which is where it converts to the oral mucosa of the vestibule, which is movable because it is not connected to the bone. The zone of attached gingiva at the labial/buccal aspect varies in height between 2 and 4 mm and is broadest at the incisors and narrowest at the premolars. Its height changes only slightly with aging. When a tooth erupts, the attached gingiva moves with it. The attached gingiva is less red than the oral mucosa.[40–42] The rigid connection prevents the gingiva from detaching from the teeth during chewing and biting and reduces the risk of lesions. A comparable situation exists at the lingual side of the mandible, where the gingiva is rigidly connected to the bone up to the point that it converts to the movable floor of the mouth. The palatal mucosa is also rigidly connected with the underlying bone.

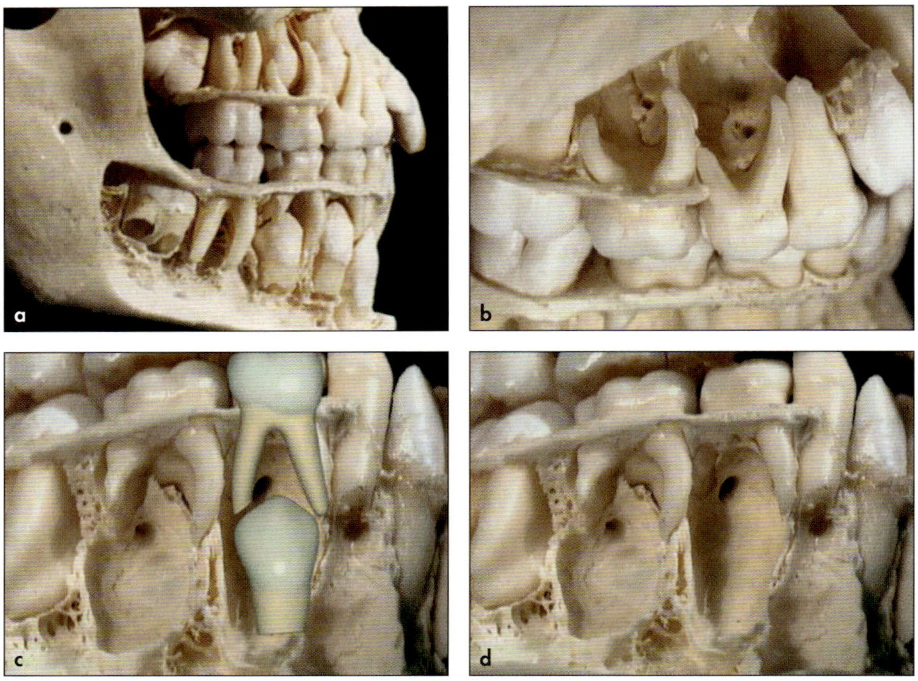

FIG 8-10 Skull section with exposed dentition. *(a)* The premolars are situated apical to and between the roots of their predecessors, which are partially resorbed. *(b and d)* The eruption of premolars is accompanied by resorption of the cementum and dentin of their predecessors as well as the surrounding alveolar bone. *(c)* Superimposed digital representation of the relationship between a premolar and deciduous molar at the beginning of resorption and eruption. *(b and d)* Note the gubernacular canal openings in the alveolar sockets.

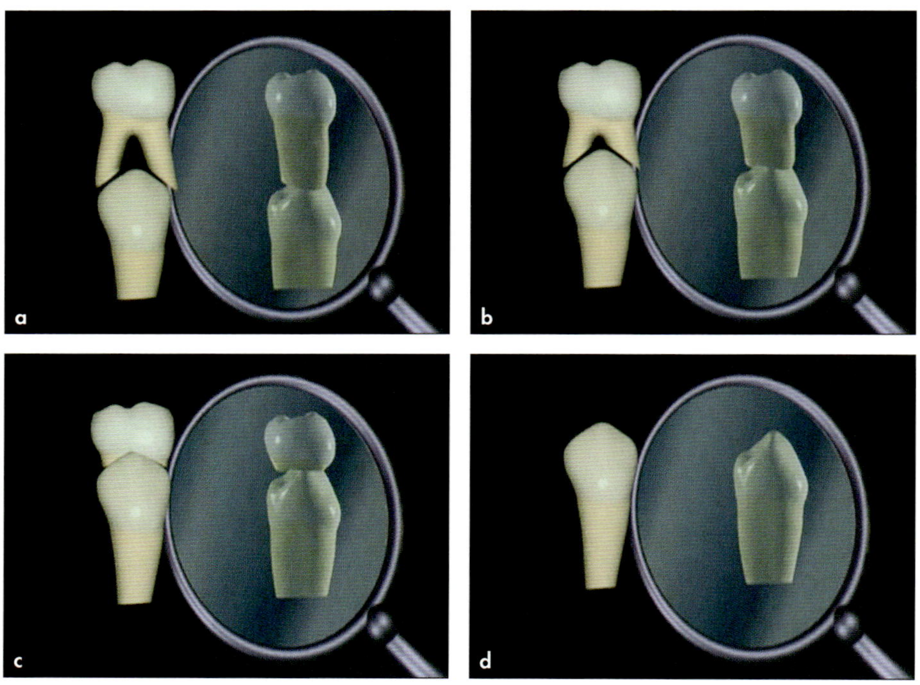

FIG 8-11 Digital representation of the replacement of a mandibular first deciduous molar. *(a to c)* The resorption of the roots of the deciduous molar starts prior to the eruption of the premolar and continues until its crown is shed. *(d)* Three-quarters of the length of the root is formed as the premolar emerges in the mouth. See video clip 23.

As stated before, deciduous molars, particularly the mandibular second molar, generally have larger crowns than their successors. Just prior to emergence, premolars are very close to the crowns of the deciduous molars (Fig 8-10). They are sometimes visible in the mouth with the crown of their predecessor looking like a hat on their head (Fig 8-11). After the loss of the deciduous crown, the opening in the gingiva is not closed. That happens only after untimely extraction.

Eruption after emergence is not a constant process; it has a day/night rhythm. It progresses the most quickly during the evening hours when the concentration of growth hormone in the blood is at its highest level. The forces of eruption are small—not more than 5 Ncm (5 g). (Note that 5 Ncm is also the magnitude of the continuous force that displaces a free-standing tooth after 6 to 8 weeks.[43]) Eruption stops when a continuous force of 5 Ncm is applied at the crown tip for 50% or more of the time. If a continuous 5-Ncm force is applied one-quarter of the time, the eruption speed is reduced. If such a force is applied 10% of the time, there is no effect. Forces applied for a short time, even if they are very heavy, have no effect on eruption[44,45] (Fig 8-12).

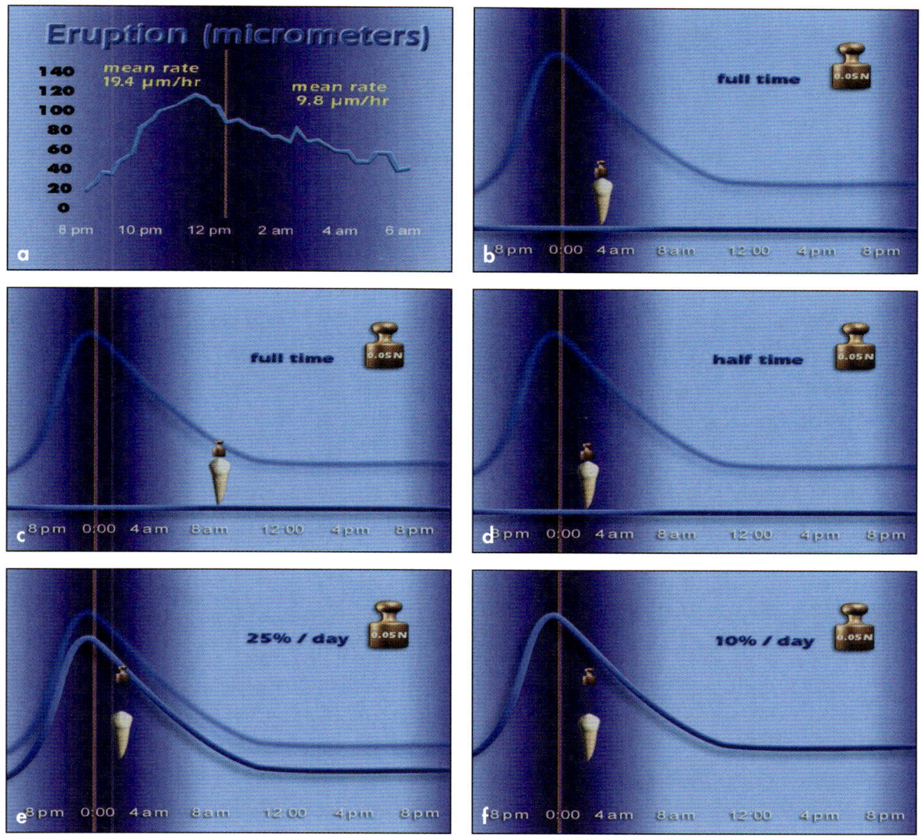

Fig 8-12 Eruption rate and effect of restricting forces. *(a)* The rate at which teeth emerge in the 4 hours before midnight is about twice as high as in the 6 hours thereafter. The average rates measured for these periods are, respectively, 19.4 and 9.8 μm per hour. From these data, it can be concluded that an active erupting premolar moves about 0.15 mm in the occlusal direction per day. During the day, the eruption rate is low. During meals and a short period thereafter, teeth do not erupt.[44] *(b and c)* If a small force (eg, 5 Ncm) is applied continuously to an erupting tooth, the eruption stops. *(d)* Eruption also ceases when that force is applied half the time. *(e)* A force applied 25% of the time has a limited effect on the eruption speed. *(f)* If the time of force application is limited to 10%, the eruption is not affected. See video clip 24. (Printed from Van der Linden and Proffit[46] with permission.)

Phases of eruption

The eruption process can be divided into a pre-emergence and a postemergence phase.[46] The postemergence phase can be differentiated further into a period of rapid eruption (prefunctional spurt) and a subsequent period of slow eruption. The latter begins when the functional position (occlusion) is reached and is related to the increase in jaw height, which mainly takes place during the adolescence growth spurt.[47] With much vertical jaw growth, the forming parts of not-yet-completed teeth do not move in an apical direction; with little growth they do. In addition, teeth can move in a sagittal direction as a consequence of jaw growth. Furthermore, as already mentioned, slow eruption compensates for the loss in height caused by occlusal attrition.[26]

In the pre-emergence eruption phase, different mechanisms are involved than in the postemergence eruption phase.[48] Several theories have been presented to explain the pre-emergence eruption, such as root lengthening, hydrostatic pressure of blood and tissue fluids, cell proliferation, and apposition of bone at the apex. However, animal experiments have demonstrated that none of these assumptions are true. Teeth in which the apical part of the root has been removed still erupt.[49] If, with preservation of the follicle, the tooth bud is replaced by an acrylic substitute, the latter erupts also, and the eruption path is cleared by resorption of bone.[50] Local increase or decrease of blood pressure has no effect.[51] After fixation of the tooth bud to the surrounding bone with a metal ligature, which stops the eruption, bone still resorbs occlusally, and an eruption path is cleared.[52,53]

It becomes increasingly clear that activities in and at the occlusal aspect of the follicle and in the epithelium that covers the crown of the developing tooth lead to the local expression of growth factors and cytokines, which trigger the differentiation, migration, and activation of macrophages and osteoclasts. This results in degradation of extracellular matrix as well as resorption of bone and roots of predecessors. Also for the apical side of the tooth bud, such local control systems resulting in bone deposition have been described.[54,55] However, none of this answers the question as to which mechanism actually causes the displacement of a tooth to the occlusal prior to emergence.

There is more clarity regarding postemergence eruption. During and after emergence, the periodontal ligament develops from the follicular tissue. The mechanism that subsequently causes further eruption is probably generated by metabolic activity in the periodontal ligament. Its collagen fibers become oriented to resist the forces of occlusion. With the maturation of the collagen fibers, cross-links are formed, and the fibers become shorter. This, together with the turnover of the fibers, might explain the mechanism of postemergence eruption. The pulling force, generated by the contraction of fibroblasts, probably plays a role as well. The mechanism is assumed to be activated by the increase in the number of fibers and their changing orientation, as the tooth becomes exposed to oral forces.[56] The explanations given above for the mechanism of postemergence eruption are also based mainly on animal experiments.

Disturbed eruption

The rate of eruption differs not only during various phases of the process. There is also a difference in the rate of eruption among individual teeth.[57] Eruption can be disturbed or even stopped by several factors. A maxillary first permanent molar can erupt too far to the mesial, leading to the resorption of the distal root of the adjacent second deciduous molar. The eruption of the permanent molar is stopped by the distal part of the crown of the deciduous molar in which it is caught. This phenomenon is called ectopic eruption, for which a genetic component has been demonstrated. It occurs more often when the maxillary first permanent molar has a large crown.[58] Ectopic eruption is shown to occur in Sweden in 4.3% of children and five times as often in children with a cleft lip and/or palate.[59,60] When the second deciduous molar is shed after the remaining roots have been resorbed, the first permanent molar continues to erupt.

Ankylosis has already been mentioned as a cause of disturbed eruption. It occurs more often with deciduous than permanent teeth, most frequently with mandibular second deciduous molars. The cause is probably a disturbance in the continuous remodeling of the periodontal ligament.[60,61] Also supernumerary teeth, cysts, and tumors can block the eruption of teeth that are not yet emerged.[62] Trauma to a maxillary central deciduous incisor can lead to marked displacement of its successor. After canting, the tooth continues its formation at the original location. The result is a bend in the root (ie, dilaceration). The angle of the deformation depends on the degree of displacement. With a severe bend, eruption stops, and the tooth becomes impacted. An abnormal location of tooth formation can also cause impaction. Maxillary permanent canines are impacted in 1.5% to 2% of the Western population.[63,64] Teeth can also be impacted because of a lack of space to erupt. This often happens with mandibular third molars.

Some syndromes, such as cleidocranial dysostosis are associated with multiple impaction. A genetic disturbance of bone resorption has been suggested as a cause.[65] There is a rare condition in which the eruption of premolars and permanent molars stops without the occurrence of ankylosis. This phenomenon is called primary failure of eruption.[66] The cause is not known; however, it is clear that a genetic factor is involved.[53,67–70]

Concluding Remarks

The development of the dentition is complex and differs from that of other structures and parts of the body. Tooth crowns are formed at their ultimate dimensions and are stored for years before they emerge. In addition, the large crowns of the permanent teeth are situated in the jaws together with the roots of the deciduous teeth. This is particularly complicated in the anterior region, the size of which is designed to ultimately contain only the roots of the permanent teeth.

For an overview of the normal development of the dentition, see video clip 23. The presentation begins with the formation of the deciduous incisors and ends with the completed adult dentition. It is shown in a rotating mode.

References

1. Clinch LM. Variations in the mutual relationship of the maxillary and mandibular gum pads in the new-born child. Int J Orthod 1934;20:359–372.
2. Van der Linden FPGM. Interrelated factors in the morphogenesis of teeth, the development of the dentition and craniofacial growth. Schweiz Monatschr Zahnheilk 1970;80:518–526.
3. Clinch LM. An analysis of serial models between three and eight years of age. Dent Rec 1951;71:61–72.
4. Moorrees CFA. The Dentition of the Growing Child: A Longitudinal Study of Dental Development Between 3 and 18 Years of Age. Cambridge: Harvard University Press, 1959.
5. Sillman JH. Dimensional changes of the dental arches: Longitudinal study from birth to 25 years. Am J Orthod 1964;50:824–842.
6. Moyers RE, Van der Linden FPGM, Riolo ML, McNamara JA Jr. Standards of Human Occlusal Development, monograph 5, Craniofacial Growth Series. Ann Arbor: University of Michigan, 1976.
7. Heikinheimo K, Nyström M, Heikinheimo T, Pirttiniemi P, Pirinen S. Dental arch width, overbite, and overjet in a Finnish population with normal occlusion between the ages of 7 and 32 years. Eur J Orthod 2012;34:418–426.
8. Farsi NMA, Salama FS. Characteristics of primary dentition occlusion in a group of Saudi children. Int J Paediatr Dent 1996;6:253–259.
9. Marshall SD, Caspersen M, Hardinger RR, Franciscus RG, Aquilino AS, Southard TE. Development of the curve of Spee. Am J Orthod Dentofac Orthop 2008;134:344–352.
10. Saitoh I, Hayasaki H, Inada E, Maruyama T, Takemoto Y, Yamasaki Y. Overlap of the primary dentition in children. J Clin Pediatr Dent 2009;33:269–274.
11. Björk A. The face in profile. Svensk Tandläk Tidskr 1947:40(suppl 5B):30–35.
12. Björk A. Variability and age changes in overjet and overbite. Am J Orthod 1953;39:779–801.
13. Fleming HB. An investigation of the vertical overbite during the eruption of the permanent dentition. Angle Orthod 1961;31:53–62.
14. Lande MJ. Growth behavior of the human bony facial profile as revealed by serial cephalometric roentgenology. Angle Orthod 1952;22:78–90.
15. Baccetti T, Franchi L, McNamara Jr JA. Longitudinal growth changes in subjects with deepbite. Am J Orthod Dentofac Orthop 2011;140:202–209.
16. Jonsson T, Karlsson KO, Ragnarsson B, Magnusson TE. Long-term development of malocclusion traits in orthodontically treated and untreated subjects. Am J Orthod Dentofac Orthop 2010;138:277–284.
17. Baume LJ. Physiological tooth migration and its significance for the development of occlusion. III. The biogenesis of the successional dentition. J Dent Res 1950;29:338–348.
18. Jonsson T, Magnusson TE. Crowding and spacing in the dental arches: Long-term development in treated and untreated subjects. Am J Orthod Dentofac Orthop 2010;138:384.e1–384.e7.
19. Eslambolchi S, Woodside DG, Rossouw PE. A descriptive study of mandibular incisor alignment in untreated subjects. Am J Orthod Dentofac Orthop 2008;133:343–353.
20. Jonsson T, Arnlaugsson S, Saemundsson SR, Magnusson TE. Development of occlusal traits and dental arch space from adolescence to adulthood: A 25-year follow-up study of 245 untreated subjects. Am J Orthod Dentofac Orthop 2009;135:456–462.
21. Sinclair PM. Maturation of untreated normal occlusions. Am J Orthod 1983;83:114–123.
22. Berg RE, Stenvik A, Espeland L. A 57-year follow-up study of occlusion. Part 2: Oral health and attitudes to teeth among individuals with deep overbite at the age of 8 years. J Orofac Orthop 2008;69:309–324.
23. Bishara SE, Treder JE, Damon P, Olsen M. Changes in the dental arches and dentition between 25 and 45 years of age. Angle Orthod 1996;66:417–422.
24. Dager MM, McNamara Jr JA, Bracetti T, Franchi L. Aging in the craniofacial complex. Angle Orthod 2008;78:440–444.
25. Behrents RG. Growth in the Aging Craniofacial Skeleton, monograph 17, Craniofacial Growth Series. Ann Arbor: University of Michigan, 1985.
26. Tallgren A. Changes in adult face height due to aging, wear, and loss of teeth and prosthetic treatment. Acta Odontol Scand 1957;15:1–22.
27. Leighton BC, Adams CP. Incisor inclination in Class 2 division 2 malocclusions. Eur J Orthod 1986;8:98–105.
28. Hotz R. Orthodontie in der täglichen Praxis: Möglichkeiten und Grenzen im Rahmen der Kinderzahnheilkunde, ed 4. Bern: Huber, 1970.
29. Van der Linden FPGM. Orthodontic Concepts and Strategies. Chicago: Quintessence, 2004.
30. Van der Linden FPGM. Simultaneous removal of first deciduous molars and first premolars [abstract]. Eur J Orthod 1996;18:428.
31. Fanning EA. A longitudinal study of tooth calcification and root resorption [abstract]. J Dent Res 1958;74:4.
32. Fanning EA. A longitudinal study of tooth formation and root resorption. N Z Dent J 1961;57:202–217.
33. Shumaker DB, El Hadary MS. Roentgenographic study of eruption. J Am Dent Assoc 1960;61:535–541.
34. De Boer M. Aspekten van de gebitsontwikkeling bij kinderen tussen vijf en tien jaar [thesis]. Utrecht: Utrecht University, 1970.
35. Giles NB, Knott VB, Meredith HV. Increase in intraoral height of selected permanent teeth during the quadrennium following gingival emergence. Angle Orthod 1963;33:195–206.
36. Moyers RE. Handbook of Orthodontics, ed 4. Chicago: Year Book, 1988.
37. Haavikko K. Correlation between the root resorption of deciduous teeth and the formation of the corresponding permanent teeth. Proc Finn Dent Soc 1973;69:191–201.
38. Korf SR. The eruption of permanent central incisors following premature loss of their antecedents. J Dent Child 1965;32:39–44.
39. Sahara N, Okafuji N, Toyoki A, et al. A histological study of the exfoliation of human deciduous teeth. J Dent Res 1993;72:634–640.
40. Ainamo A, Ainamo J. The width of attached gingiva on supraerupted teeth. J Periodontal Res 1978;13:194–198.
41. Ainamo J, Talari A. Eruptive movements of teeth in human adults. In: Poole DFG, Stack MV (eds). The Eruption and Occlusion of Teeth [Proceedings of the 27th Symposium of the Colston Research Society, 3–7 Apr 1975, Bristol, UK]. London: Butterworth, 1976:97–107.
42. Beertsen W, Quirynen M, Van Steenberghe D, Van der Velden U. Parodontologie. Houten: Bohn Stafleu van Loghum, 2009.
43. Weinstein S, Haack DC, Morris LY, Snyder BB, Attaway HE. On an equilibrium theory of tooth position. Angle Orthod 1963;33:1–11.
44. Lee CF, Proffit WR. The daily rhythm of tooth eruption. Am J Orthod Dentofac Orthop 1995;107:38–47.

45. Proffit WR, Prewitt JR, Baik HS, Lee CF. Video microscope observations of human premolar eruption. J Dent Res 1991;70:15–18.
46. Van der Linden FPGM, Proffit WR. Dynamics of Orthodontics: Orofacial Functions [DVD 4]. Berlin: Quintessence, 1999.
47. Siersbæk-Nielsen S. Rate of eruption of central incisors at puberty: An implant study on eight boys. Tandlægebladet 1971;75:1288–1295.
48. Craddock HL, Youngson CC. Eruptive tooth movement—The current state of knowledge. Br Dent J 2004;197:385–391.
49. Berkovitz BKB. The effect of root transection and partial root resection on the unimpeded eruption rate of the rat incisor. Arch Oral Biol 1971;16:1033–1043.
50. Marks SC Jr, Cahill DR. Experimental study in the dog of the non-active role of the tooth in the eruptive process. Arch Oral Biol 1984;29:311–322.
51. Cheek CC, Paterson RL, Proffit WR. Response of erupting human second premolars to blood flow changes. Arch Oral Biol 2002;47:851–858.
52. Cahill DR, Marks SC Jr. Tooth eruption: Evidence for the central role of the dental follicle. J Oral Pathol 1980;9:189–200.
53. Proffit WR, Frazier-Bowers SA. Mechanism and control of tooth eruption: Overview and clinical implications. Orthod Craniofac Res 2009;12:59–66.
54. Thesleff I. Does epidermal growth factor control tooth eruption? J Dent Child 1987;54:321–329.
55. Wise GE. Cellular and molecular basis of tooth eruption. Orthod Craniofac Res 2009;2:67–73.
56. Moxham BJ, Berkovitz BKB. The mobility of the lathritic rabbit mandibular incisor in response to axially directed extrusive loads. Arch Oral Biol 1984;29:773–778.
57. Shinji H, Kumasaka S, Matsubara S, Yang J, Ozawa N, Uchimura N. Study on eruption of deciduous teeth. Pediatr Dent J 1998:8:113–118.
58. Bjerklin K, Kurol J. Ectopic eruption of the maxillary first permanent molars: Etiologic factors. Am J Orthod 1983;84:147–155.
59. Bjerklin K, Kurol J, Paulin G. Ectopic eruption of maxillary first permanent molars in children with cleft lip and/or palate. Eur J Orthod 1993;15:535–540.
60. Raghobar GM, Boering G, Jansen HWB, Vissink A. Secondary retention of permanent molars: A histologic study. J Oral Pathol Med 1989;18:427–431.
61. Raghobar GM, Boering G, Stegenga B, Vissink A. Secondary retention in the primary dentition. J Dent Child 1991;58:17–22.
62. Duterloo HS. An Atlas of Dentition in Childhood. Orthodontic Diagnosis and Panoramic Radiology. London: Wolfe, 1991.
63. Bachmann H. Die Häufigkeit von Nichtanlagen bleibender Zähne (ausgenommen der Weisheitszähne). Ergebnisse der Auswertung von 8694 Orthopantogrammen 9-10 jähriger Schulkinder aus Zürich [thesis]. Zürich: University of Zürich, 1974.
64. Thilander B, Myrberg N. The prevalence of malocclusion in Swedish schoolchildren. Scand J Dent Res 1973;81:12–21.
65. Jensen BL, Kreiborg S. Craniofacial growth in cleidocranial dysplasia–A roentgencephalometric study. J Craniofac Genet Dev Biol 1995;15:35–43.
66. Proffit WR, Vig KWL. Primary failure of eruption: A possible cause of posterior open bite. Am J Orthod 1981;80:173–190.
67. Dibiase AT, Leggat TG. Primary failure of eruption in the permanent dentition of siblings. Int J Paediatr Dent 2000;10:153–157.
68. Frazier-Bowers SA, Simmons D, Koehler K, Zhou J. Genetic analysis of familial non-syndromic primary failure of eruption. Orthod Craniofac Res 2009;12:74–81.
69. Rose E. Die primäre Zahneruptionsstörung. Inf Orthod Kieferorthop 2009;41:13–17.
70. Stellzig-Eisenhauer A, Decker E, Meyer-Marcotty P, et al. Primary failure of eruption (PFE)–Clinical and molecular genetics analysis. J Orofac Orthop 2010;71:6–16.

9

Growth and Development of the Facial Complex: Interactions Among the Dentition, Skeleton, and Function

This chapter begins with an explanation of interactions in the development of the facial complex with emphasis on functional aspects. Thereafter, the growth of the facial skeleton is presented, and the variation in growth patterns is illustrated. The contribution to growth of bone, cartilage, and the associated remodeling of bony surfaces is discussed. Finally, the functional factors acting in the orofacial region are described, with indications given regarding which ones are relevant for the development of the facial complex and which ones are not.

Interactions in the Development of the Facial Complex

Interactions among the skeleton, dentition, and function play an essential role in the growth and development of the facial complex. In Fig 9-1, the facial complex is presented as a system with skeleton, dentition, and function as entities. Each is assigned its own range of variation. For example, the range of variation of the skeleton allows for various growth patterns. The dentition, which involves a great diversity in tooth positions, occlusal patterns, and orthodontic deviations, is assigned the largest range in variation. The function is dominant in the system and has the smallest range of variation.

The skeleton has a greater influence on the dentition than vice versa, and function has a greater influence on the skeleton and dentition than either entity has on it. The most important components of function are the soft tissues, particularly the musculature. They affect the growth of the bony structures, which initially determines the position of the teeth. After emergence, the arrangement of the teeth also becomes influenced by the musculature. The occlusion takes care of the fine-tuning of the positions of antagonists. The process described here is based on interactions between all three entities.

An example of the interaction between function and the dentition is the stabilization of opposing posterior teeth. The ultimate positions of premolars and molars are determined by intercuspation. By this mechanism, the posterior teeth maintain their position, even in cases of periodontal breakdown and mobility.

Another example of interaction between function and the dentition is the occurrence of irregularities in the mandibular anterior region after the development of the dentition is completed. Anterior teeth do not interdigitate and are not fixed three-dimensionally by the occlusion. The incisal edges of the mandibular incisors mostly contact only the marginal ridges at the palatal surfaces of the maxillary incisors (Fig 9-2). In addition, the mandibular incisors have small labiolingual dimensions and narrow interproximal contacts.[4] This combination results in an unstable equilibrium. Late displacement of mandibular incisors, and to a lesser degree sometimes maxillary incisors, is quite common.

A third example of interaction between function and the dentition is the phenomenon that adjacent teeth stay in contact when their width reduces by interproximal attrition. This loss of tooth material can amount to more than 6 mm per quadrant.[5,6] In the maintenance of the continuity of the dental arch, three functional aspects play a role: the anterior component of occlusal force,[7,8] the pressure of the labial and buccal musculature, and the traction of the supra-alveolar fibers[9] (Fig 9-3).

The cone-funnel mechanism is an example of interaction among the three entities. The size and relation of the jaws (skeleton), the initial location of the posterior teeth in the jaws (dentition), and the alteration of the eruption direction as soon as contact is reached (function) result in the final position of the posterior teeth (Fig 9-4).

Another example of interaction among the three entities is the rail mechanism. With more anterior growth of the mandible than the maxilla, the mandibular teeth gradually occlude slightly more mesially, leading to some widening of the maxillary dental arch (Fig 9-5).

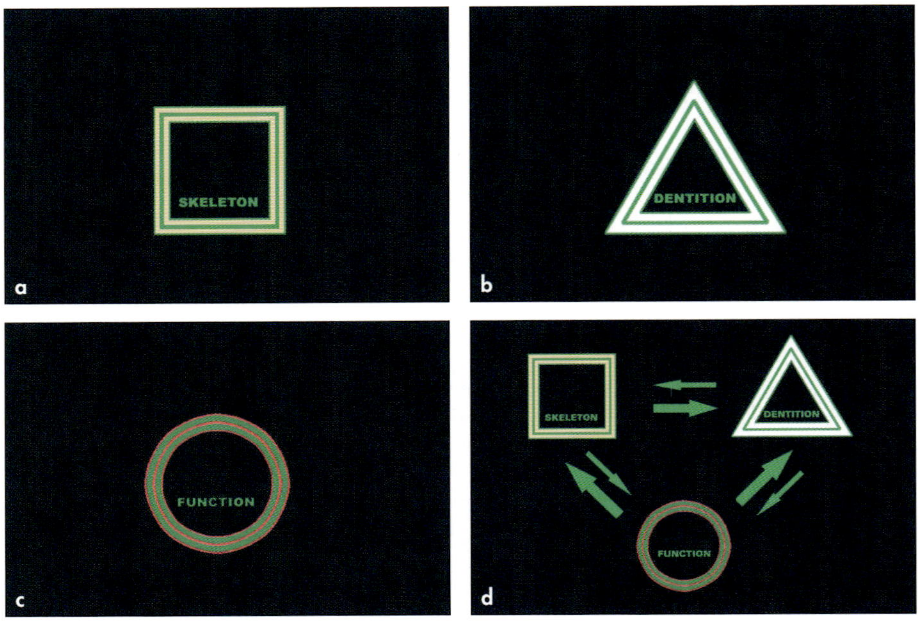

Fig 9-1 System of the facial complex. *(a to c)* In descending order, the largest range of variation (expressed in the distance between the inner and outer lines) is assigned to the dentition, skeleton, and function. Each of them will develop in its own way and at its own pace within its given range of variation. *(d)* Because of this, there is a degree of flexibility in their interactions. The thickness of the arrows indicates the intensity of the interactions.

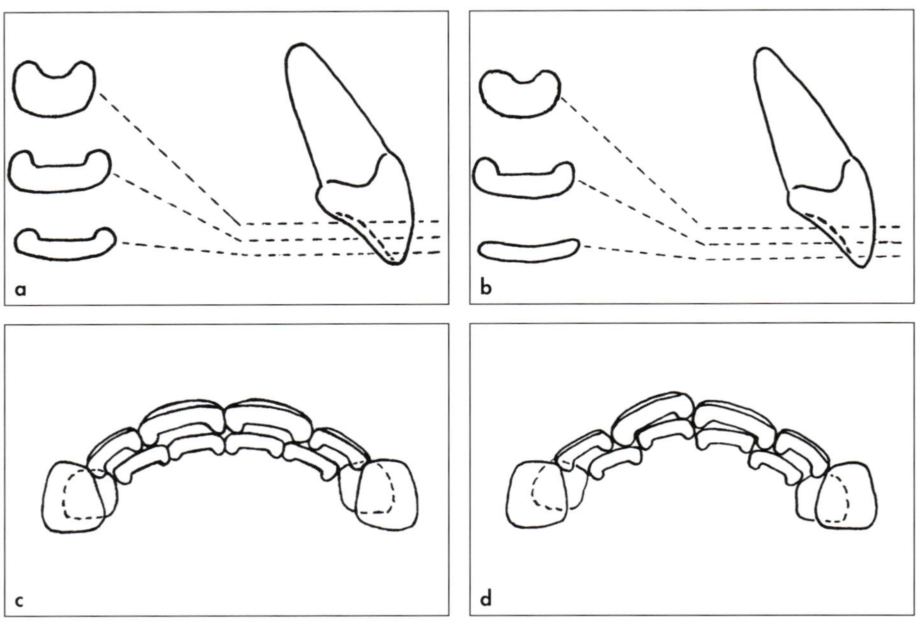

Fig 9-2 Effect of marginal ridges on the occlusal contact between incisors. More than half of the Western population has marginal ridges of varying thicknesses at the palatal surfaces of incisors. In the Asian population, it is common to have prominent marginal ridges (shovel-shaped teeth).[1,2] *(a)* Marginal ridges can extend to the incisal edge. *(b)* They can also stop short of the incisal edge. *(c)* Marginal ridges interfere with the realization of broad occlusal contacts. *(d)* An irregular arrangement is usually associated with broader occlusal contacts. Maxillary incisors may become malpositioned due to the occlusion.[3]

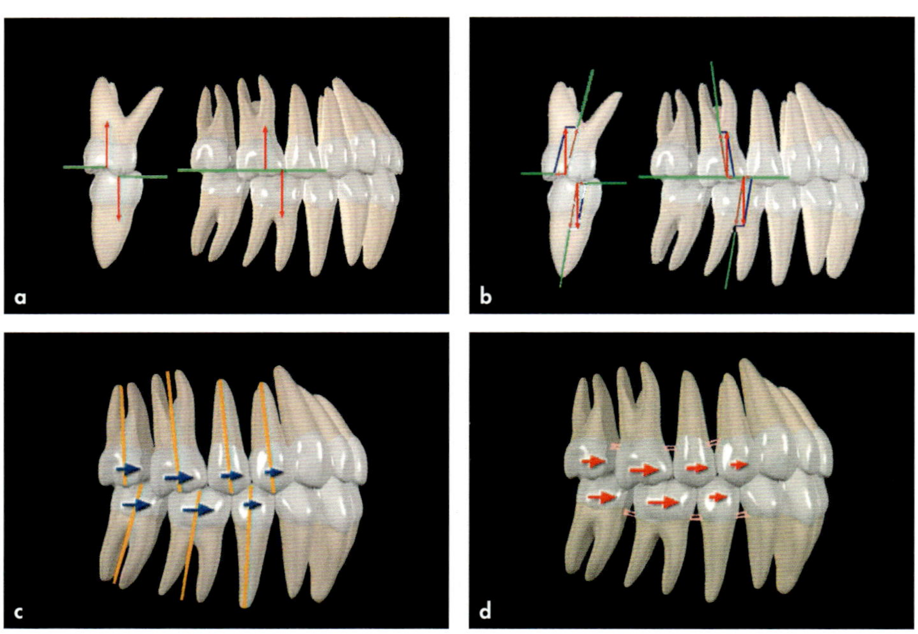

Fig 9-3 Preservation of the continuity of dental arches. *(a)* Teeth stay in contact during the gradual reduction of their crown widths. This phenomenon is based partly on forces caused by biting (anterior component of occlusal force). *(b)* These forces can be resolved in vectors perpendicular to the occlusal plane and in mesial and transverse directions. *(c)* This resolution corresponds to the mesial angulation of most posterior teeth, the lingual inclination of the mandibular teeth, and the buccal inclination of the maxillary teeth.[7] *(d)* In addition, the vestibular musculature and the traction of the supra-alveolar fibers contribute.[9]

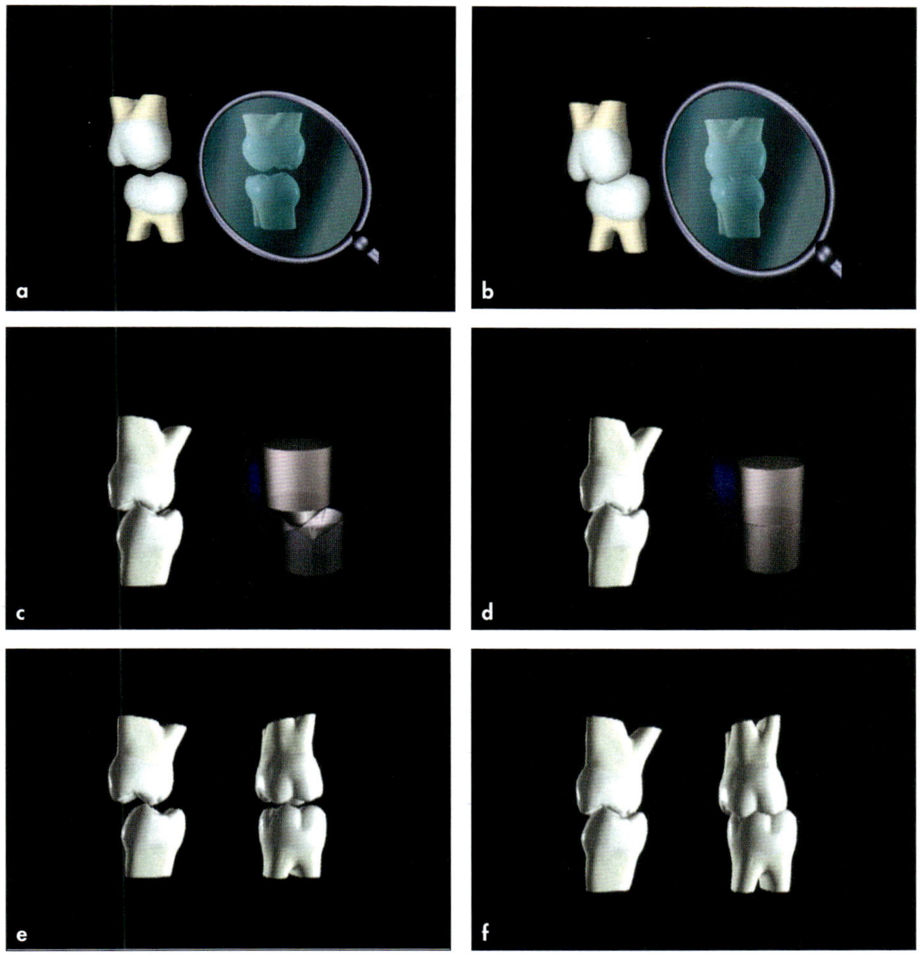

Fig 9-4 Cone-funnel mechanism. *(a and b)* Opposing posterior teeth rarely erupt in the precise position and orientation for intercuspation. Instead, they are guided into an optimal intercuspation by the cone-funnel mechanism, which comes into play for the first time when the first deciduous molars start to contact each other. *(c and d)* This occurs every time that opposing posterior teeth reach the stage of contact. *(e and f)* The maxillary teeth probably move more than the mandibular teeth. If the eruption is hindered, as in lateral tongue interpositions, the cone-funnel mechanism does not work. See video clip 26. (Printed from Van der Linden et al[10] with permission.)

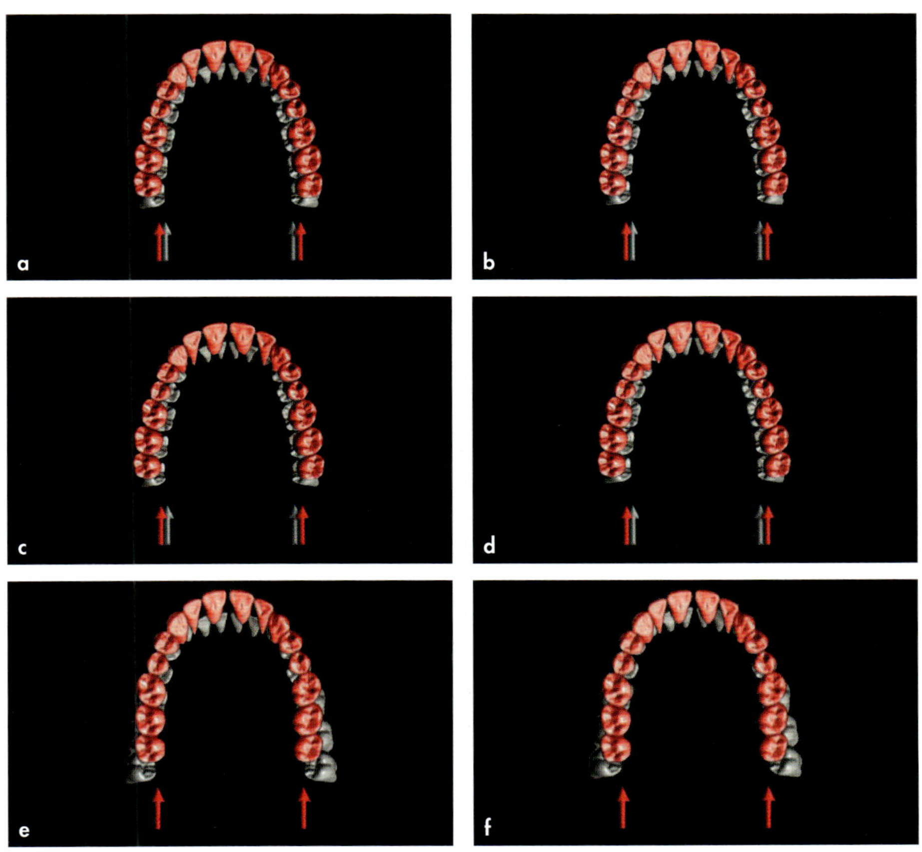

Fig 9-5 Rail mechanism. With more anterior growth of the mandible than the maxilla, intercuspation adapts the width of the maxillary dental arch to the mandibular dental arch. In that context, the mandibular dental arch can be imagined as a rail on which the maxillary dental arch rides. The mandibular base does not widen; the space within the cortical walls is limited. The roots of the mandibular molars and premolars can move only slightly to the buccal. The maxillary dental arch can still widen by bone growth at the median suture and apposition of bone buccally at the alveolar processes. *(a to d)* The rail mechanism functions only in situations with adequate transverse intercuspation. *(e and f)* In lateral open bites and nonocclusions, the maxillary dental arch does not widen. See video clip 22. (Printed from Van der Linden et al[10] with permission.)

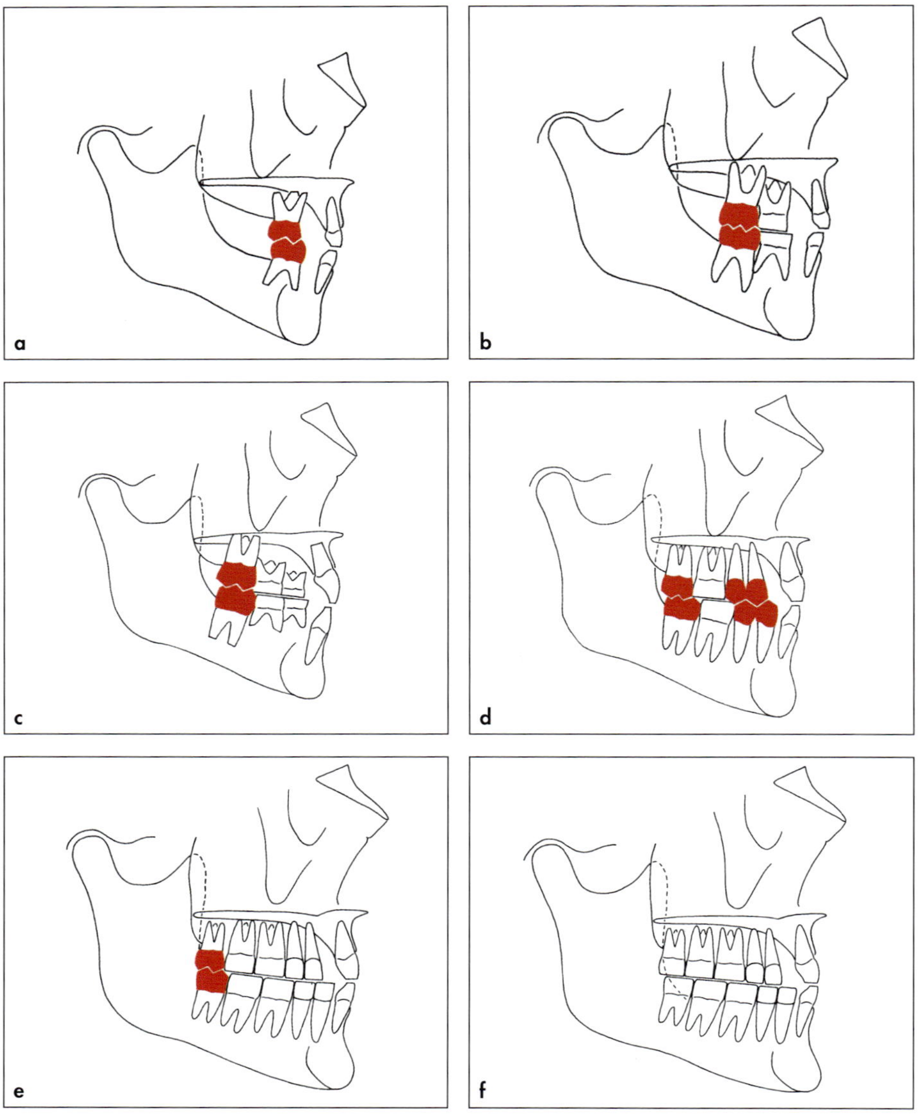

Fig 9-6 Guiding role of intercuspation in the maintenance of occlusion, illustrated in a situation with excessive attrition. *(a)* After the first deciduous molars have reached occlusion at 16 months of age, the anteroposterior relationship between the dental arches is confirmed every time the molars are put together. *(b)* When the second deciduous molars have reached occlusion at 28 months of age, they will, together with the remaining cusps of the first deciduous molars, fulfill that role. *(c)* At 8 years of age, the first permanent molars, which emerged 2 years earlier, are only slightly worn. Their intercuspation secures the continuation of its role. *(d)* At 14 years of age, the task is taken over by the second permanent molars and premolars, which emerged about 2 years before. *(e)* Finally, the third molars perform the function. *(f)* After a number of years, all intercuspation has faded.

In the context of the interactions just described, it is obvious that intercuspation plays an essential role in the maintenance of the occlusion in the growing face.[11] That role begins when the first deciduous molars reach occlusion. When they become worn down, the second deciduous molars take over the task. Subsequently, the first permanent molars perform the task. Six years later, in the period of significant jaw growth, the second permanent molars, together with the premolars, do the work. Another 6 years later, the third molars make their contribution (Fig 9-6).

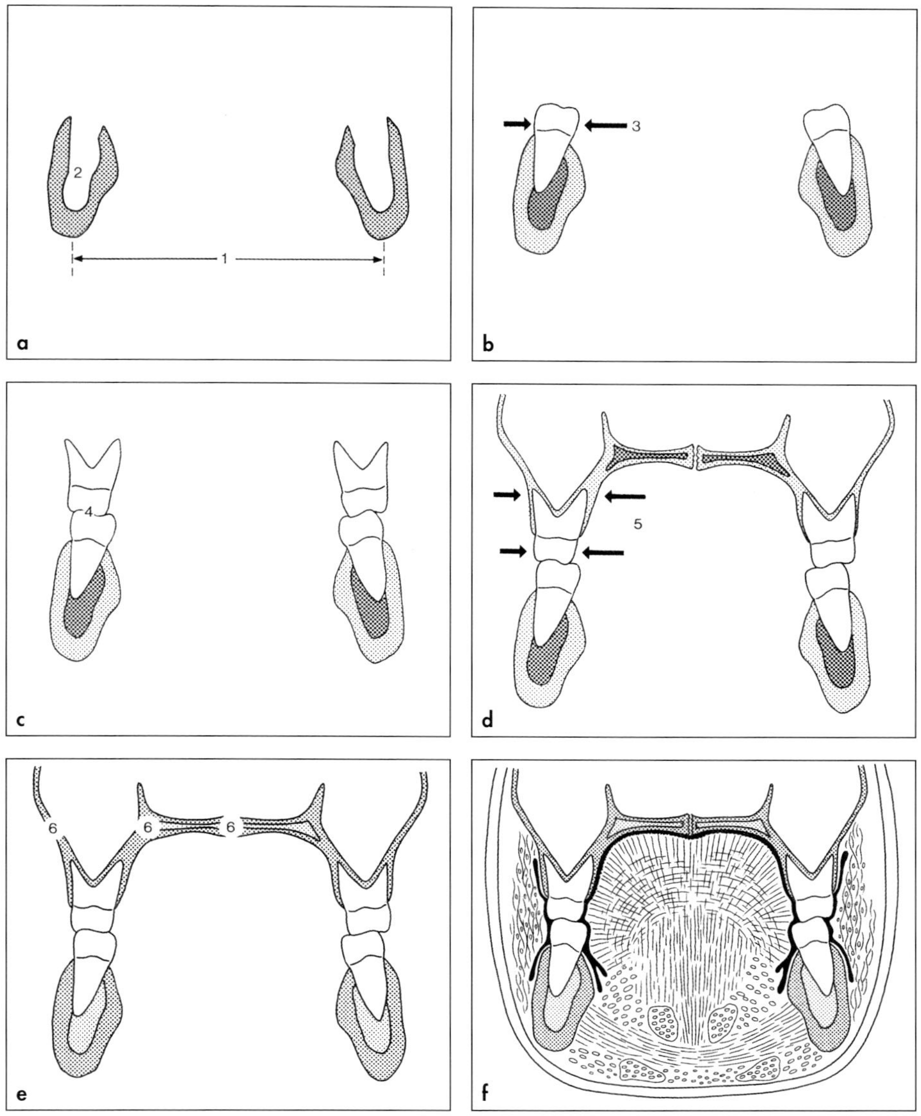

FIG 9-7 Transverse development of the jaws and the position of the first permanent molars. *(a)* The mandibular base does not change in width (1). There is little room within the cortical walls (2) for the localization of the apices. *(b)* The roots of the molars (3) are close to the buccal cortical walls. *(c)* The localization of the maxillary molar crowns depends on their intercuspation (4) with the mandibular crowns. *(d)* The occlusion with the maxillary molars and the pressure of the tongue and cheeks affect the inclination of the mandibular molars. That also applies to the maxillary molars (5). The occlusion together with the pressure of the tongue against the palate leads to broadening of the maxilla. *(e)* Through growth at the median suture and bone apposition buccally accompanied by resorption palatally (6), the maxillary apices can move buccally. This leads to an alteration in inclination. *(f)* The tongue and cheeks press against the molar crowns and alveolar processes. There are no data that indicate that the mandibular base increases in width by bone reconstruction. However, it has been shown that the mandibular canal displaces to the lateral by internal bone resorption and apposition.[12]

The adjustment in transverse development is based on a complex interaction of the three entities (Fig 9-7). It depends on the intercuspation in the posterior regions. A limited number of teeth are sufficient, as is also the case in the sagittal adjustment. However, if occlusal contact is not reached, as in lateral tongue interposition, the inclination of the teeth and the width of the dental arches are not adapted. The tongue is positioned low in the mouth and covers the linguo-occlusal margins of the mandibular teeth. The cone-funnel mechanism will not work. The mandibular posterior teeth remain perpendicularly positioned in the jaw, and the mandibular dental arch is wide. The maxillary dental arch is too narrow.

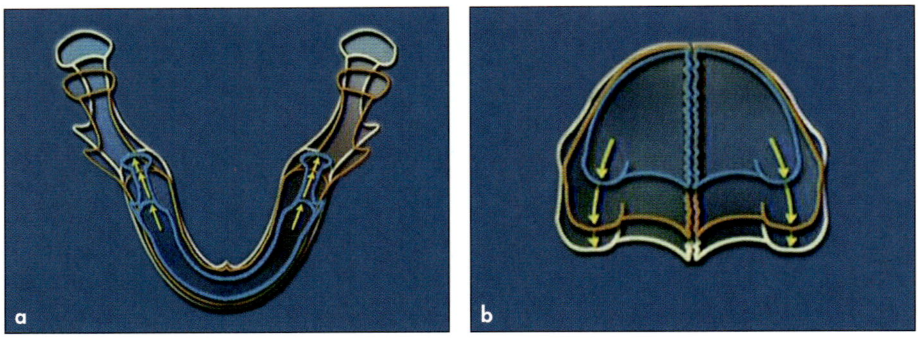

Fig 9-8 Contours of the jaws in three developmental stages. *(a)* The base of the mandible becomes broader by bone apposition at the inner and outer surfaces. *(b)* The maxilla widens. The majority of the enlargement of both jaws is growth to the posterior.

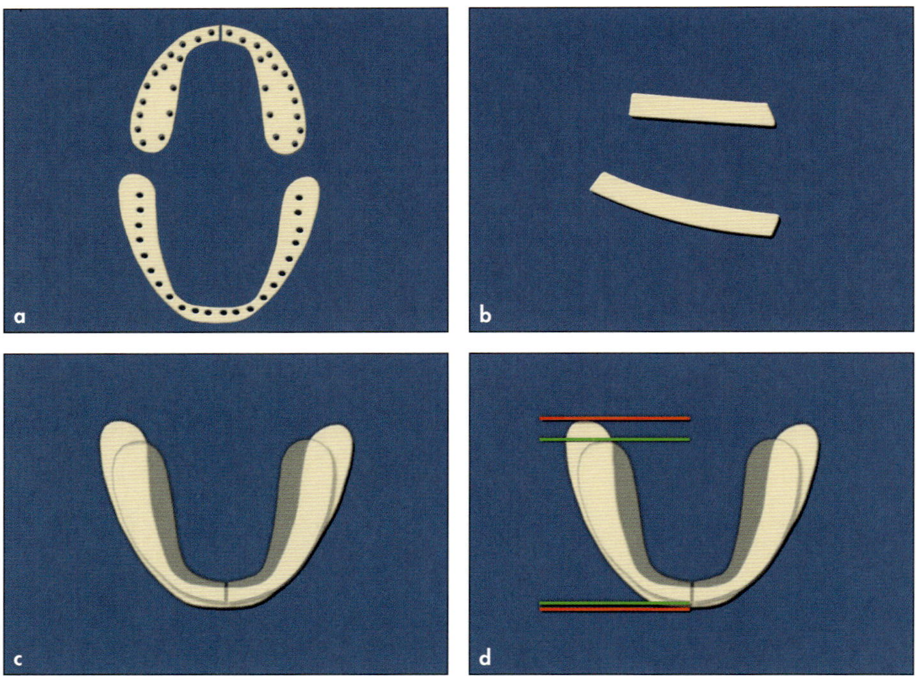

Fig 9-9 Size and relationship of the apical areas. *(a)* Apical areas vary in size and shape and in localization of apices. *(b)* Sagittal and vertical orientation of apical areas. *(c)* Superposition shows the more buccal position of the apical area in the mandibular molar region. *(d)* The apical area in the maxilla is shorter than that in the mandible, which extends farther anteriorly and posteriorly. The inclination and angulation of the teeth depend on the relation between the opposing apical areas.

In a growing face, teeth migrate within the jaws. The intercuspation ensures that the teeth in both jaws are displaced in a coordinated way. In the absence of solid intercuspation, opposing teeth move independently of each other, and their position and inclination are not reciprocally adjusted. This applies to both the sagittal and transverse directions.

When all teeth, except the third molars, have attained occlusion, the permanent dentition is complete. However, the face still continues to grow the most during puberty and adolescence, particularly in boys. The soft tissues are the last to mature.[13] These differences in timing and rate of growth and development of the various structures lead to specific interactions among the three entities. Through these interactions during the outgrowth of the jaws, the incisors upright and attain a more posterior position in the face. The pressure exerted by the lips increases.

The interaction between the skeleton and the dentition is demonstrated by means of the apical areas, which increase in size mainly by overall vertical growth and posterior growth at the maxillary and lingual tuberosities (Fig 9-8). Not only their size and shape, but also the spatial relationship between the two apical areas is of importance. This relationship is the starting point for the inclination and angulation of the teeth (Fig 9-9). The division of the apical areas into anterior, middle, and posterior sections specified earlier is defined and illustrated in Fig 9-10.

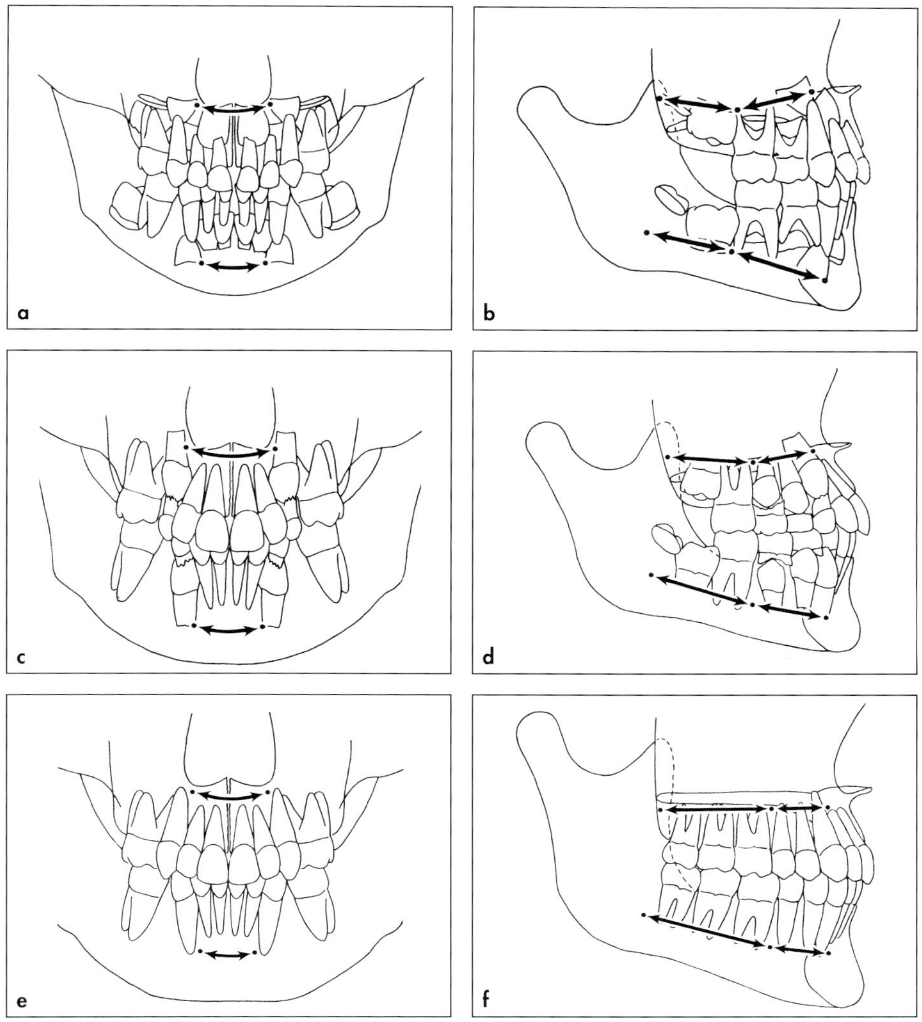

Fig 9-10 Apical areas in three stages. *(a and b)* In a 4-year-old child, the anterior section of the apical area *(a, arrows)* is the region between the mesial sides of the forming parts of the permanent canines. The middle section *(b, top and bottom right arrows)* lies between the demarcation of the anterior section and the mesial side of the forming part of the first permanent molar. The posterior section *(b, top and bottom left arrows)* lies behind the middle section and extends to the posterior side of the maxillary tuberosity and the mandibular lingual tuberosity. *(c and d)* For a 10-year-old child, basically the same demarcations apply as outlined for the 4-year-old, with modifications for the vertical displacement of the canines and first permanent molars. *(c, arrows)* Anterior section of the apical area. *(d, top and bottom right arrows)* Middle section of the apical area. *(d, top and bottom left arrows)* Posterior section of the apical area. *(e and f)* In a 21-year-old, the demarcations are slightly mesial of the roots of the canines and of the third molars. *(e, arrows)* Anterior section of the apical area. *(f, top and bottom right arrows)* Middle section of the apical area. *(f, top and bottom left arrows)* Posterior section of the apical area.

The dentoalveolar compensatory mechanism is an important phenomenon of interaction among the skeleton, dentition, and function (Fig 9-11). It is defined by Solow as "a system that attempts to maintain normal interarch relations under varying jaw relationships."[15] This mechanism works only if eruption proceeds normally and functional conditions do not deviate. Then the occlusion and pressure of tongue, lips, and cheeks will lead to adequate contacts between the opposing teeth. Variations in the anteroposterior relationship within the anterior sections of apical areas can be adjusted by the inclination of the incisors. With a relatively receding maxillary anterior section of the apical area, the maxillary incisors are more labially inclined, and the interincisal angle is smaller. The inclination of the canines, premolars, and molars varies in a comparable way.[16] The dentoalveolar compensatory mechanism functions mainly in the permanent dentition but little in the deciduous dentition.[17,18]

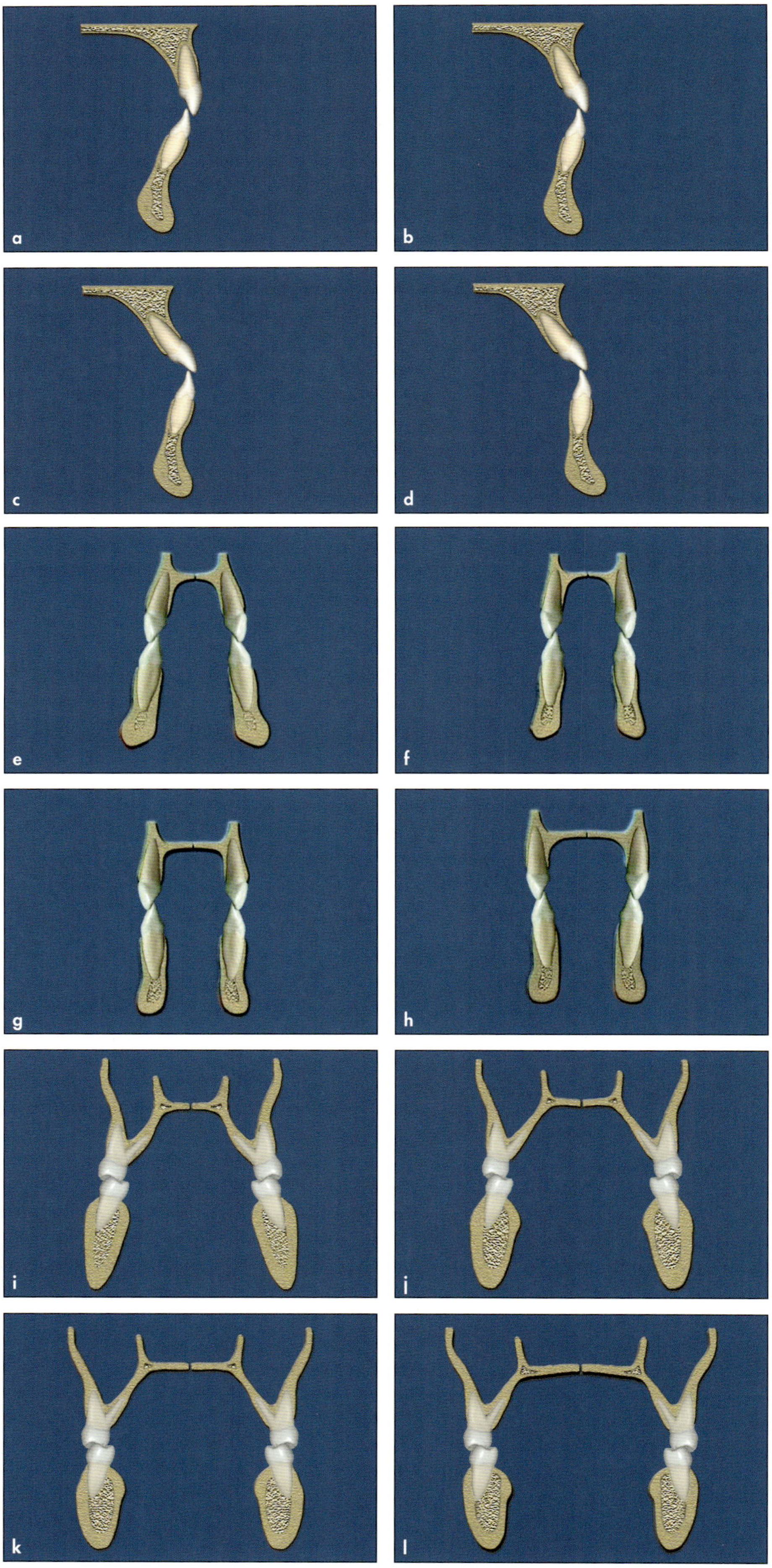

Fig 9-11 The dentoalveolar compensatory mechanism. *(a to d)* Depending on the anteroposterior relationship of the anterior sections of the apical areas, the inclination of the incisors varies. *(e to h)* The apices of the maxillary canines are located laterally and close to the piriform aperture, which can vary considerably in width, as can the mandibular base in the canine region. The inclination of the canines adapts to the transverse relation of the apical areas. *(i to l)* The adaptation in width of the maxilla to the width of the mandible is limited. The inclination of the molars depends on the transverse relationship of the apical areas, which varies greatly. The dentoalveolar compensatory mechanism is based on the reconstruction and adaptation of the alveolar processes. If the discrepancy in position of the opposing apical areas is too large, adequate occlusion cannot be realized. The dentoalveolar compensatory mechanism is not effective in open bites and nonocclusions.[14]

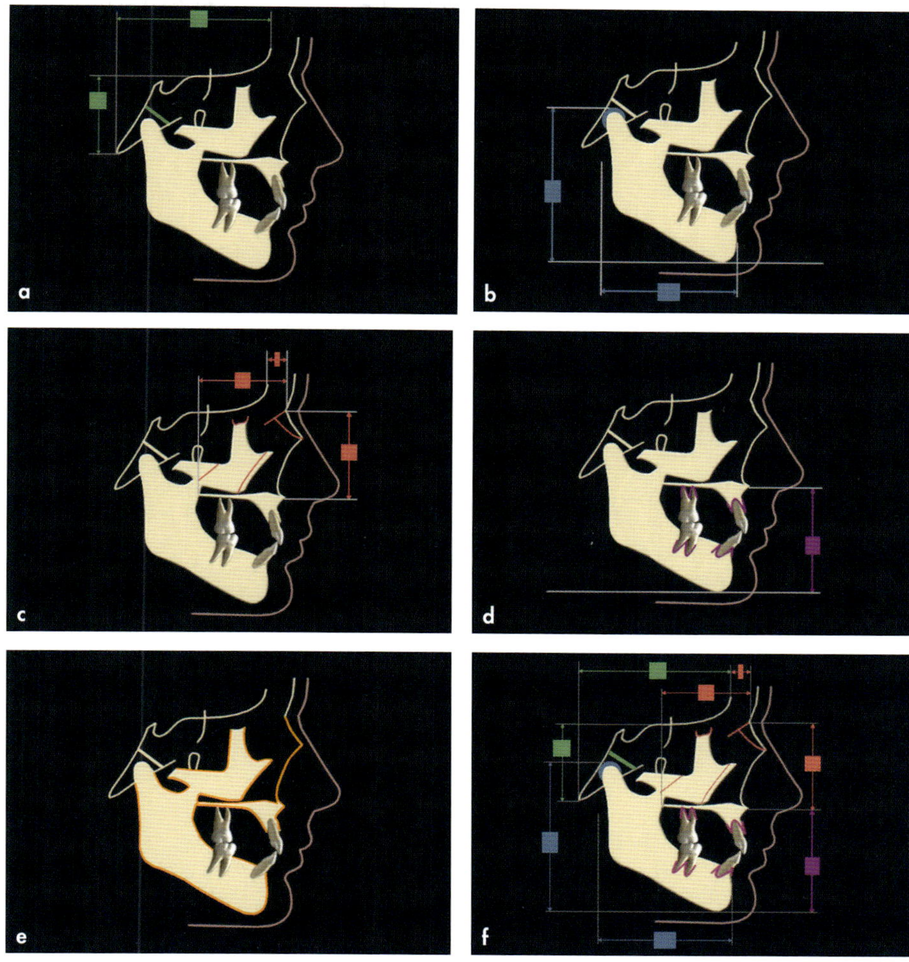

Fig 9-12 Growth sites of the facial skeleton differentiated in type and direction. *(a)* The spheno-occipital synchondrosis takes care of a large part of the sagittal and vertical growth of the upper part of the facial skeleton. *(b)* The condyles perform the same function for the lower part of the facial skeleton, but their larger contribution is the lengthening and anterior displacement of the mandible. *(c)* In addition, the inferior extension of the temporal bones and the associated downward displacement of the mandibular fossae contribute to the increase in height of the posterior part[19] (not shown in figure). The vertical and sagittal growth of the upper part is realized largely by growth at the sutures.[20] *(d)* The vertical growth of the anterior part of the lower face is mainly realized by bone apposition at the alveolar processes.[21] *(e)* Bone apposition at the outer surfaces of the facial bones also contributes to vertical growth of the anterior part of the lower face. *(f)* Indeed, the enlargement of the facial skeleton is realized by fast-growing cartilage and by apposition and resorption of bone at sutures and at internal and external surfaces, accompanied by remodeling (see Fig 9-21). The size of the colored blocks represents the assumed amount contributed by the various structures.

Growth of the Facial Skeleton

The growth sites of the facial skeleton are illustrated in Fig 9-12. The interaction among the three entities regarding the increase in height of the lower face is revealed in the growth of the mandibular condyle and the eruption of the teeth with the associated increase in height of the alveolar processes. The individual bones become larger, and they change in shape in accordance with the functional requirements through the combined action of the growth of cartilage and bone.

As explained above, functional aspects play an important role in facial growth. It is assumed that the vertical development of the face, and especially of its lower part, is largely determined by the interaction between internal and external functional components. Internal functional components involve not only the intraoral structures but also the nasal and pharyngeal structures and spaces. The external functional components include the muscles and soft tissues outside of the facial skeleton. Not only their volume and shape but also their activities are influential. However, it is not the incidental muscle contractions, but the situation at rest that is decisive. The large quantity of soft tissues present anteriorly with a closed mouth will have a different effect than the thin, weak coverage that occurs with an open mouth.

Normally, a balance exists between internal and external functional components (Fig 9-13a). However, if internal functional components dominate, facial growth is inferiorly directed (Fig 9-13b). A restricted nasal passage, a large tongue, and hypertrophic adenoids and tonsils can generate the need for more space. These conditions are often combined with tongue interposition, an open mouth, increased lower facial height, a receding chin, and labially tipped incisors. If external functional components dominate (Figs 9-13c and 9-13d), facial growth is anteriorly directed, and the height of the lower face increases only slightly.[22,23]

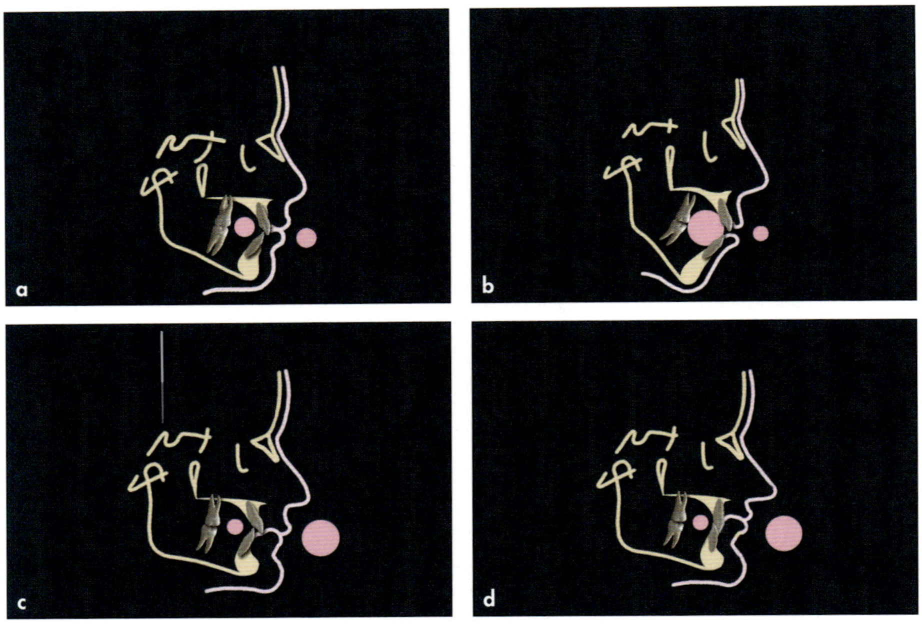

FIG 9-13 Variations in growth direction through functional influences. *(a)* When there is an equilibrium between internal and external functional components, a favorable growth direction and facial pattern result. *(b)* Dominance of internal functional components will lead to more vertical growth. *(c)* If external functional components dominate, and excess room exists for internal components, the height of the lower face will increase only slightly, and growth will be directed primarily anteriorly. This happens in Class II, division 1 malocclusions with excess external functional components. *(d)* Dominance of external functional components is also characteristic for Class II, division 2 malocclusions and Class I malocclusions with overerupted and palatally tipped maxillary incisors (total complete overbite).

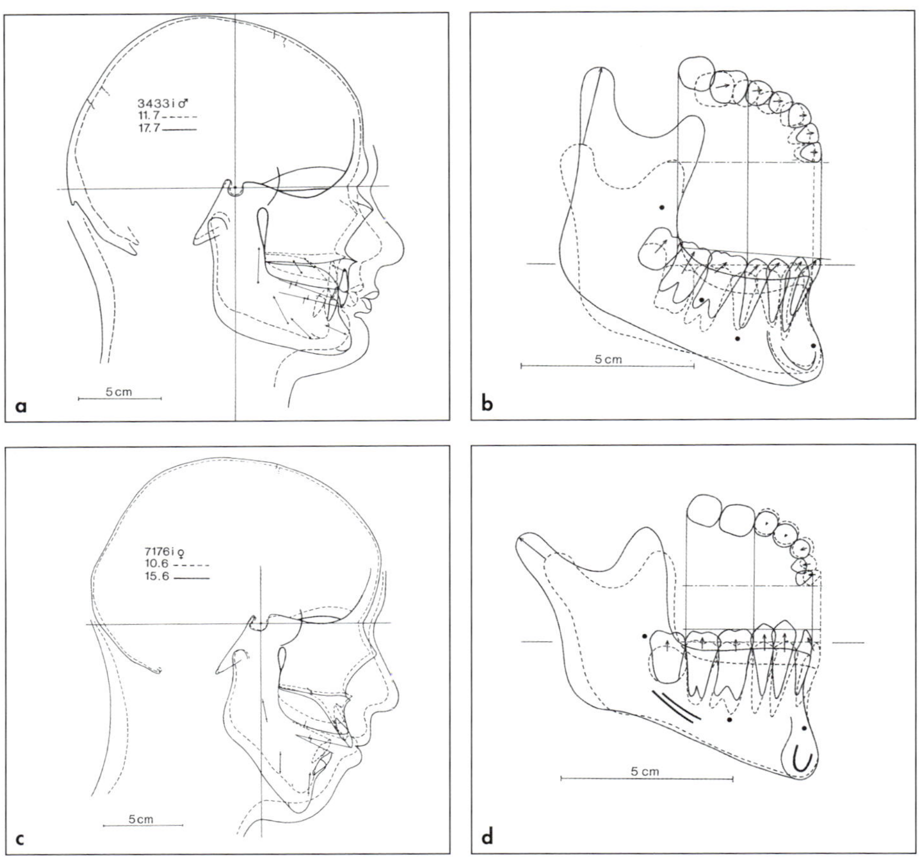

FIG 9-14 Tracings of cephalometric radiographs of a boy and a girl in whom metal implants were placed. The images in *a* and *c* are superimposed on the anterior cranial base; those in *b* and *d* are superimposed on the implants. The displacements of implants are indicated with *arrows*. *(a)* The boy has a short lower facial height; a Class II, division 2 malocclusion; a total complete overbite and excess external soft tissues. The mandible has rotated forward, and the chin has moved anteriorly. *(b)* The growth at the condyles was substantial and directed anteriorly. The mandibular teeth have migrated mesially. *(c)* The girl has a Class II, division 1 malocclusion with an anterior open bite, an increased lower facial height, and a shortage of external soft tissues. The mandible rotated posteriorly and came down. The chin moved straight down. *(d)* Condylar growth was to the posterior. The mandibular teeth are displaced perpendicularly to the occlusal plane. (Reprinted from Björk[26] with permission.)

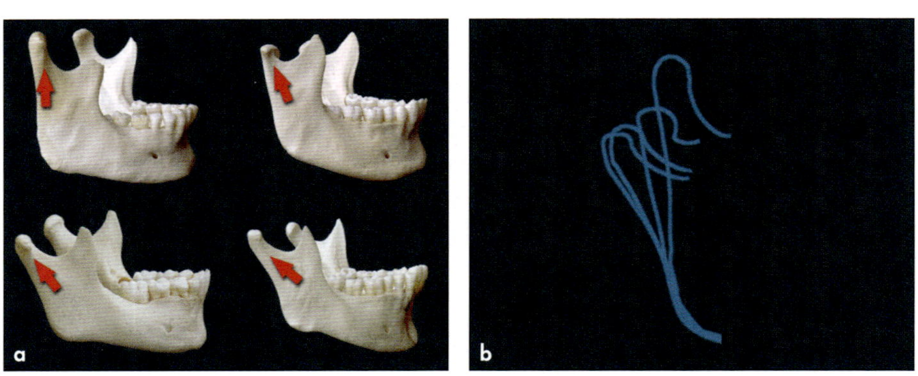

FIG 9-15 Growth at the condyles and diversity in mandibular shape. *(a)* Through local differences in mitotic activity of the chondrocytes and endochondral ossification, the condyle can grow *(red arrows)* in various directions. *(b)* This, in combination with external remodeling, results in a variety of mandibular shapes.

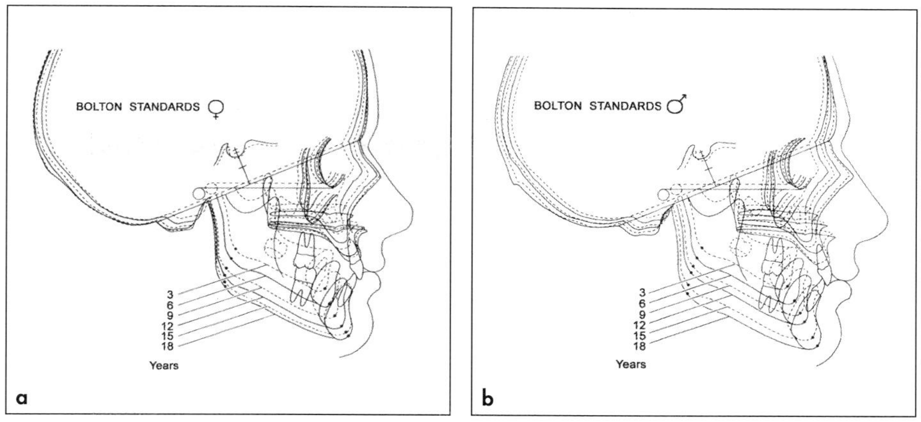

Fig 9-16 Growth of the facial skeleton. Girls *(a)* grow less than boys *(b)*, have an earlier and smaller adolescence growth spurt, and undergo less marked changes in appearance such as anterior movement of the chin, straightening of the profile, and enlargement of the nose. Nowadays, growth is completed in girls at 15 years of age or earlier; in boys it is completed around 20 years of age. These drawings are based on the averages of 20 normal individuals, 10 boys and 10 girls, with similar facial configurations. Because the drawings are based on averages, the adolescence growth spurts are smoothed and reduced (see chapter 17, Fig 17-11). The underlying data were collected starting in 1930 and were published in 1975. Today, adolescence growth spurts occur 1 to 2 years earlier, and growth in girls is completed at a younger age.[27] (Reprinted from Broadbent et al[28] with permission.)

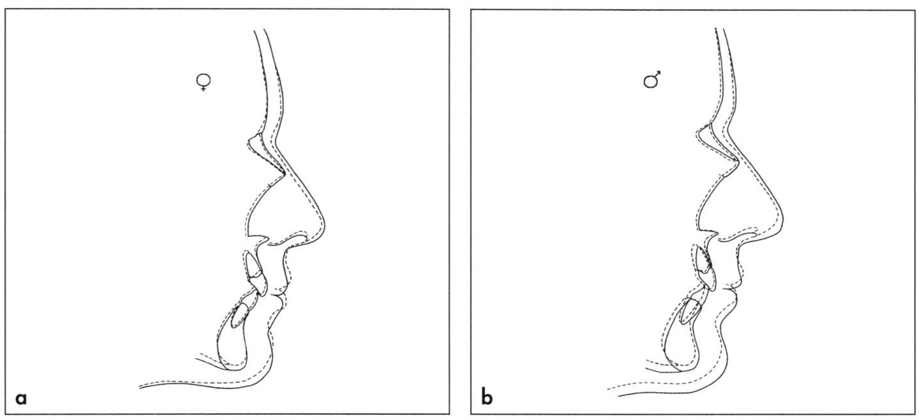

Fig 9-17 Average changes from 20 *(dashed lines)* to 50 *(solid lines)* years of age of 34 women *(a)* and 79 men *(b)*. Facial height increases. The mandible rotates posteriorly in women and anteriorly in men, in whom the chin moves forward. In both sexes, the nose becomes larger, moves inferiorly, and gets sharper. The lip line descends, the upper lip becomes longer and thinner, and the lower lip is more anteriorly positioned. (Reprinted from Behrents[32] with permission.)

There is a large variation in the size and shape of human heads and faces. In newborns, the variation is less than in adults, although prior to birth different facial patterns already exist (McNamara JA Jr and Van der Linden FPGM, unpublished data, 1970). The growth of the facial skeleton after birth varies considerably among individuals.[24,25] The diversity in postnatal development of the facial skeleton is demonstrated with two examples in Fig 9-14.

Individual differences in growth at the condyle after birth result in variations in mandibular shape and size (Fig 9-15). There is little difference in the shape of the mandible in newborns, whose ramus is only minimally developed. The superior side of the ramus is at the same level as that of the mandibular body.

Facial growth differs between boys and girls. In boys, growth continues longer. Their adolescent growth spurt occurs later, is greater, and lasts longer than that of girls. They develop a larger and straighter face (Fig 9-16). The individual variation in facial growth is great, not only in direction but also in the rate over the years.[29] After adulthood is reached, a small amount of facial growth still occurs.[30,31] There is also a difference between the sexes in this phase of growth (Fig 9-17).

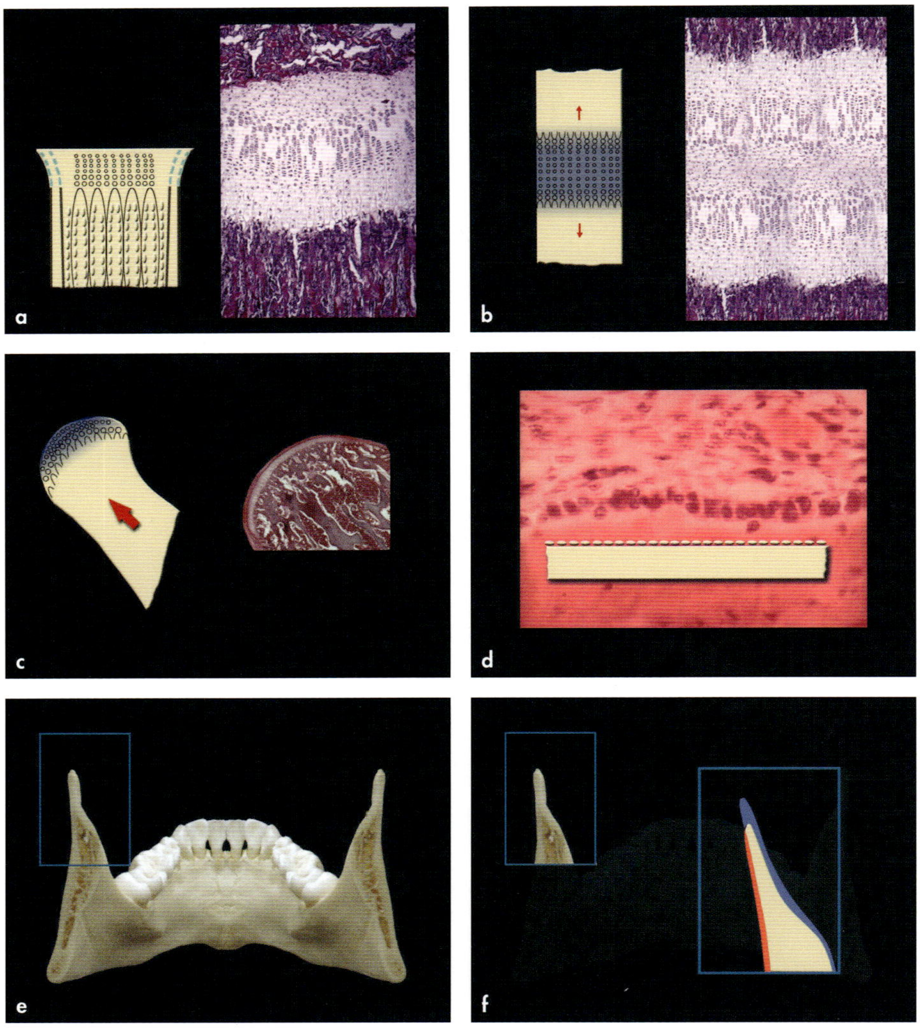

FIG 9-18 Modalities of fast elongation of bony structures. Epiphyseal disks in long bones contain chondrocytes, which can proliferate quickly. They deposit interstitial matrix, which drives the chondrocytes apart. Following hypertrophy of these cells, part of the extracellular matrix is resorbed, and only the partitions remain. Subsequently, bone is deposited on them. *(a)* This happens in an epiphyseal disk only in the direction of the diaphysis. *(b)* In a synchondrosis, it occurs in the two opposite directions. *(c)* At the condyles, the cartilage zone lies directly under the connective tissue layer that covers the half-round condylar head. *(d)* The potential for perpendicular bone growth at a surface is limited. *(e and f)* Elongation of tapering, sharp-ended structures can occur quickly because the osteoblasts are oriented at a slight angle to the growth direction. That is the case in the wedge-shaped structure of the mandibular ramus anterior to the condyle. The apposition of bone *(blue)* is accompanied by resorption *(red)*; this is the process of remodeling.

Characteristics of cartilage and bone

The growth of the skeleton is realized by chondrocytes, osteoblasts, and osteoclasts. Osteoblasts create bone. These ellipsoid-shaped surface cells have a limited capacity for matrix deposition, about 10 µm a day, which adds up to 3.6 mm a year.[33,34] Osteoclasts are large multinuclear cells that can, especially if they are numerous, break down a significant amount of bone in a short period of time. Bone is calcified and cannot grow internally, whereas cartilage can. Cartilage is not vascularized but depends on diffusion of tissue fluid.

Long bones have cartilaginous epiphyseal disks by which they can increase substantially in length in a short period of time. This occurs through interstitial growth of the cartilage by chondroblast proliferation and extracellular matrix production. Subsequently, the cartilage matrix mineralizes and is replaced by bone through endochondral ossification. This compensates for the limited capacity for bone apposition on surfaces. The same phenomenon takes place in synchondroses and the mandibular condyles (Figs 9-18a to 9-18c). Because cartilage growth is equally intensive over the whole width of an epiphyseal disk and a synchondrosis, the bone enlarges perpendicular to these structures. The situation is different in the condyles, where the growth direction can vary because of local differences in mitotic activity of the chondrocytes.

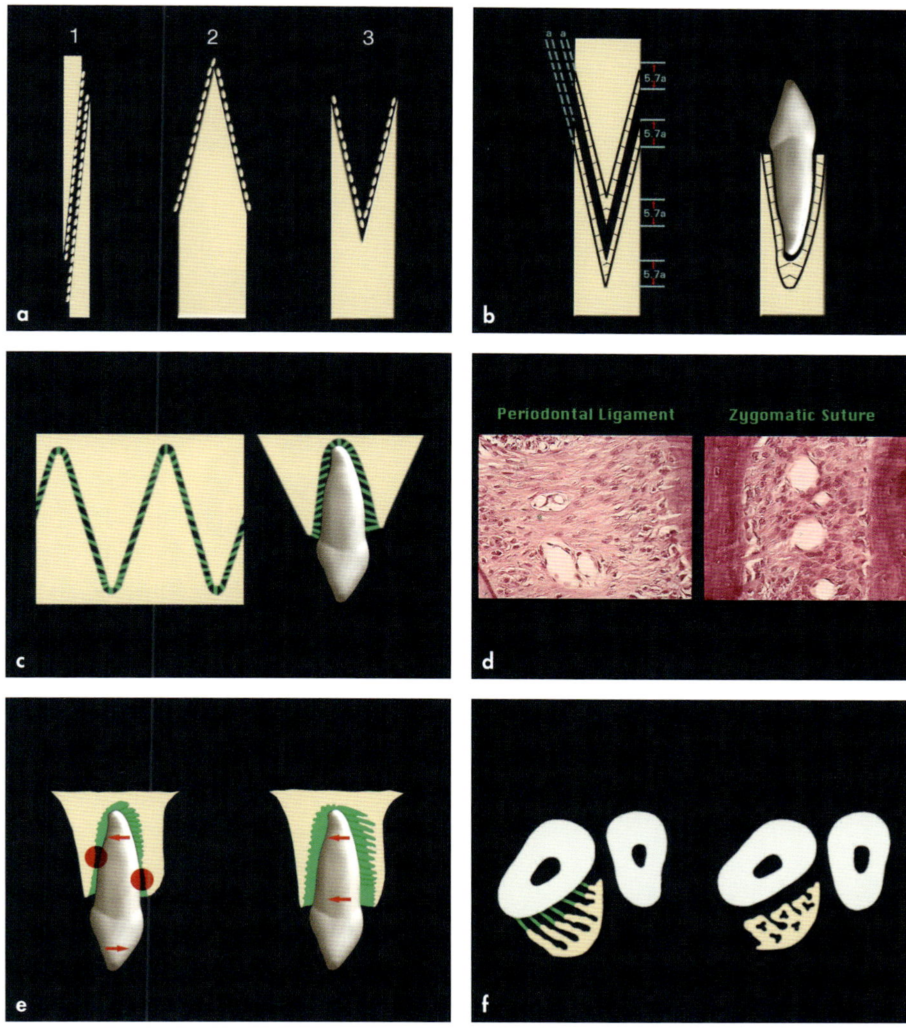

FIG 9-19 Similarities of sutures and alveoles. *(a)* Overlapping sutures can grow quickly if the bone ends lay against each other with a sharp angle (1). That also applies to tapering sharp-ended structures (2) and alveoles (3). *(b)* Osteoblasts differentiated from mesenchymal cells extend the tips of the bone. Osteoblasts arranged along the opposing surfaces fill in the space that develops when the two bones move apart lengthwise. *(c)* The orientation of the osteoblasts in a suture resembles that in a periodontal ligament, although that bone is deposited only on one side. *(d)* Sections of a periodontal ligament *(left)* and a zygomaticomaxillary suture *(right)* of a rhesus monkey demonstrate the histologic similarities. (Courtesy of B. J. Moffett). *(e)* Rapid bone formation can also occur as fibers attached to bone are stretched. Subsequently, spicules are created, which are obliquely oriented to the growth direction and on which matrix is deposited. That also happens as teeth are tipped, moved bodily, or rotated. *(f)* Subsequently the bone is reorganized, and the spaces in between are filled up.

The limited capacity for bone apposition by osteoblasts at a surface (Fig 9-18d) can also be compensated by increasing the surface area on which osteoblasts can lay down bone matrix. That is the case in tapering, sharp-ended structures such as the anterior part of the superior border of the mandibular ramus, where the osteoblasts are not oriented perpendicularly but obliquely at the growth direction (Figs 9-18e and 9-18f). It can also be effectuated by sutures that overlap over a long distance such as in the squamosal suture, between the temporal and the parietal bone, or by sutures with many sharp extensions and notches on their contact surfaces, the so-called interdigitating sutures (Figs 9-19a to 9-19d). Indeed, in interdigitating sutures, the bones are laying close together over a large surface through numerous extensions and notches. The space that otherwise should arise between the bones as the two sides of the suture shift apart is filled up by osteoblasts arranged along the opposing surfaces. The elongation of sharp ends occurs through bone formation by osteoblasts, which differentiate from mesenchymal cells. The fast eruption of teeth and the building up of alveolar processes is based on the same mechanism as the growth at sutures. That also applies to some extent to movements of teeth within the jaws (Figs 9-19e and 9-19f).

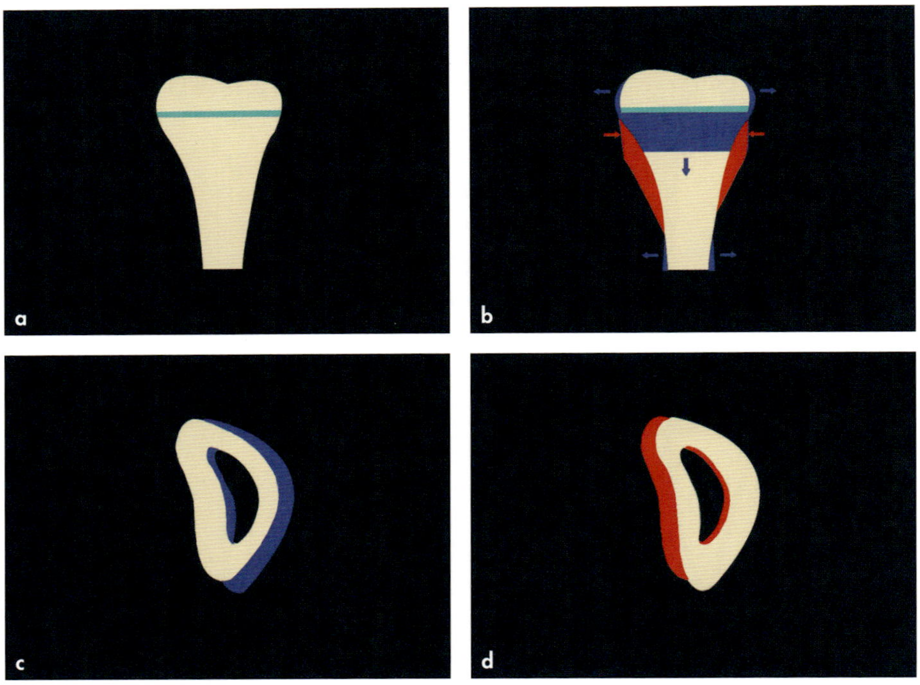

Fig 9-20 Remodeling of separate bones. *(a and b)* An epiphyseal disk of a long bone can grow rapidly *(blue)*. Resorption *(red)* takes care of the preservation of the shape. *(c and d)* Translation of skeletal parts, such as the zygomatic bone, is caused by local apposition *(blue)* and resorption *(red)*. In that way, a skeletal part can move laterally without losing its position in relation to adjacent bones, which in this case would be the maxilla and the temporal bone.

On the other hand, growth sites such as the spheno-occipital synchondrosis and the mandibular condyle rely on the potential of rapid interstitional proliferation of cartilage cells. The cartilage growth at the condyle differs from that in the synchondroses, as it is found only directly underneath the articular surface of the condyle. This enables changes in growth direction, which are not possible in synchondroses. In addition, apposition and resorption of bone at surfaces (bone remodeling) provides an important contribution to the growth of the facial skeleton.

Bone remodeling is described by Enlow as the process of local apposition and resorption of bone at outer and inner surfaces through which a bone or combination of bones can grow with preservation of shape.[35] That applies, for example, to a long bone, to the cheekbone (Fig 9-20), and to the maxilla, as well as to the facial complex as a whole (Fig 9-21). The bone remodeling of the face differs among individuals and is related to the variation in growth patterns.[37]

Position of teeth

As described previously, the growth and development of the facial complex can be considered as a system with three entities: skeleton, dentition, and function. The influence of functional components determines to a large extent the degree and direction of the growth of the facial skeleton. In combination with other functional components, this determines the position of the teeth.

Incisors have, as with all other teeth, the possibility to move slightly if they are exposed to pressure. Indeed, one of the functional features of the dentition is the physiologic movement of teeth that depends on stretching and compression of the periodontium and on bending of the marginal alveolar bone (see video clip 27).

The incisors are the teeth with the largest diversity in position. The attaining and maintaining of the position of the incisors depend on the size, shape, and position of the tongue and lips. An equilibrium exists as the forces exerted on the teeth and surrounding structures are in balance and active for a long period of time[38,39] (Fig 9-22). In that equilibrium, periodontal ligaments have a special function. They provide the extra resistance against the labial displacement of maxillary incisors that otherwise should happen because the pressure exerted by the tongue is greater than that of the lips. In situations of periodontal breakdown, the incisors become displaced (Fig 9-23).

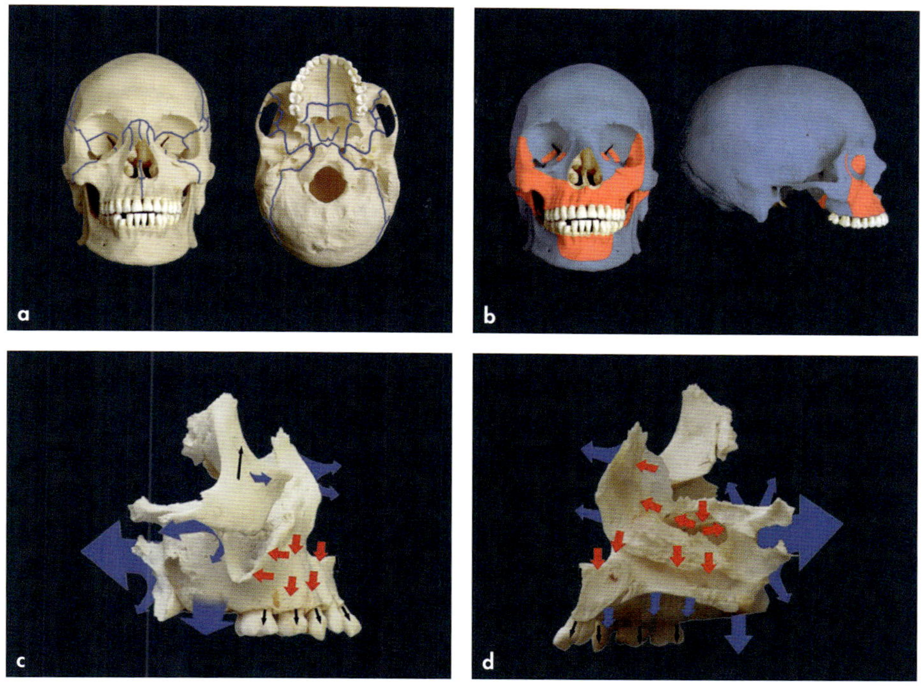

FIG 9-21 Remodeling of the craniofacial skeleton. *(a)* The skull has many bones. Between most of them are sutures where growth can take place. *(b)* Apposition *(blue)* and resorption *(red)* contribute to growth and also preserve the shape of the bone. *(c)* While the maxilla extends laterally by apposition of bone at the outer surface and resorption at the inner surface, its anterior contour moves posteriorly through resorption. *(d)* In the meantime, the maxilla as a whole translates to the anterior.[35,36]

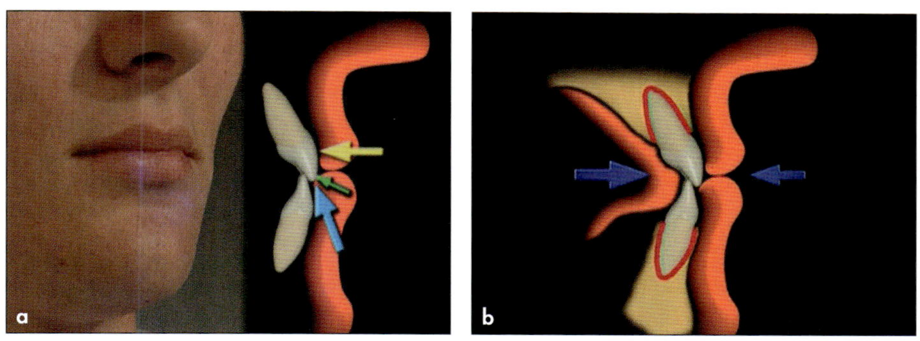

FIG 9-22 Equilibrium in the anterior region. *(a)* Normally, the lower lip covers 2 to 3 mm of the maxillary incisors and supports them vertically. The upper lip lies against the maxillary incisors. *(b)* The force of the tongue on the incisors is greater than that of the lips—approximately 15 and 5 Ncm, respectively. The periodontal ligament provides resistance against tooth displacement.[38–40]

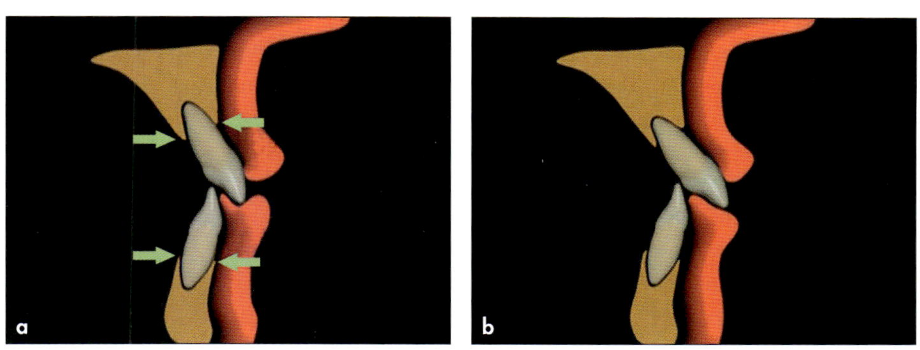

FIG 9-23 Displacement of incisors following breakdown of the periodontal ligament. *(a)* With severe loss, the maxillary incisors tip forward and elongate, and the mandibular incisors elongate. *(b)* With interposition of the lower lip, the displacements are greater. See video clips 28 and 29.

Effects of Orofacial Functional Factors on the Facial Complex

In the preceding paragraphs, it is frequently stated that functional components dominate in the growth of the face and the development of the dentition. The following text discusses the activities in the orofacial region in general and indicates which of them have an effect on facial growth and development of the dentition.

As mentioned before, there is a variation in the timing and rate at which the various structures of the facial complex grow and mature, and the same also applies to the tissues involved. For example, the lymphoid tissues of the adenoids and tonsils are large in early childhood and decrease in size during puberty. In children, the tongue is also large in comparison with the volume of the oral cavity. In babies, the tongue is positioned between the jaws and in contact with the lips and cheeks. Only after the deciduous teeth have emerged does the tongue attain a position inside the dental arches.

The most essential and vital activity of the orofacial region is breathing. Babies cannot breathe through the mouth. Instead, the position and movements of the trachea and esophagus temporarily facilitate the ability to breathe and swallow simultaneously. In children and adults, the lips are closed most of the time, and in breathing the air passes through the nose. With physical activity and increased need for oxygen in the blood, breathing will also occur through the mouth.

The size of the nostrils is the restricting factor in the amount of air that can pass through the nose.[40] Excessive mouth breathing is usually the effect of a limitation in the nasal passage, mostly due to allergies or other causes that lead to swelling of the nasal mucosa. It can also be due to a septum deviation, sometimes caused by trauma, or to nasal polyps. In young children, enlarged and infected adenoids and tonsils often limit the nasal passage. Long-lasting abnormal breathing modes affect the position of the tongue, lips, and teeth and the condition of the hard and soft tissues.

Swallowing is another highly important activity in the orofacial region. Swallowing movements can be distinguished in three modes: the infantile, the transitional, and the adult pattern. In an infantile swallow, the mouth is not closed off, and the tongue is positioned anteriorly between the jaws or teeth. In the transitional swallow, the mouth is closed and the tongue brought forward. In the adult swallow, the tongue stays inside the dental arches, and the lips do not move or only slightly. The swallowing movement is complex and can be divided into an oral phase and a pharyngeal phase[41] (Fig 9-24).

It generally holds true that to affect the morphology of the facial skeleton and the position of the teeth, a constant pressure must be exerted for at least 6 hours a day. Only then is the equilibrium of the forces exerted on the dentition disturbed. Consequently, swallowing does not affect tooth position and facial morphology. A swallowing act lasts only 1 second. With a frequency of 600 to 900 swallowing movements a day, the total time does not exceed 10 to 15 minutes,[42,43] which is not nearly enough to have any effect. Hence, a deviating swallowing mode cannot cause an open bite or nonocclusion.[44] The swallowing movement adapts to the existing morphologic situation rather than the other way around. In an open bite or nonocclusion the tongue has to be brought forward and in contact with the lips to realize the anterior sealing of the mouth, a requirement for swallowing.

Chewing, another activity of the orofacial region, also has no effect on tooth position. The forces involved are too varied and too short in duration. The same applies to speaking, a learned activity with a large variety of movements. In speaking, only incidental small forces are exerted at various points. Even in someone who speaks 6 hours a day, the tongue is only in contact with the teeth a fraction of that time. As a side note, only a small correlation exists between the morphology of the dentoalveolar structures and the quality of speech. Individuals with excellent occlusion may have impaired speech, and those with severe malocclusion do not necessarily have speech problems.

Habits such as digit sucking, if practiced 6 to 10 hours a day, lead to deviations in tooth positions and in the shape and position of the maxilla. However, if these habits are discontinued in due time, the deviations correct spontaneously, unless another factor prevents it.

Indeed, the equilibrium in the orofacial region, particularly the position of the teeth, depends on long-lasting factors. The position of the tongue at rest is the most important element in this regard, directly followed by the lips and cheeks—although the forces they exert are relatively minor. Together with the morphology of the facial skeleton and the occlusion, they determine to a large extent the position of the teeth.

An exception to the rule that a small force can alter the position of a tooth only if it lasts 6 to 10 hours a day[39] is the guiding of the eruption direction by the cone-funnel mechanism. That also applies to the rail mechanism. Another exception is an erupting tooth that has to avoid an obstacle in the dental arch, ie, when there is a shortage of space that results in tooth rotations and positions outside the dental arch. For the guidance of the eruption direction, incidental occlusal contacts are sufficient as they occur at every swallow and bite. That also applies to the migration of teeth in the preservation of the relation between the dental arches in growing jaws. In the absence of eruption, only long-lasting forces result in tooth displacements.

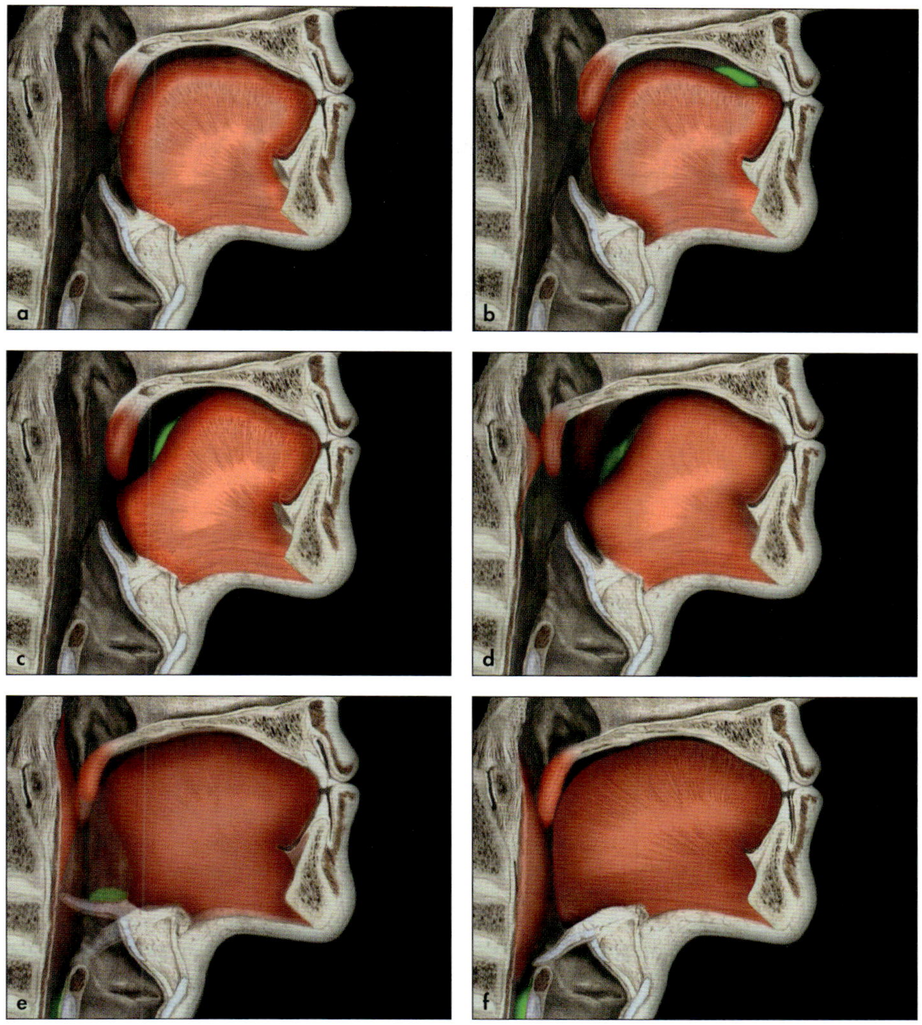

Fig 9-24 When a normal adult swallows, the lips move only slightly or not at all, and the tongue stays inside the dental arches. *(a and b)* The movement starts with the tongue behind the maxillary incisors and against the palate. *(c and d)* Subsequently, the dental arches are occluded, and the posterior part of the tongue starts the reflective movement that transports the bolus in the direction of the esophagus. *(e and f)* The oral phase is followed by the pharyngeal phase. Surrounding and more inferiorly located structures are also involved in the swallowing act. See video clip 30.

In Fig 9-25, the influence of the various factors described above is summarized and expressed on a time scale. Interposition of the tongue at rest lasts longer than 17 hours a day and hence affects tooth position and facial morphology and results in lack of adequate occlusal contact in the involved region. The lip position plays a comparable role; the lips are at rest more than 17 hours and exert a continuous pressure.

It is evident that a disturbance in the balanced interplay of forces, as in long-lasting digit sucking, has an unfavorable effect on the development of the dentition and on facial growth.[45] That also applies to a lesser extent to the continuous restriction of the nasal passage as caused by enlarged adenoids.[46–49]

In conclusion, in the short term, functional activities in the oral cavity adapt to form; in the long term, functional activities affect the structural form through long-lasting pressures on teeth and bony structures.

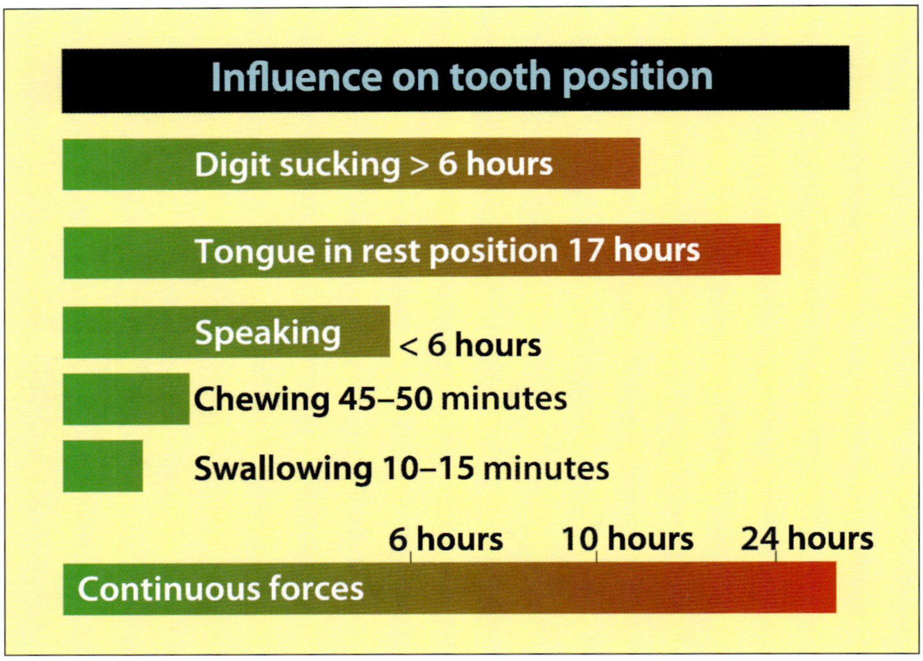

FIG 9-25 The influence of various activities on the position of teeth and on the morphology of the facial skeleton, expressed in terms of the length of duration. The tongue and lip position at rest is the most important factor. If the tongue lies between opposing teeth, an open bite and/or nonocclusion will result. Other activities, with the exception of long-lasting digit sucking, have no effect.

Concluding Remarks

Indeed, the development of the dentition and facial growth are complex processes. That applies particularly to the phase of ontogenesis and to a lesser extent to the subsequent growth and development. Within the growing face, the dentition develops in its typical way. The teeth are the hardest structures in the body and take the longest time to form. The permanent incisors mineralize before the deciduous ones start to erupt. The skeletal changes are realized by proliferation of cartilage and apposition and resorption of bone at surfaces. These changes are initiated primarily by functional factors, which also are partly responsible for the variations encountered in facial size and shape. The space available for the development of the two sets of teeth is confined to the apical areas. Under favorable conditions, the development of the dentition proceeds harmoniously and ends with satisfactory alignment and occlusion of the permanent teeth. However, the size of the skeletal structures is often too small to allow favorable development of the dentition, with malocclusion as a result.

Functional aspects play a major role in the development of the dentition and in facial growth. The interactions of functional components with the skeleton and dentition largely determine the end product. With solid intercuspation, the opposing dental arches shift in coordination within the growing face. If such intercuspation is missing, the opposing dental arches shift independently.

References

1. Hrdlička A. Shovel-shaped teeth. Am J Phys Anthropol 1920;3:429–465.
2. Peck S, Peck H. Orthodontic aspects of dental anthropology. Angle Orthod 1975;45:95–102.
3. Van der Linden FPGM. The future of orthodontics: Overview and discussion. In: Carels C, Willems G (eds). The Future of Orthodontics. Leuven, Belgium: Leuven University Press, 1998:273–281.
4. Peck H, Peck S. An index for assessing tooth shape deviations as applied to the mandibular incisors. Am J Orthod 1972;61:384–401.
5. Begg PR. Stone Age man's dentition. Am J Orthod 1954;40:298–312,373–383,462–475,517–531.
6. Corruccini RS. Australian aboriginal tooth succession, interproximal attrition, and Begg's theory. Am J Orthod Dentofacial Orthop 1990;97:349–357.
7. Moore AW. The mechanism of adjustment to wear and accident in the dentition and periodontium. Angle Orthod 1956;26:50–58.
8. Southard TE, Behrents RG, Tolley EA. The anterior component of occlusal force. I. Measurement and distribution. Am J Orthod Dentofacial Orthop 1989;96:493–500.
9. Picton DC, Moss JP. The part played by the trans-septal fibre system in experimental approximal drift of the cheek teeth of monkeys *(Macaca irus)*. Arch Oral Biol 1973;18:669–680.
10. Van der Linden FPGM, Radlanski RJ, McNamara JA Jr. Dynamics of Orthodontics: Normal Development of the Dentition [DVD 3A]. Berlin: Quintessence, 2000.
11. Brace CL. Occlusion to the anthropological eye. In: McNamara JA Jr (ed). The Biology of Occlusal Development, monograph 7, Craniofacial Growth Series. Ann Arbor: University of Michigan, 1977:179–209.
12. Krarup S, Darvann TA, Larsen P, Marsh JL, Kreiborg S. Three-dimensional analysis of mandibular growth and tooth eruption. J Anat 2005;207:669–682.
13. Vig PS, Cohen AM. Vertical growth of the lips: A serial cephalometric study. Am J Orthod 1979;75:405–415.
14. Ostyn JM, Maltha JC, Van 't Hof MA, Van der Linden FPGM. The role of intercuspation in the regulation of transverse maxillary development in *Macaca fascicularis*. Angle Orthod 1995;65:215–222.
15. Solow B. The dentoalveolar compensatory mechanism: Background and clinical implications. Br J Orthod 1980;7:145–161.
16. Solow B. Die dentoalveoläre Kompennsation: Grundlagen und klinische Bedeutung. Inf Orthod Kieferorthop 2006;38:148–162.
17. Ishikawa H, Nakamura S, Iwasaki H, Kitazawa S, Tsukada H, Chu S. Dentoalveolar compensation in negative overjet cases. Angle Orthod 2000;70:145–148.
18. Tollaro I, Baccetti T, Defraia E. Dentoalveolar compensation to sagittal skeletal discrepancies in the primary dentition. Eur J Paediatr Dent 2000;1:21–25.
19. Jensen BL, Kreiborg S. Craniofacial growth in cleidocranial dysplasia—A roentgencephalometric study. J Craniofac Genet Dev Biol 1995;15:35–43.
20. Björk A. Sutural growth of the upper face studied by the implant method. Trans Eur Orthod Soc 1964;40:48–64.
21. Björk A, Skieller V. Facial development and tooth eruption. Am J Orthod 1972;62:339–383.
22. Van der Linden FPGM. The development of long and short faces, and their limitations in treatment. In: McNamara JA Jr (ed). The Enigma of the Vertical Dimension, monograph 36, Craniofacial Growth Series. Ann Arbor: University of Michigan, 2000:61–73.
23. McNamara JA Jr, Van der Linden FPGM. Vertical dimension. In: McNamara JA Jr, Brudon WL. Orthodontics and Dentofacial Orthopedics. Ann Arbor: Needham, 2001:111–148.
24. Björk A. Facial growth in man, studied with the aid of metallic implants. Acta Odontol Scand 1955;13:9–34.
25. Björk A. Variations in the growth pattern of the human mandible: Longitudinal radiographic study by the implant method. J Dent Res 1963;42:400–411.
26. Björk A. Kæbernes relation til det øvrige kranium. In: Lundström A (ed). Nordisk Lärobok i Orthodonti, ed 4. Stockholm: Sveriges Tandläkarforbunds Förlagsförening, 1975:69–110.
27. Fredriks AM, Van Buuren S, Burgmeijer RJF, et al. Continuing positive secular growth change in the Netherlands 1955-1997. Pediatr Res 2000;47:316–323.
28. Broadbent BH Sr, Broadbent BH Jr, Golden WH. Bolton Standards of Dentofacial Developmental Growth. St Louis: Mosby, 1975.
29. Buschang PH. Craniofacial growth and development. In: English JD, Peltomäki T, Pham-Litschel K (eds). Mosby's Orthodontic Review. St Louis: Mosby, 2008:1–12.
30. Forsberg CM. Facial morphology and ageing: A longitudinal cephalometric investigation of young adults. Eur J Orthod 1979;1:15–23.
31. West KS, McNamara JA Jr. Changes in the craniofacial complex from adolescence to midadulthood: A cephalometric study. Am J Orthod Dentofacial Orthop 1999;115:521–532.
32. Behrents RG. Growth in the Aging Craniofacial Skeleton, monograph 17, Craniofacial Growth Series. Ann Arbor: University of Michigan, 1985.
33. Baylink D, Morey E, Rich C. Effect of calcitonin on the rates of bone formation and resorption in the rat. Endocrinology 1969;84:261–269.
34. Baylink D, Wergedal J, Thompson E. Loss of proteinpolysaccharides at sites where bone mineralisation is initiated. J Histochem Cytochem 1972;20:279–292.
35. Enlow DH. Handbook of Facial Growth. Philadelphia: Saunders, 1975.
36. Enlow DH, Bang S. Growth and remodeling of the human maxilla. Am J Orthod 1965;51:446–464.
37. Kurihara S, Enlow DH, Rangel RD. Remodeling reversals in anterior parts of the human mandible and maxilla. Angle Orthod 1980;50:98–107.
38. Proffit WR. Equilibrium theory revisited: Factors influencing position of the teeth. Angle Orthod 1978;48:175–186.
39. Weinstein S, Haack DC, Morris LY, Snyder BB, Attaway HE. On an equilibrium theory of tooth position. Angle Orthod 1963;33:1–11.
40. Proffit WR. Contemporary Orthodontics, ed 4. St Louis: Mosby, 2008.
41. Proffit WR. Lingual pressure patterns in the transition from tongue thrust to adult swallowing. Arch Oral Biol 1972;17:555–563.
42. Lear CSC, Flanagan JB, Moorrees CFA. The frequency of deglutition in man. Arch Oral Biol 1965;10:83–99.
43. Neff CW. Frequency of Deglutition of Tongue Thrusters Compared to a Sample Population of Normal Swallowers [thesis]. Seattle: University of Washington, 1964.
44. Mason RM, Proffit WF. The tongue thrust controversy: Background and recommendations. J Speech Hear Disord 1974;39:115–132.
45. Moore MB, McDonald JP. A cephalometric evaluation of patients presenting with persistent digit sucking habits. Br J Orthod 1997;24:17–23.

46. Linder-Aronson S. Adenoids. Their effect on mode of breathing and nasal airflow and their relationship to characteristics of the facial skeleton and dentition. A biometric, rhino-manometric and cepahlometro-radiographic study on children with and without adenoids. Acta Otolaryngol Scand Suppl 1970;265:1–132.
47. Linder-Aronson S. Respiratory function in relation to facial morphology and the dentition. Br J Orthod 1979;6:59–71.
48. McNamara JA. Influences of respiratory pattern on craniofacial growth. Angle Orthod 1981;51:269–300.
49. Vig KWL. Nasal obstruction and facial growth: The strength of evidence for clinical assumptions. Am J Orthod Dentofacial Orthop 1998;113:603–611.

10

Abnormalities of the Dental Arches

Arch Length Discrepancy

A difference between the needed and available arch length, called arch length discrepancy (ALD), is the most common abnormality of the dental arches. It may manifest as either crowding or spacing. In crowding, the teeth are too large or the dental arch is too small to allow satisfactory alignment of the teeth. In spacing, the opposite situation exists. The terms crowding and spacing apply regardless of whether it is the teeth or the arch (or both) that contribute to the abnormality.

Crowding

Symptoms of crowding are deviating tooth positions such as rotated and overlapping teeth, tooth emergence inside or outside the dental arch, and impaction due to lack of space (Fig 10-1). Crowding is rare in the deciduous dentition, but quite frequent in later phases of development. In adults crowding in the mandibular anterior region is not uncommon.

Crowding is distinguished into three types: primary, secondary, and tertiary.[1] Primary crowding refers to the crowding caused by the genetically determined size discrepancy between the teeth and the jaw that contains them. Secondary crowding is the shortage of space that can manifest after extraction of deciduous teeth through migration of neighboring teeth into the open space. It also includes crowding caused by deviating functional conditions. Tertiary crowding refers to irregularities developing in the mandibular—and sometimes slightly in the maxillary—anterior region during early adulthood and later.

Spacing

Spacing is characterized by diastemata and is usually not accompanied by misalignment of teeth. In contrast to crowding, spacing does not occur often, and when it does, it is seen mostly in the anterior regions (Fig 10-2).

Deviations in number, size, and shape of teeth

Teeth can be large or small in relation to the size of head. When teeth are relatively large, there will be crowding or a domination of the dentition in the face, ie, protrusion of the incisors, or a combination of both. With relatively small teeth, there will be spacing or retrusion of the anterior teeth, resulting in a posterior position of the lips in relation to the nose and chin (ie, a dished-in profile), or a combination of both.

There can be too few or too many teeth formed, and crown size and shape can be abnormal. In the deciduous dentition, deviations in tooth number are rare; in the permanent dentition, they happen quite often and more in women than in men.[2] Third molars in both jaws are the teeth most often not formed, followed by mandibular second premolars and maxillary lateral incisors[3] (Fig 10-3). Agenesis of other teeth also may occur. In some cases, more than one tooth may be missing. The prevalence of ageneses is presented in chapter 17, Table 17-31. Deciduous teeth without successors, such as mandibular second molars, resorb little and can be preserved until old age.[5]

If more than six teeth are missing, it is called oligodontia; if all are missing, the term anodontia is used. The prevalence of oligodontia is 0.14%; that of anodontia is much lower.[2,6,7] Anodontia is accompanied by a "sunken-in" face and reduced anterior facial height.[8,9] Supernumerary teeth (Fig 10-4) can occur in any region, but especially in the anterior maxilla, and more often in the permanent than the deciduous dentition.[13,14] In some syndromes, such as cleidocranial dysostosis, multiple supernumerary teeth are present. The most frequently appearing supernumerary tooth is a small, cone-shaped tooth that is present in various orientations between the maxillary central incisors (mesiodens).[15] In some cases, two mesiodentes may develop.[10,11,16] A mesiodens can lead to delayed emergence and deviating positions of central incisors and to a large central diastema.[17]

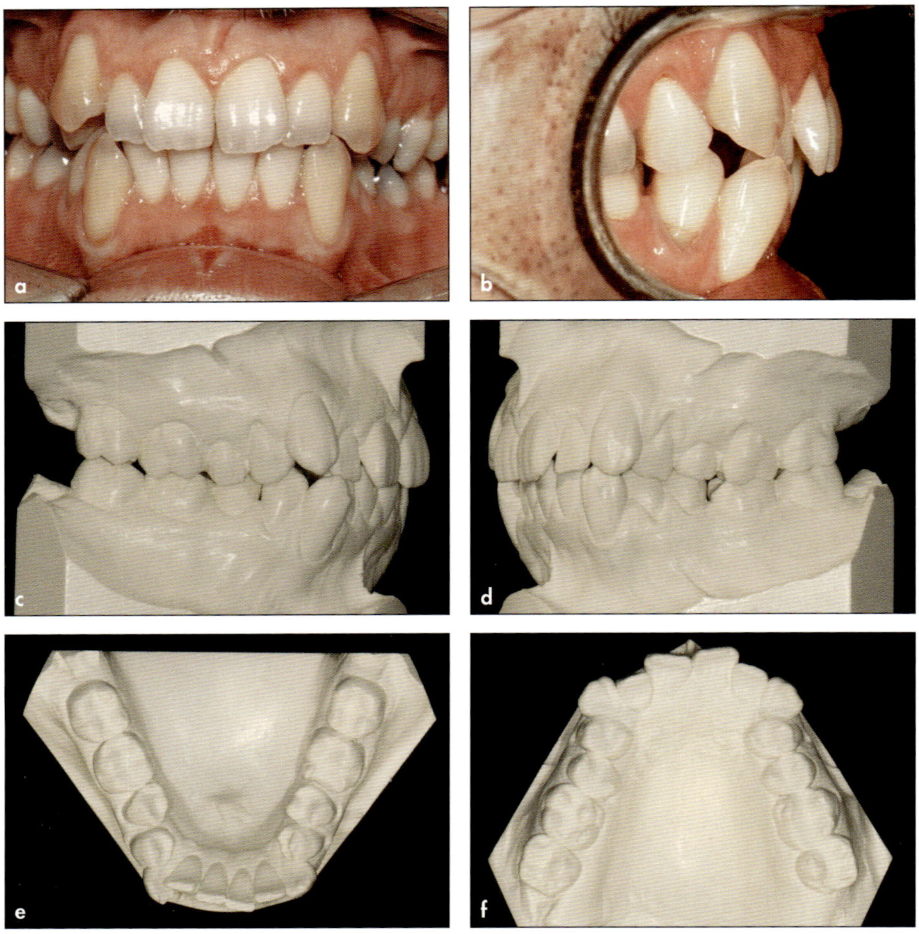

Fig 10-1 *(a to f)* Crowding in both dental arches. Crowding is mainly concentrated in the anterior parts of the dental arches and in the third molar region.

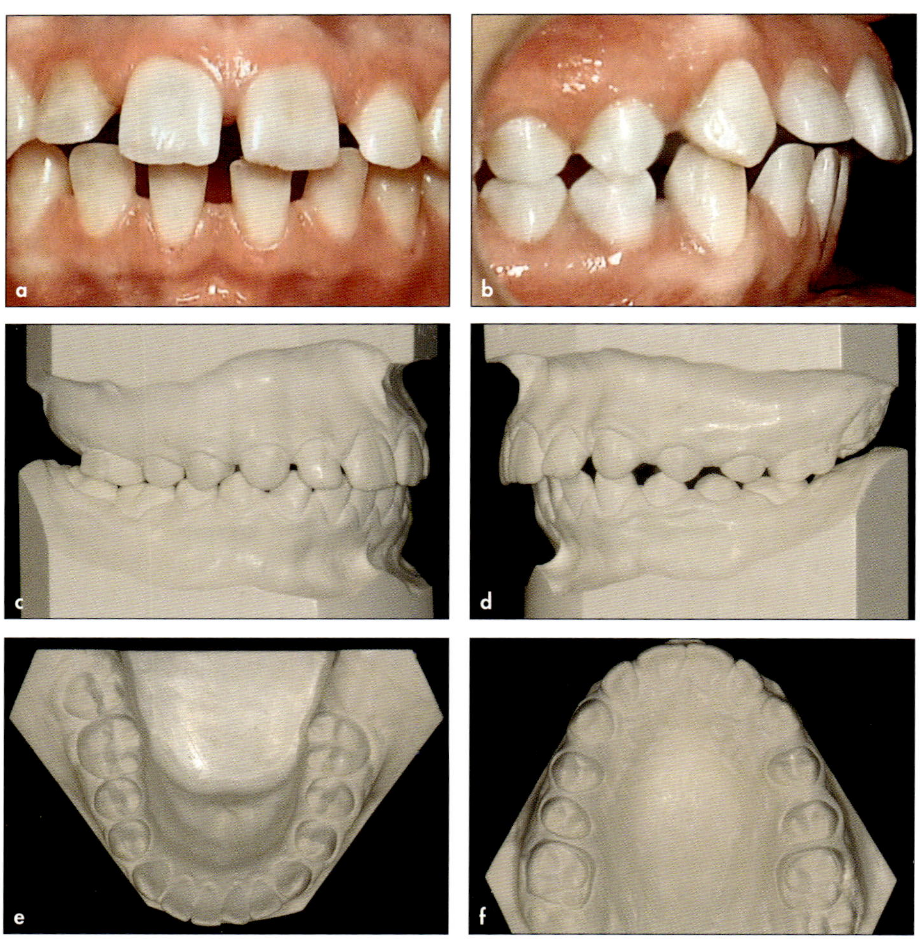

Fig 10-2 *(a to f)* Spacing in both dental arches. Spacing occurs most frequently in the maxillary anterior region and to a lesser degree in the mandibular anterior region. Diastemata between all teeth are rare.

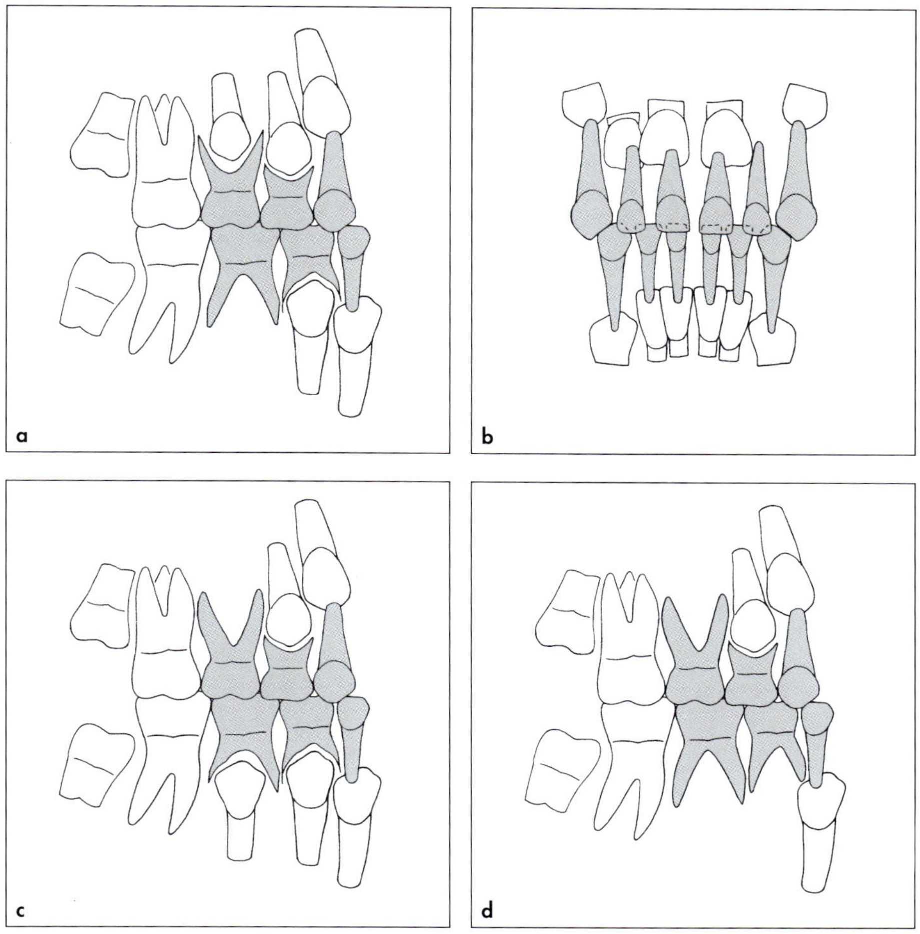

FIG 10-3 Agenesis of permanent teeth. *(a)* In the mandible, the third molar is most frequently not formed (20%), followed by the second premolar (4.4%). *(b and c)* In the maxilla, the third molar is also most frequently not formed (21%), followed by the lateral permanent incisor (1.7%) and second premolar (1.6%).[3,4] *(d)* Example of multiple ageneses.

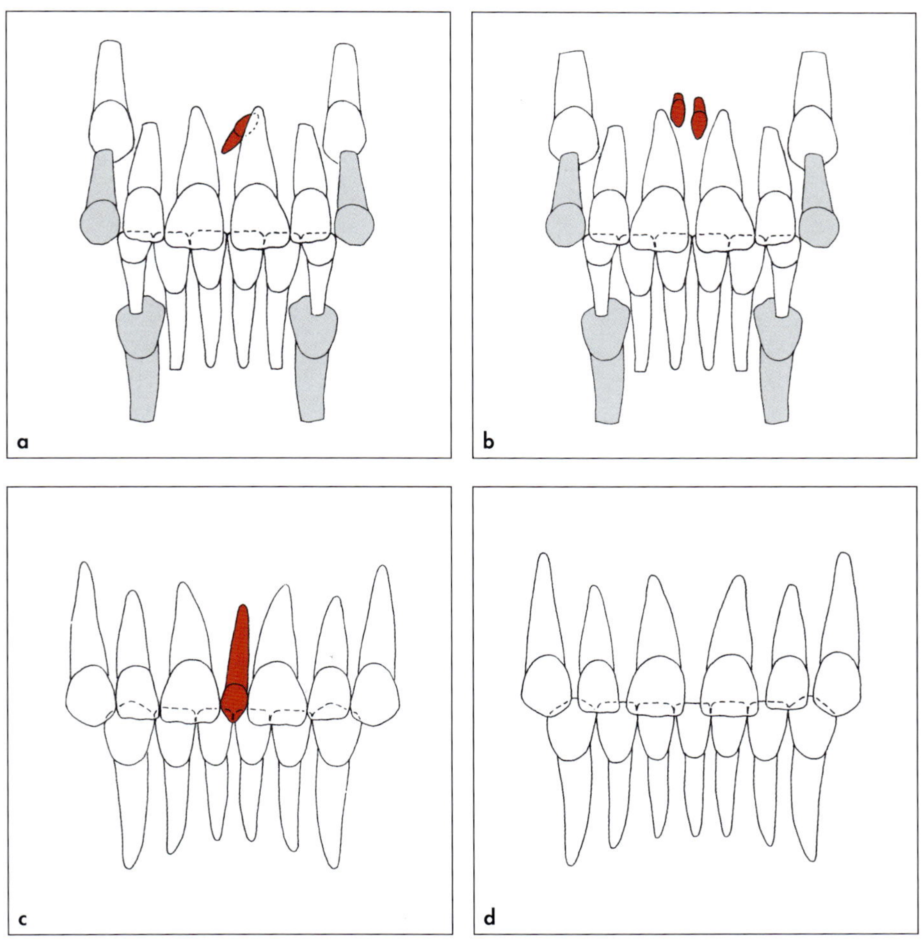

FIG 10-4 Supernumerary teeth. In about 1% of the population, twice as often in men than in women, an extra tooth is formed in the median region of the maxilla.[10–12] *(a)* A small, cone-shaped mesiodens situated partially palatal to the maxillary left central incisor. *(b)* Two mesiodentes. *(c)* An extra maxillary central incisor, deviating in size and shape but emerging normally. *(d)* Five mandibular incisors, all normal in size and shape.

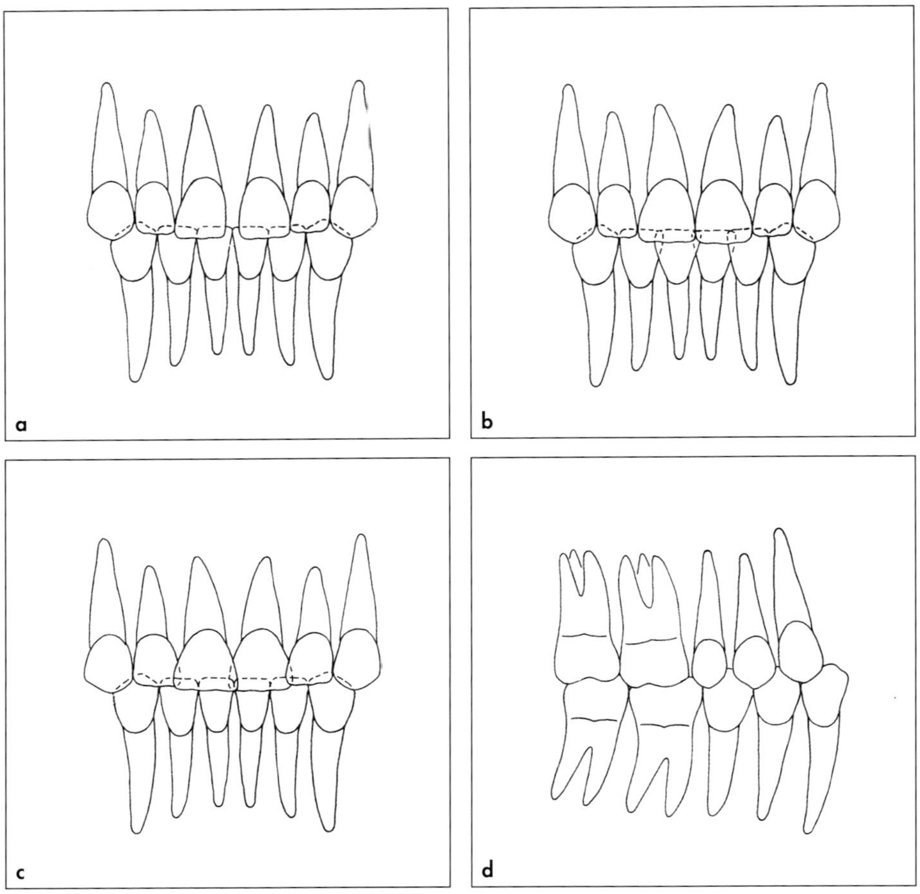

FIG 10-5 Examples of TSD. *(a)* Relatively narrow maxillary incisors (or broad mandibular incisors). *(b)* Crowding of mandibular incisors, which are too broad in comparison with the maxillary incisors. *(c)* Crowded, relatively broad maxillary incisors. *(d)* Diastema due to a narrow maxillary premolar. TSD occurs in 20% of the population, usually involving the incisors. It is more common to have relatively narrow maxillary teeth (or relatively broad mandibular teeth) than vice versa.[22]

Tooth size discrepancy

A maxillary lateral incisor crown that is too small is the most frequent deviation in tooth size. If one or more teeth in one dental arch are too wide or too narrow without compensation in the other arch, diastemata or crowding will result. This condition is called tooth size discrepancy (TSD)[18–21] (Fig 10-5). Deviations in crown shape usually only cause problems in the anterior region. Maxillary lateral incisors can have tapering, overly narrow crowns (ie, peg-shaped).

Disturbed Eruption and Nonemergence of Teeth

Disturbances in eruption such as ankylosis and primary failure of eruption can lead to specific anomalies (Fig 10-6). Ankylosis of deciduous molars can appear at an early stage.[23] Their eruption can be delayed to the point that they become squeezed in by adjacent teeth.[24] The resorption of the roots of ankylosed deciduous teeth is not affected. When the ankylosed region is resorbed, the tooth will erupt again unless it is squeezed in. Permanent teeth can also become ankylosed. Little is known about what causes ankylosis[23]; however, for permanent teeth, trauma has been suggested.[24]

In addition, permanent teeth can be impacted or retained. Third molars are the most frequently impacted teeth; this occurs because of shortage of space. Impacted teeth also can be caused by formation in an abnormal position, spontaneous migration, or displacement caused by trauma to their predecessor, which sometimes happens with maxillary central incisors. The maxillary permanent canine is the most frequently impacted tooth, occurring in 1.0% to 1.5% of the Western population.[15] There is a large variation in the position and orientation of impacted canines. They usually are situated palatally but sometimes may be buccally located. Their predecessors resorb little and can be maintained for many years. In addition to impaction, there are other reasons that teeth do not emerge,[25,26] some of which are demonstrated in the radiographs shown in Fig 10-7.

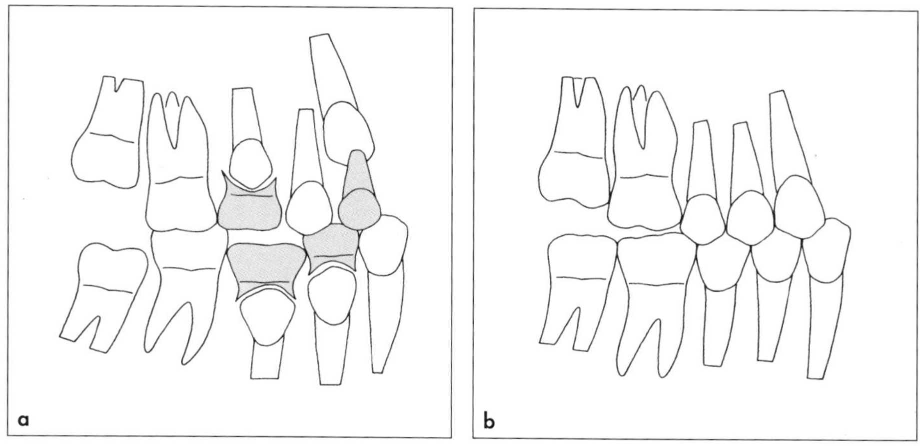

FIG 10-6 Teeth with arrested eruption. *(a)* The mandibular second deciduous molar is ankylosed and becomes submerged with the eruption of the adjacent teeth. *(b)* Primary failure of eruption of maxillary permanent molars.

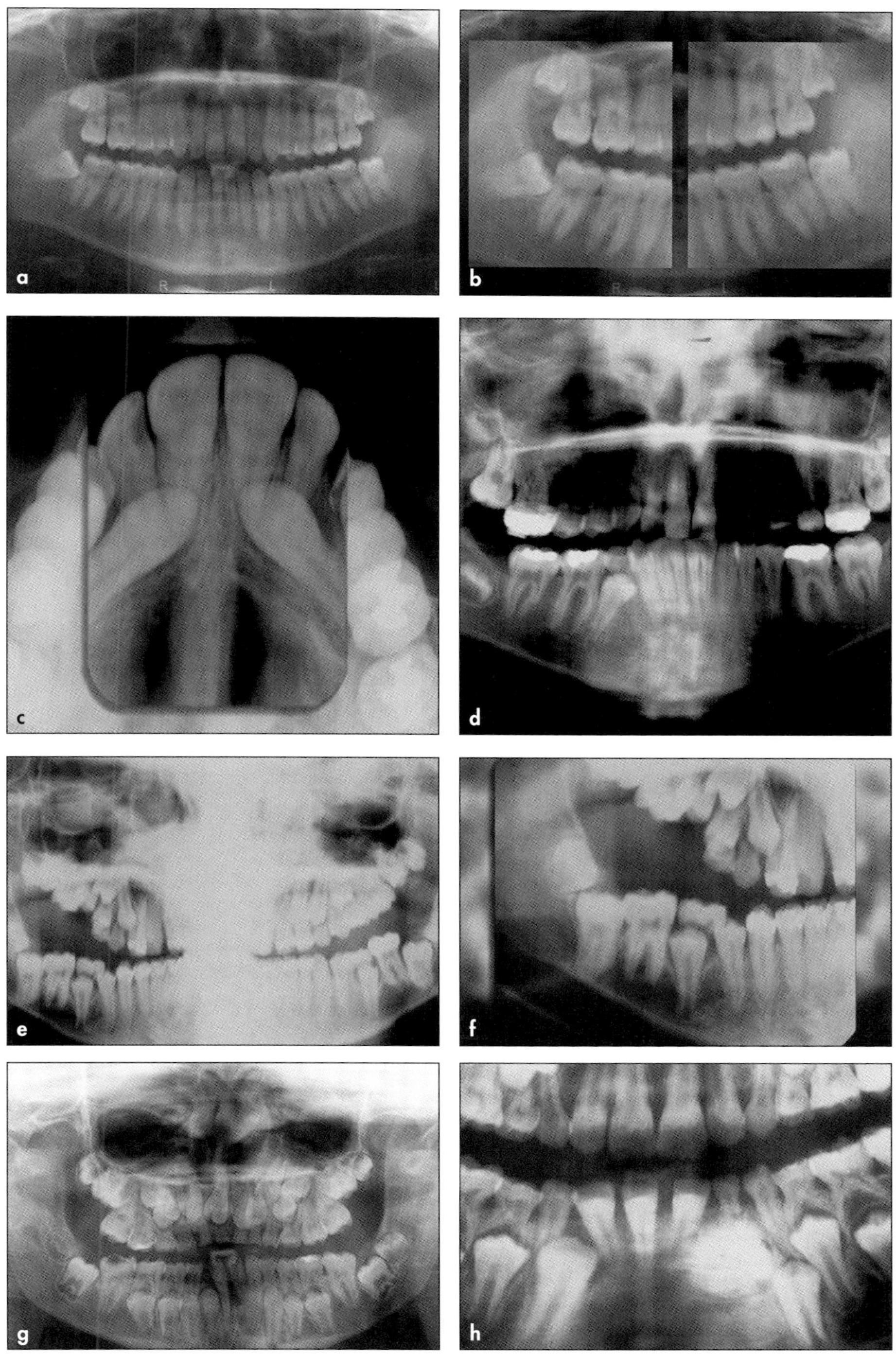

FIG 10-7 Radiographs of impacted and retained teeth. *(a and b)* Impaction of mandibular third molars due to lack of space. *(c)* Impacted maxillary canines, horizontally situated in the palate. *(d)* Retained mandibular right second premolar, caused by migration of adjacent teeth after premature loss of its predecessor. *(e and f)* Sometimes premolars and molars stop erupting even though they are not ankylosed, ie, primary failure of eruption. *(g)* Retarded eruption, late emergence, and supernumerary teeth in a case of cleidocranial dysostosis. *(h)* Odontogenic tumor blocking eruption. In addition, deficient bone resorption and supernumerary teeth can disturb eruption.

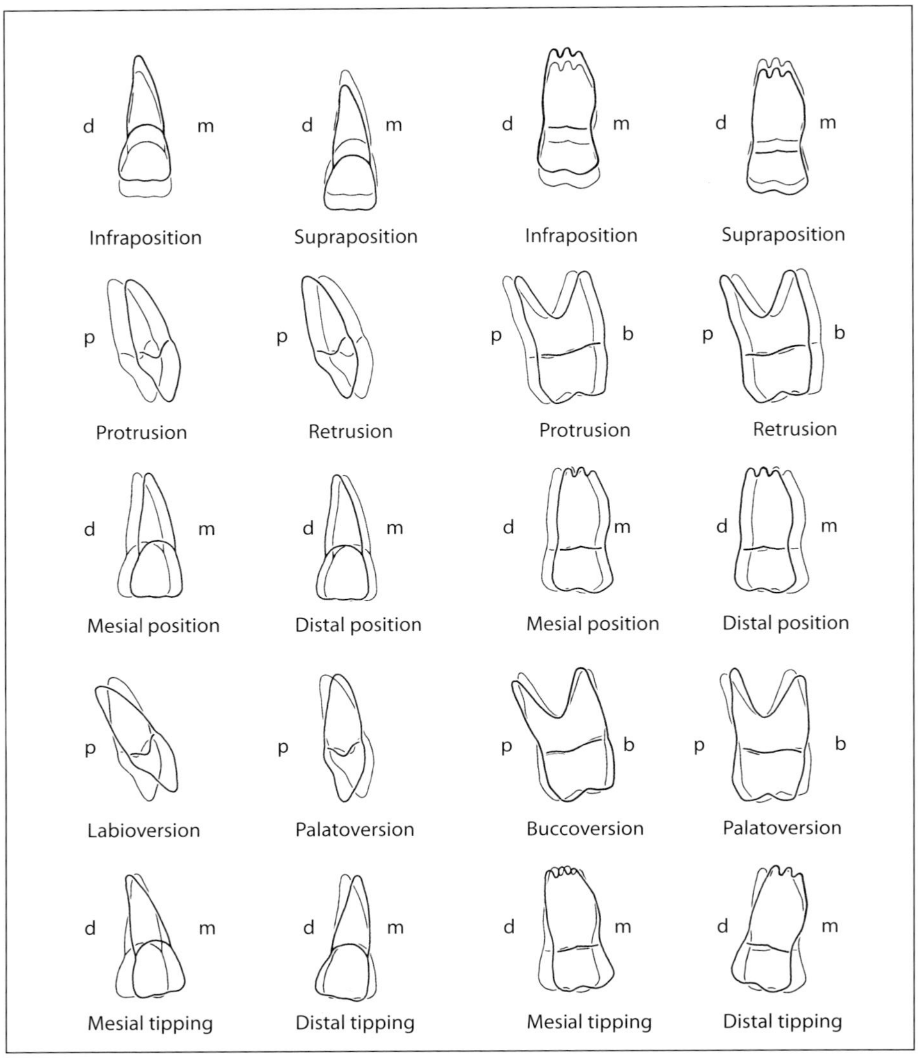

FIG 10-8 Variations and deviations in tooth positions and occlusion with accompanying terms. Teeth can be positioned too far away from the occlusal plane (infraposition) or be overerupted (supraposition). Deviations in axial orientation and their position in relation to other teeth can be distinguished in various directions. Various positions are presented for the maxillary right central permanent incisor and first molar; however, the same terminology is used for the other teeth. The normal position is drawn with a *thin line*, the deviating one with a *thick line*. b, buccal; d, distal; l, labial; m, mesial; p, palatal.

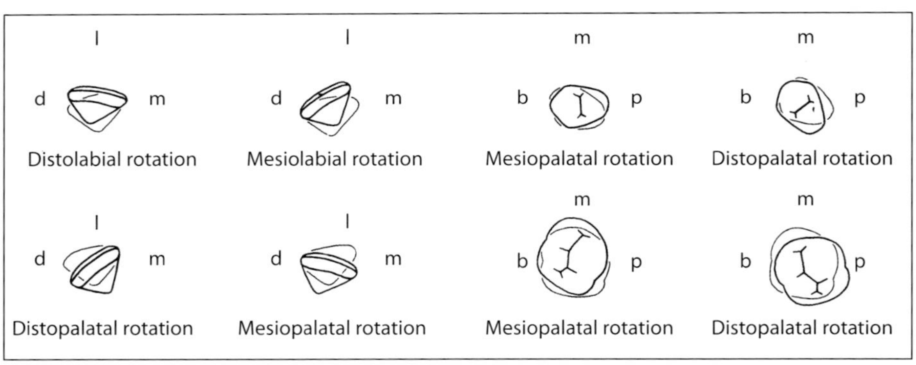

FIG 10-9 Rotations of teeth. Drawn are the maxillary right central permanent incisor, first premolar, and first permanent molar. The normal position is drawn with a *thin line*, the deviating one with a *thick line*. The description of the rotations is in reference to the normal crown positions. b, buccal; d, distal; l, labial; m, mesial; p, palatal

Variations and Deviations in Tooth Position and Occlusion

An overview of the various ways in which tooth positions may deviate is given in Figs 10-8 and 10-9. Box 10-1 provides a list of equivalent terms used to describe variations and deviations in tooth position and occlusion.

Box 10-1 Equivalent terms for variations and deviations in tooth position and occlusion*

- Labial inclination, buccal inclination, proclination, labioversion, buccoversion
- Lingual inclination, palatal inclination, retroclination, linguoversion, palatoversion
- Prognathism, protrusion
- Retrognathism, retrusion
- Sagittal overbite, overjet
- Vertical overbite, overbite
- Class I occlusion, neutroclusion
- Class II occlusion, distoclusion, postnormal occlusion
- Class III occlusion, mesioclusion, prenormal occlusion

*Note that there is a slight difference in the meaning of some of the terms listed as equivalent. *Labial* is used to refer to the anterior region, and *buccal* is used for the posterior region; *lingual* is used for the mandible, and *palatal* is used for the maxilla.

References

1. Van der Linden FPGM. Theoretical and practical aspects of crowding in the human dentition. J Am Dent Assoc 1974;89:139–153.
2. Polder BJ, Van't Hof MA, Van der Linden FPGM, Kuijpers-Jagtman AM. A meta-analysis of the prevalence of dental agenesis of permanent teeth. Community Dent Oral Epidemiol 2004;32:217–226.
3. Bachmann H. Die Häufigkeit von Nichtanlagen bleibender Zähne (ausgenommen der Weisheitszähne). Ergebnisse der Auswertung von 8694 Orthopantogrammen 9-10 jähriger Schulkinder aus Zürich [thesis]. Zürich: University of Zürich, 1974.
4. Bredy E, Erbring C, Hübenthal B. The incidence of hypodontia with the presence and absence of wisdom teeth [in German]. Dtsch Zahn Mund Kieferheilkd Zentralbl 1991;79:357–363.
5. Bjerklin K, Al-Najjar M, Kårestedt H, Andrén A. Agenesis of mandibular second premolars with retained primary molars. A longitudinal radiographic study of 99 subjects from 12 years of age to adulthood. Eur J Orthod 2008;30:254–261.
6. Mattheeuws N, Dermaut L, Martens G. Has hypodontia increased in Caucasians during the 20th century? A meta-analysis. Eur J Orthod 2004;26:99–103.
7. Thompson GW, Popovich F. Probability of congenitally missing teeth: Results in 1,191 children in the Burlington Growth Centre in Toronto. Community Dent Oral Epidemiol 1974;2:26–32.
8. Ben-Bassat Y, Brin I. Skeletal and dental patterns in patients with severe congenital absence of teeth. Am J Orthod Dentofacial Orthop 2009;135:349–356.
9. Nomura S, Hasegawa S, Noda T, Ishioka K. Longitudinal study of jaw growth and prosthetic management in a patient with ectodermal dysplasia and anodontia. Int J Paediatr Dent 1993;3:29–38.
10. Russell KA, Folwarczna MA. Mesiodens-diagnosis and management of a common supernumerary tooth. J Can Dent Assoc 2003;69:362–366.
11. Stellzig A, Basdra EK, Komposch G. Mesiodentes: Incidence, morphology, etiology. J Orofac Orthop 1997;58:144–153.
12. Asaumi JI, Shibata Y, Yanagi Y, et al. Radiographic examination of mesiodens and their associated complications. Dentomaxillofac Radiol 2004;33:125–127.
13. De Oliveira Gomes C, Drummond SN, Jham BC, Abdo EN, Mesquita RA. A survey of 460 supernumerary teeth in Brazilian children and adolescents. Int J Paediatr Dent 2008;18:98–106.
14. Rajab LD, Hamdan MAM. Supernumerary teeth: Review of the literature and a survey of 152 cases. Int J Paediatr Dent 2002;12:244–254.
15. Thilander B, Myrberg N. The prevalence of malocclusion in Swedish schoolchildren. Scand J Dent Res 1973;81:12–21.
16. Baart JA, Groenewegen BT, Verloop MA. Correlations between the presence of a mesiodens and position abnormalities, diastemas, and eruption disturbances of maxillary frontal teeth [in Dutch]. Ned Tijdschr Tandheelkd 2009;116:399–402.
17. Gregg TA, Kinirons MJ. The effect of the position and orientation of unerupted premaxillary supernumerary teeth on eruption and displacement of permanent incisors. Int J Paediatr Dent 1991;1:3–7.
18. Bolton WA. Disharmony in tooth size and its relation to the analysis of malocclusion. Angle Orthod 1958;38:113–130.
19. Crosby DR, Alexander CG. The occurrence of tooth size discrepancies among different malocclusion groups. Am J Orthod 1989;95:457–461.
20. Freeman JE, Maskeroni AJ, Lorton L. Frequency of Bolton tooth size discrepancies among different malocclusion groups. Am J Orthod 1996;110:24–27.
21. Santoro M, Ayoub ME, Pardi VA, Cangialosi TJ. Mesiodistal crown dimensions and tooth size discrepancy of the permanent dentition of Dominican Americans. Angle Orthod 2000;70:303–307.
22. Manke M, Miethke R-R. Size of the anterior Bolton Index and frequency of the Bolton discrepancy in the anterior tooth segment in untreated orthodontic patients [in German]. Fortschr Kieferorthop 1983;44:59–65.
23. Kjær I, Fink-Jensen M, Andreasen JO. Classification and sequelae of arrested eruption of primary molars. Int J Paediatr Dent 2008;18:11–17.
24. Kurol J. Infra-occlusion of primary molars. An epidemiological, familial, longitudinal, clinical, and histological study. Swed Dent J Suppl 1984;21:1–67.
25. Dibiase D. Dental abnormalities affecting eruption. In: Poole DFG, Stack MV (eds). The Eruption and Occlusion of Teeth [Proceedings of the 27th Symposium of the Colston Research Society, 3–7 Apr 1975, Bristol, UK]. London: Butterworth, 1976:156–158.
26. Duterloo HS. An Atlas of Dentition in Childhood. Orthodontic Diagnosis and Panoramic Radiology. London: Wolfe, 1991.

11

Class II, Division 1 Malocclusions

A malocclusion is usually not a pathologic condition but rather a disharmonious combination of variables in the dentition and face that on their own do not exceed the normal range of variation. Individuals with a malocclusion are not sick, have no pain, and mostly do not experience physical discomfort.[1] The term malocclusion literally indicates that the occlusion is bad.

Angle Classification of Malocclusion

In 1899, Edward H. Angle introduced a classification to create order among the large diversity of malocclusions. The Angle classification is based on, and limited to, the occlusion and is purely descriptive. The term *occlusion* refers to the relationship between mandibular and maxillary teeth in functional contact.[2] The Angle classification only considers the sagittal aspect of the occlusion. Other aspects, such as open and deep bites, are not included. Despite its limitations, the Angle classification is generally accepted and used worldwide.

A normal sagittal relationship of the dental arches (ie, neutroclusion) is called Class I. If the position of the mandibular dental arch is too posterior in relation to the maxillary dental arch (ie, distoclusion), it is called a Class II malocclusion. If the reverse situation exists—the mandibular dental arch is too far anterior in relation to the maxillary dental arch (ie, mesioclusion)—it is called a Class III malocclusion. The terms Class II and Class III do not indicate whether the abnormality lies in the mandible or the maxilla or in both. In fact, nothing is suggested regarding the cause of the malocclusion.

In addition, Angle categorized the Class II malocclusions as either Class II, division 1 or Class II, division 2. In Class II, division 1 malocclusions, the maxillary incisors are inclined normally or too far labially. In Class II, division 2 malocclusions, to be discussed in the next chapter, two or more maxillary incisors are palatally inclined. In severe Class II, division 1 malocclusions, the lower lip is positioned between the mandibular and maxillary incisors. In Class II, division 2 malocclusions, the lips are closed.

Malocclusions in which the sagittal occlusion differs between the left and right sides were named subdivisions by Angle. A Class II subdivision means that a normal occlusion (ie, neutroclusion) exists on one side and a distoclusion on the other side. The Class II subdivision is discussed in chapter 15 together with the Class III subdivision. This chapter also does not cover the deviations in the dental arches that can complicate a Class II, division 1 malocclusion. However, it is important to understand that all of the abnormalities mentioned in chapter 10 can occur in Class II, division 1; Class II, division 2; and Class III malocclusions.

Characteristics of Class II, Division 1 Malocclusions

It also holds true in Class II malocclusions that the mandible cannot grow further in the transverse plane after 6 months of age, while the maxilla can. The rule that the mandibular dental arch serves as a mold for the transverse positioning of the maxillary posterior teeth also applies to Class II malocclusions.

For this discussion of the development of Class II, division 1 malocclusions, it is assumed that no abnormalities were initially present in the dental arches. Rather, deviations developed secondary to the distoclusion.

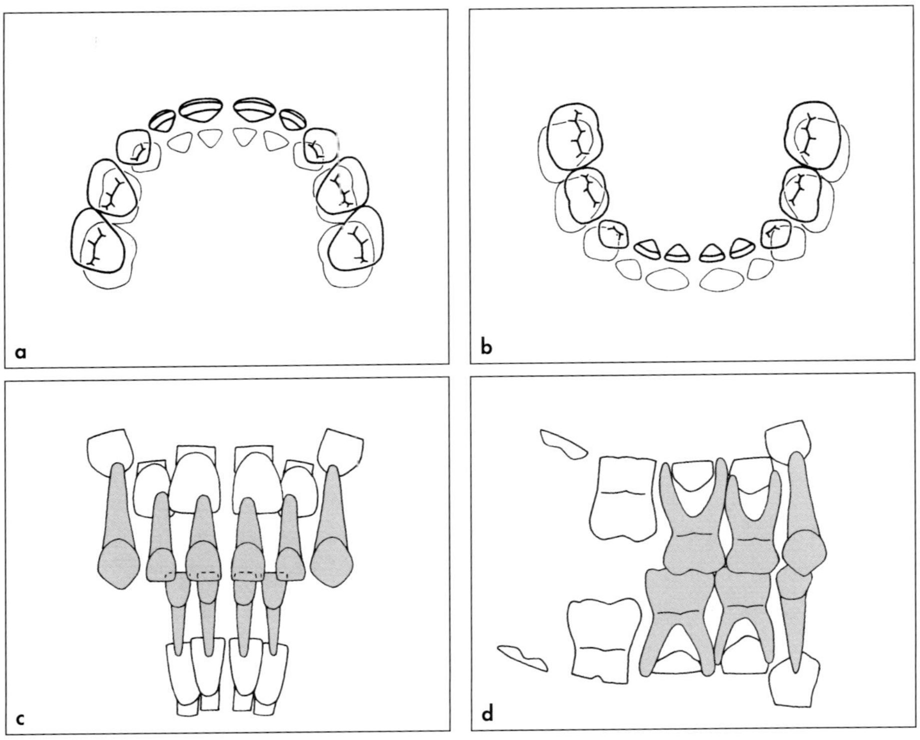

FIG 11-1 Class II, division 1 malocclusion in the deciduous dentition (compare with Fig 2-26). *(a and b)* The position of the mandibular dental arch is too far posterior in relation to the maxillary dental arch. The deciduous molars are in adequate transverse occlusion. The mandibular dental arch has a normal width; the maxillary dental arch is slightly too narrow. *(b)* The overjet is too large. *(c)* The overbite is small. *(d)* The mandibular posterior teeth occlude too far to the distal. The terminal plane of the deciduous dentition has a distal step.

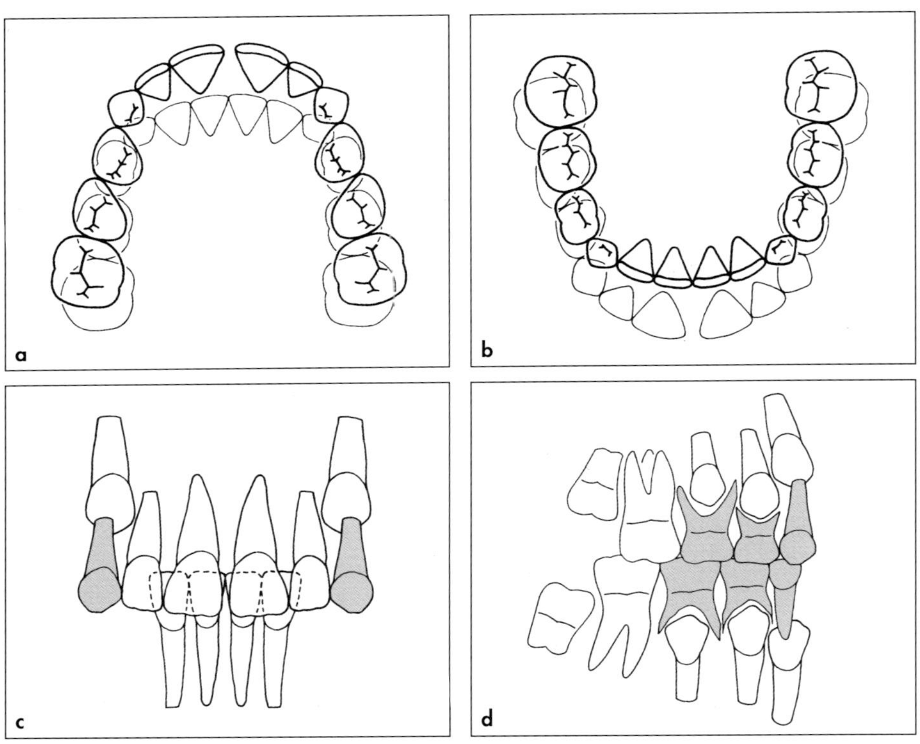

FIG 11-2 Class II, division 1 malocclusion in the intertransitional period (compare with Fig 4-1). *(a and b)* The distoclusion coincides with an abnormally large overjet, a small and tapering maxillary dental arch, and an adequate transverse occlusion. *(c)* The permanent incisors erupt until they are vertically supported. There is a large overbite. The edges of the mandibular incisors may be in contact with the palate. *(d)* The mandibular permanent molars occlude too far to the distal.

Because the mandibular dental arch position is too posterior in relation to the maxillary dental arch, the latter will have a smaller width than normal. This results in the permanent dentition being housed in a narrower and sometimes more tapering maxillary dental arch. This is not a primary aspect of the Class II, division 1 malocclusion but a secondary effect of the distoclusion.

A comparable phenomenon occurs in the anterior region. Due to the distoclusion, the permanent incisors will not end up in normal, reciprocally supported contact. The mandibular and maxillary incisors will continue to erupt until they are slowed down and stopped by the occlusal contact, lip, tongue, or palate. This results in an enlarged overjet and overbite. Furthermore, the overeruption of the mandibular anterior teeth leads to a deepening of the curve of Spee (Figs 11-1 to 11-9). Note that many illustrations in this chapter are based on a distoclusion of one premolar crown width; however, most Class II, division 1 malocclusions show distoclusion of one-third to two-thirds of a premolar crown width.

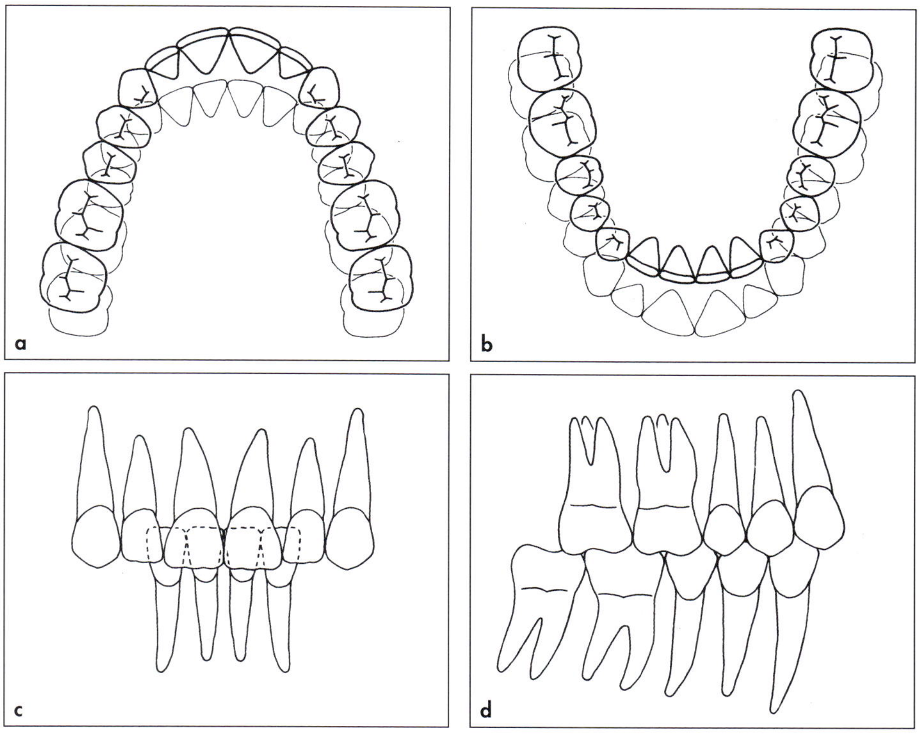

Fig 11-3 Class II, division 1 malocclusion in the permanent dentition with a distoclusion of one premolar crown width (compare with Fig 7-1). *(a and b)* The mandibular dental arch is positioned too far to the posterior in relation to the maxillary dental arch. There is a large overjet and an adequate transverse occlusion. The mandibular dental arch has a normal form; the maxillary dental arch is narrow and tapering. *(c)* The overbite is large, and the mandibular incisors touch the palate. *(d)* All posterior teeth occlude one premolar crown width too far to the distal. They interdigitate with a large part of their occlusal surfaces in contact.

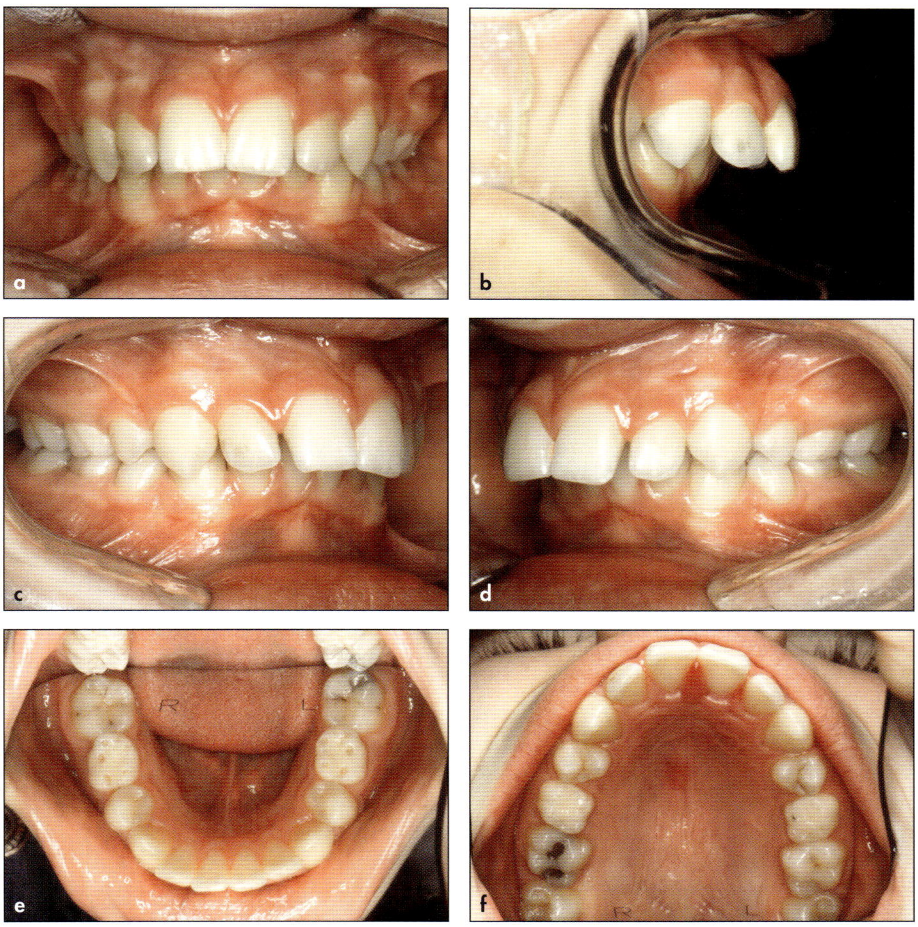

Fig 11-4 Class II, division 1 malocclusion. *(a to f)* The lower lip is positioned behind the maxillary incisors and does not support them vertically. The mandibular incisors have erupted far, and the curve of Spee has deepened. There is an adequate transverse occlusion. The mandibular dental arch has a normal width; the maxillary dental arch is narrow.

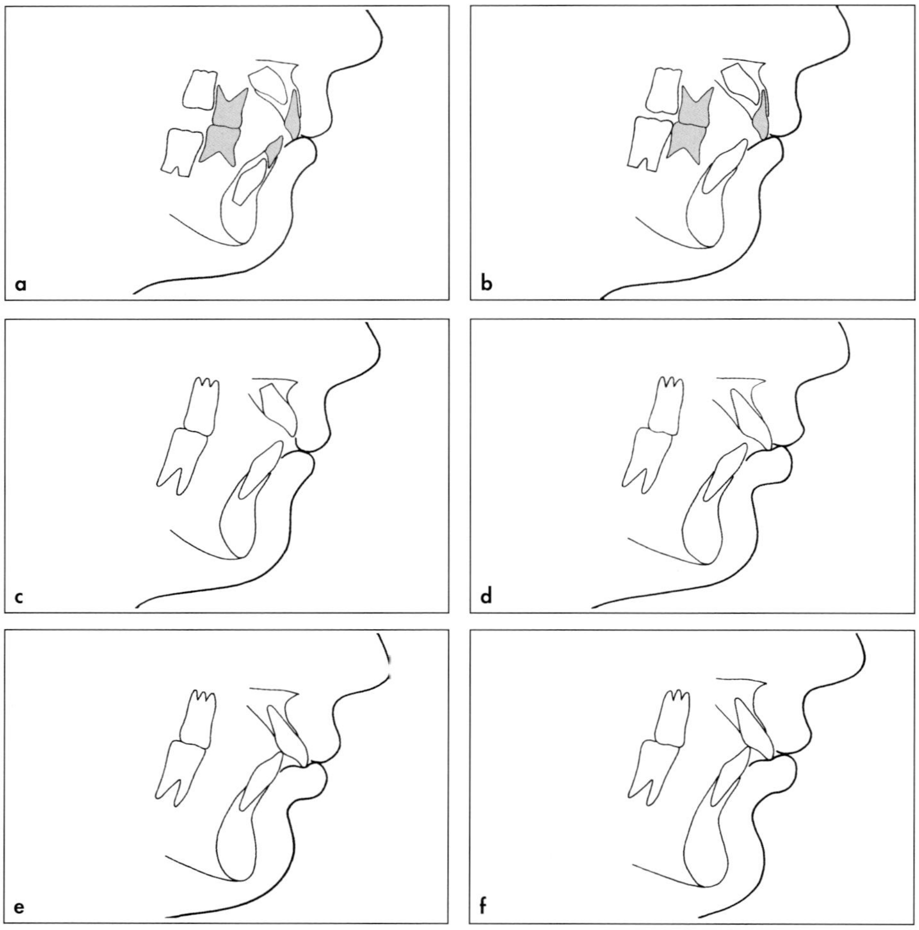

Fig 11-5 Development of a Class II, division 1 malocclusion with a distoclusion of half a premolar crown width (compare with Fig 3-4). *(a)* The deciduous dentition has an enlarged overjet and a terminal plane with a distal step. The lower lip is more posteriorly positioned than normal. *(b)* The mandibular central permanent incisor emerges first. The maxillary central deciduous incisor is in vertical contact with the lower lip. The first permanent molars emerge next in distoclusion and will make contact over a large part of their occlusal surfaces. *(c)* The maxillary central permanent incisor emerges in line with its position within the jaw. *(d)* It is arrested in its eruption by the lower lip, which supports it vertically. *(e)* The mandibular central permanent incisor attains contact with the cervical aspect of the maxillary central permanent incisor. *(f)* The amount of lip material is greater in the adult stage than during the intertransitional and second transitional periods. The mouth is closed at rest.

The width and form of the maxillary dental arch and the size of the overjet and overbite are related to the degree of distoclusion. A small deviation leads to limited secondary changes; a large deviation results in significant secondary changes.

In Class II, division 1 malocclusions, the sagittal and transverse occlusion in the posterior region is reached through the cone-funnel mechanism. Thereafter, the occlusion is reinforced every time the teeth are brought into habitual contact.

In a Class II, division 1 malocclusion without further complications, the mandibular dental arch will look normal from the occlusal perspective. However, Class II, division 1 malocclusions also often have some of the dental arch abnormalities described in chapter 10. In addition, the risk for trauma to the maxillary anterior teeth is higher.[4]

FIG 11-6 Development of the incisors in relation to the lips in a severe Class II, division 1 malocclusion (compare with Fig 3-5). *(a)* In the deciduous dentition, there is a large overjet, incompetent lips, and an open mouth. *(b)* The transition proceeds normally. *(c and d)* After the mandibular central deciduous incisor is lost, its successor will erupt more labially. *(e and f)* That is also the case in the maxilla, where the position of the central permanent incisor is affected unfavorably by the lips. *(g)* The lower lip becomes positioned behind the maxillary incisors, which leads to their further labial tipping. Consequently, the maxillary central incisors are not supported vertically by the lower lip or by the mandibular incisors. The maxillary central and lateral incisors overerupt. The mandibular anterior teeth also overerupt. *(h)* Because of the positioning of the lower lip behind the maxillary incisors, they will not upright with the maturation of the face. The mandibular incisors will be pushed lingually by the lower lip and become more upright than normal. See video clip 31. Note that the tongue and palate are not shown in these illustrations. If the tongue is positioned at rest within the dental arches, the mandibular incisors continue to erupt until they reach the palate. If the tongue rests on top of the mandibular incisors, vertical contact is not reached, and nonocclusion results in the anterior region. (Printed from Van der Linden et al[3] with permission.)

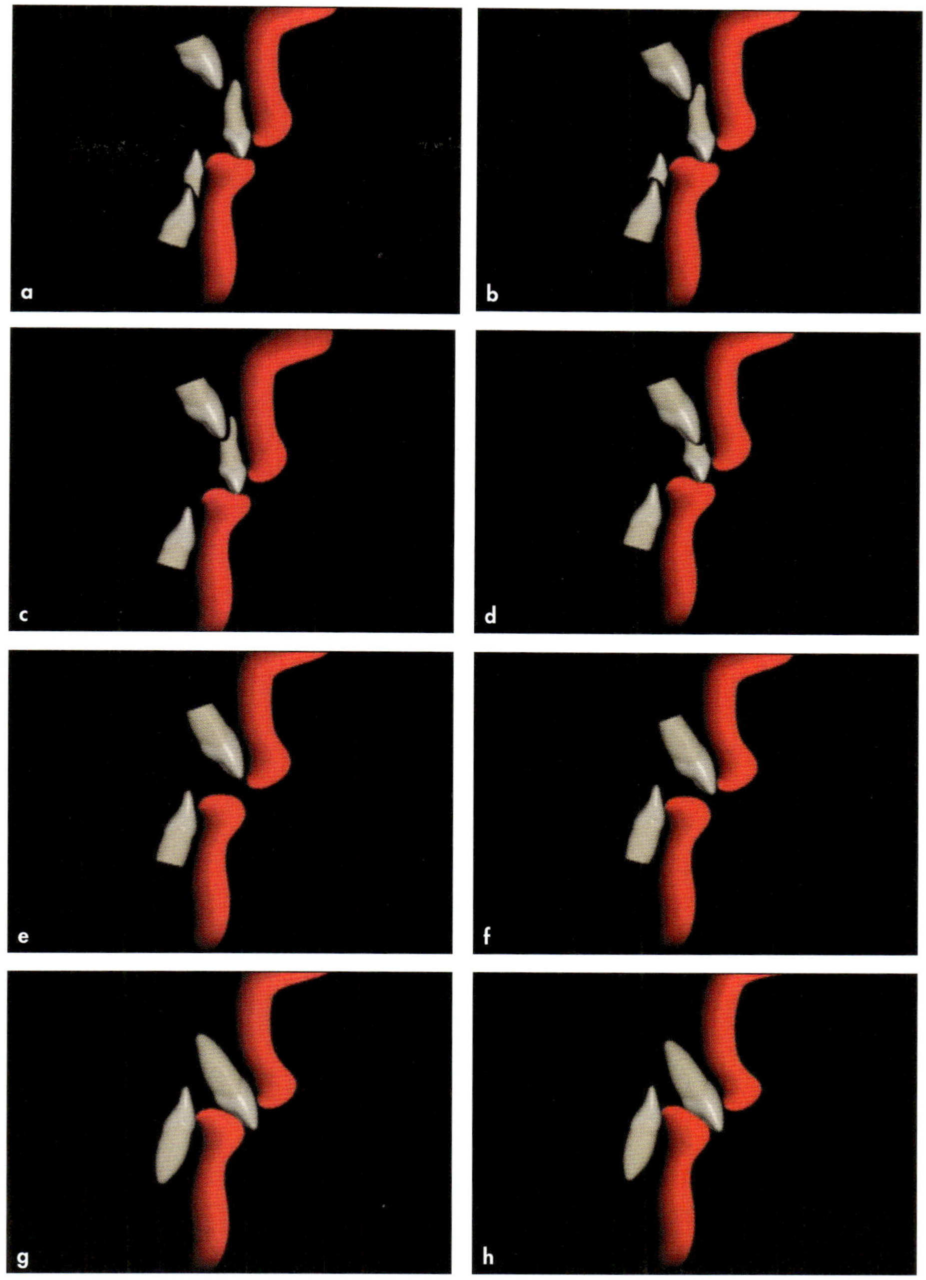

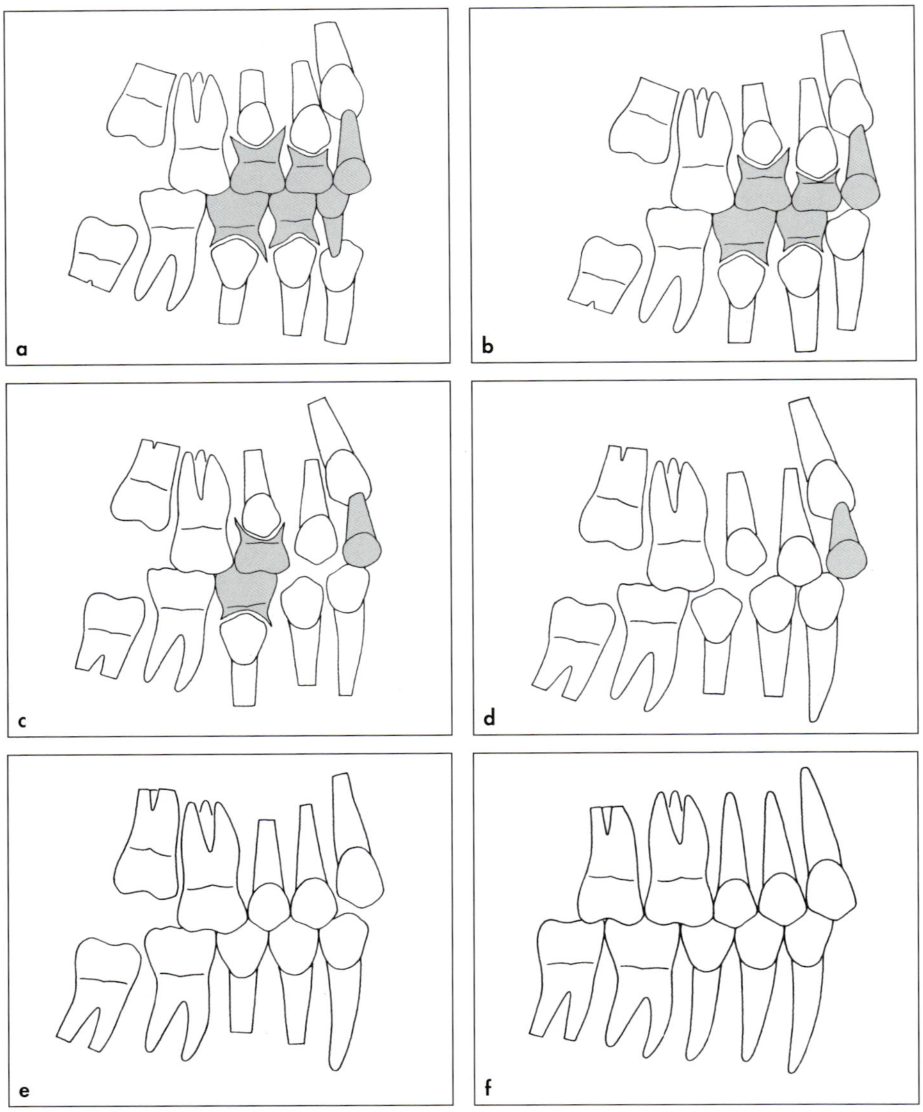

Fig 11-7 Transition of the canines and deciduous molars/premolars and emergence of the second permanent molars in a Class II, division 1 malocclusion (compare with Fig 5-1). *(a)* In the posterior regions, all mandibular teeth occlude distal to the maxillary teeth, and the not-yet-emerged second permanent molars are positioned accordingly. *(b)* The resorption of the roots of the deciduous teeth and the eruption of their successors proceed undisturbed. *(c and d)* Upon emergence, the permanent canines and premolars will interdigitate and consolidate the distoclusion. *(e)* The mandibular permanent canine occludes distal, rather than mesial, to the maxillary permanent canine. Subsequently, the second permanent molars emerge. *(f)* The distal surface of the mandibular second molar is too far distal in relation to that of the maxillary second molar. The distoclusion shown measures one premolar crown width. In such cases, adequate occlusion can result. The teeth fit together like gears, albeit one cusp too far to the distal.

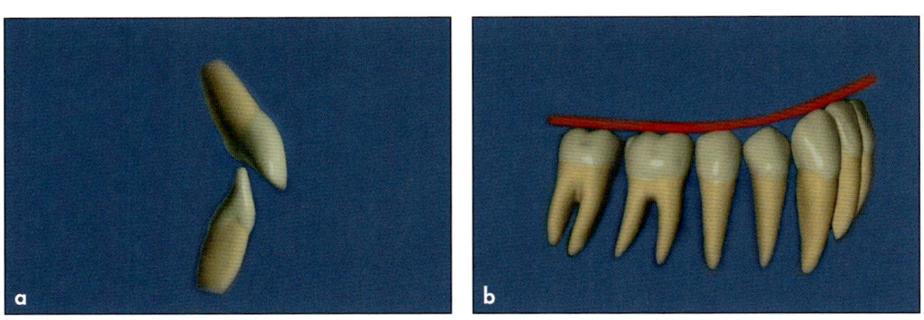

Fig 11-8 Overeruption of the mandibular anterior teeth. *(a)* Depending on the sagittal relationship, the size of the overjet and overbite varies. *(b)* The mandibular anterior teeth overerupt, and the curve of Spee deepens.

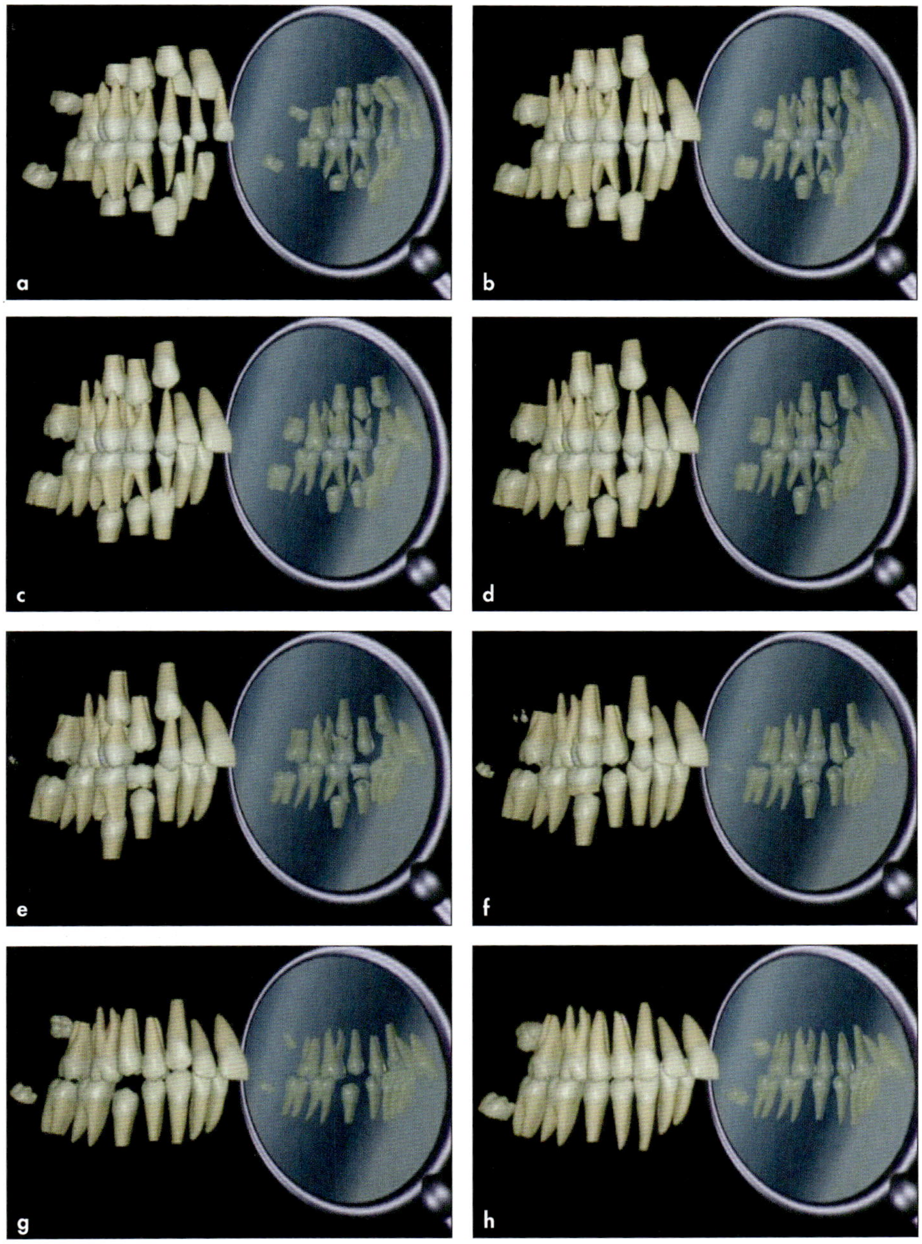

FIG 11-9 Development of a severe Class II, division 1 malocclusion. *(a)* The distoclusion of the dental arches already exists in the deciduous dentition. *(b and c)* The permanent incisors erupt until they meet resistance. *(d)* The result is a large overjet and overbite. *(e to g)* The transition of the canines and deciduous molars/premolars is not affected by the distoclusion. After emergence, the premolars and permanent molars are guided into distoclusion by the cone-funnel mechanism. *(h)* The degree of distoclusion determines the contact between opposing teeth. The maxillary incisors are not supported by the lower lip in a severe Class II, division 1 malocclusion and will overerupt. See video clip 32. (Printed from Van der Linden et al[3] with permission.)

Class II, division 1 malocclusions vary from mild to severe (distoclusion of one premolar crown width) (Fig 11-10). The development of a Class II, division 1 malocclusion, as presented in this chapter, is based on the assumption that the distoclusion did not increase, which is usually the case.[5] However, a Class II, division 1 malocclusion can also worsen or improve during further development.[6]

As stated previously, Class II, division 1 malocclusions develop because the mandibular dental arch is positioned too posterior in relation to the maxillary dental arch. The other symptoms that characterize a Class II, division 1 malocclusion are the result of the distoclusion (Fig 11-11). Whether a normal lip relation prevails or the lower lip becomes positioned behind the maxillary incisors depends on the degree of the distoclusion.

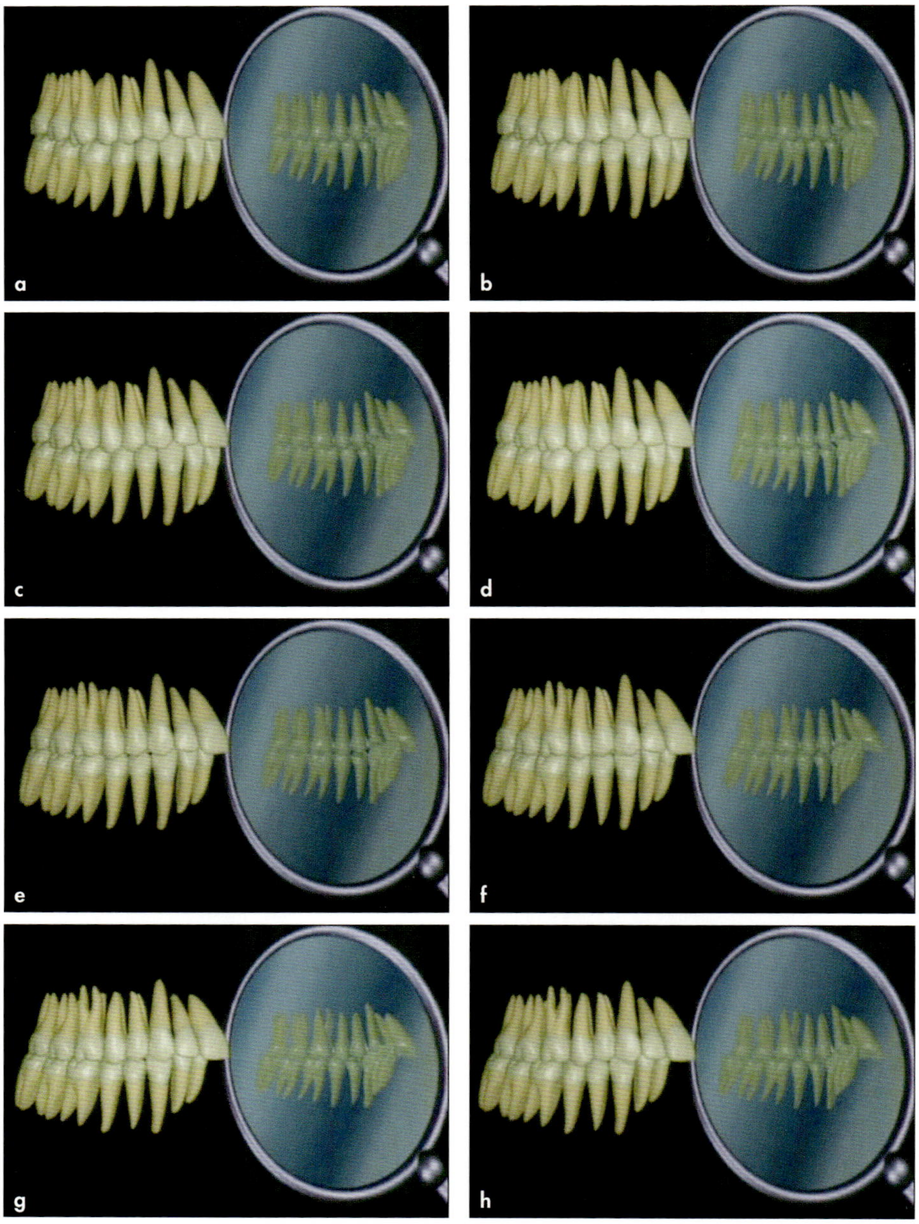

Fig 11-10 Spectrum of severity of a Class II, division 1 malocclusion, from neutroclusion to distoclusion by one premolar crown width. *(a)* Normal occlusion in the permanent dentition. *(b and c)* Slight distoclusion results in small secondary deviations. *(d)* With increasing distoclusion, the incisors will erupt farther. *(e)* The overjet and overbite enlarge. *(f to h)* The distoclusion increases and ultimately reaches one premolar crown width. See video clip 33. (Printed from Van der Linden et al[3] with permission.)

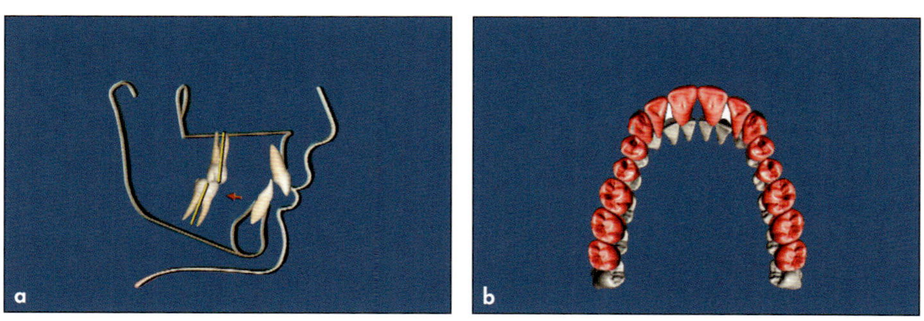

Fig 11-11 Secondary effects of a Class II, division 1 malocclusion. *(a)* The distoclusion is the primary factor. The enlarged overjet and overbite as well as the deepened curve of Spee are secondary effects. *(b)* The narrow maxillary dental arch is another secondary effect.

References

1. Van der Linden FPGM, Boersma H. Diagnosis and Treatment Planning in Orthodontics. Chicago: Quintessence, 1987.
2. Daskalogianakis J. Glossary of Orthodontic Terms. Chicago: Quintessence, 2000.
3. Van der Linden FPGM, Radlanski RJ, McNamara JA Jr. Dynamics of Orthodontics: Malocclusions and Interventions [DVD 3B]. Berlin: Quintessence, 2000.
4. Lewis TE. Incidence of fractured anterior teeth as related to their protrusion. Angle Orthod 1959;29:128–131.
5. Baccetti T, Stahl F, McNamara JA Jr. Dentofacial growth changes in subjects with untreated Class II malocclusion from late puberty through young adulthood. Am J Orthod Dentofacial Orthop 2009;135:148–154.
6. Berg R. Dento-facial Development Between 6 and 12 Years of Age [thesis]. Oslo: University of Oslo, 1983.

12

Class II, Division 2 Malocclusions

Characteristics of Class II, Division 2 Malocclusions

Class II, division 2 malocclusions are characterized by distoclusion, palatal tipping of two or more maxillary permanent incisors, and lingual tipping of the mandibular incisors. They are differentiated into three types (Fig 12-1). In Type A, all four maxillary permanent incisors are tipped palatally, and the maxillary canines are well aligned in the dental arch. In Type B, the maxillary central permanent incisors are palatally tipped, and the lateral incisors are labially tipped. In Type C, all four maxillary permanent incisors are tipped palatally, and the canines are buccally located, outside the dental arch. However, the essential characteristic of Class II, division 2 malocclusions is the high position of stomion. Stomion is the most anterior point of contact between the upper and lower lips at rest in the midsagittal plane.[1] In Class II, division 2 malocclusions, stomion, which is normally located 1 to 3 mm superior to the incisal edges of the maxillary central incisors, is instead at their cervical borders.

Class II, division 2 malocclusions differ from Class II, division 1 malocclusions not only in terms of appearance but also because of etiology. Under highly similar circumstances, either malocclusion can develop (Fig 12-2).

Class II, division 2 malocclusions, and also Class I occlusions with symptoms of Class II, division 2 malocclusions, are called *total complete overbite*. They are caused by excessive coverage of the maxillary incisors by the lower lip. The risk for this is greater with a short upper lip, a reduced lower anterior facial height, and excess external soft tissues. The lips recede, which increases the force exerted by the lower lip on the maxillary incisors[2] (Fig 12-3). However, a total complete overbite can also develop with thin lips, if the coverage of the maxillary incisors by the lower lip is excessive.

Shortly after the emergence of the maxillary central permanent incisors in Class II, division 1 malocclusions, it becomes clear to the casual observer that they are positioned too far to the anterior, particularly if a competent lip seal is lost. The dental characteristics of Class II, division 2 malocclusions show up rather late; initially there may seem to be no problems.

In the deciduous dentition phase, there is little variation in the labiopalatal inclination of the maxillary incisors. They are oriented nearly perpendicular to the occlusal plane since their successors are situated apical and lingual to their roots.

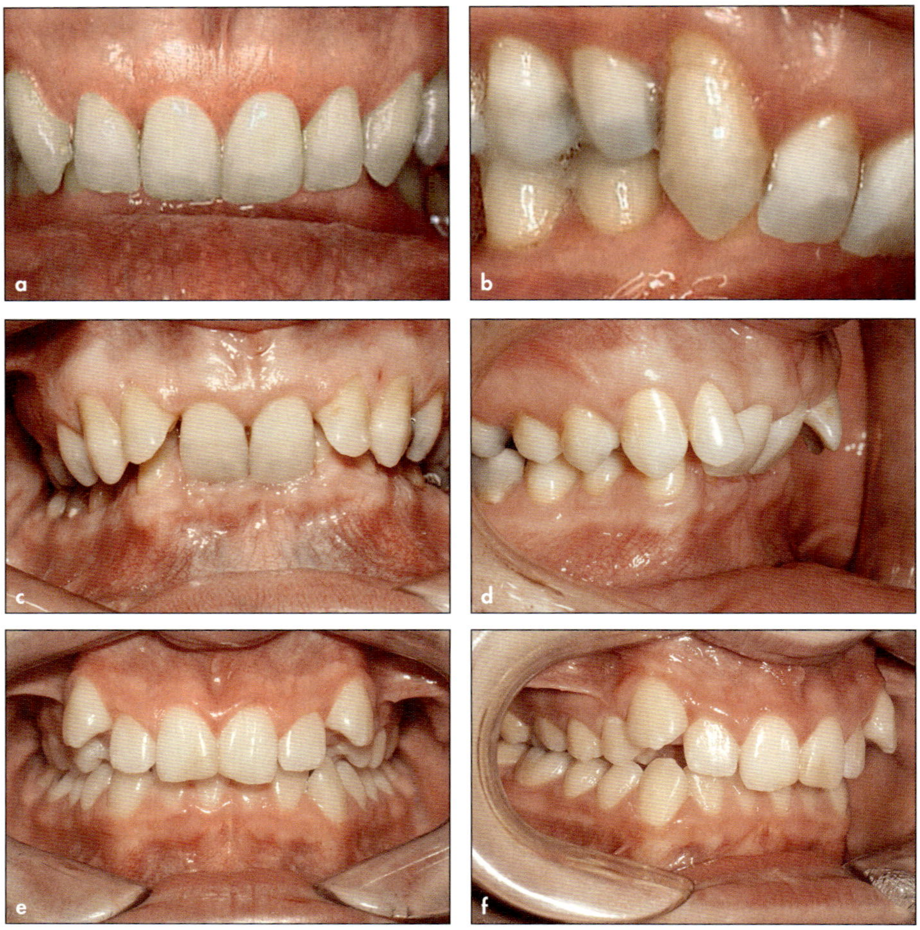

FIG 12-1 Class II, division 2 malocclusions. *(a and b)* Type A. With excess space in the maxillary dental arch, all four maxillary incisors can tip palatally, and the canines attain a correct position in the dental arch. *(c and d)* Type B. With limited space, the maxillary central incisors tip palatally, and the lateral incisors tip labially. *(e and f)* Type C. With marked shortage of space, the four maxillary incisors tip palatally, and the canines emerge buccally outside the dental arch.

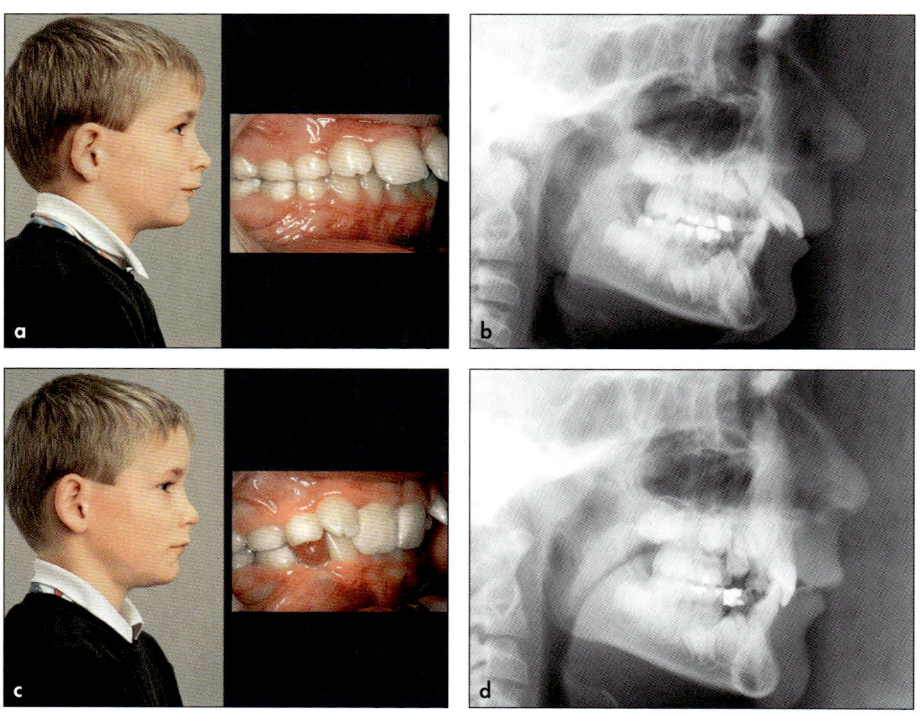

FIG 12-2 Monozygotic twins. *(a and b)* Class II, division 1 malocclusion. The lower lip is situated behind the maxillary incisors. *(c and d)* Class II, division 2 malocclusion. The lower lip coverage of the maxillary incisors is excessive. *(b and d)* The configuration of the facial skeleton is almost identical. (Courtesy of Dr S. Ruf.)

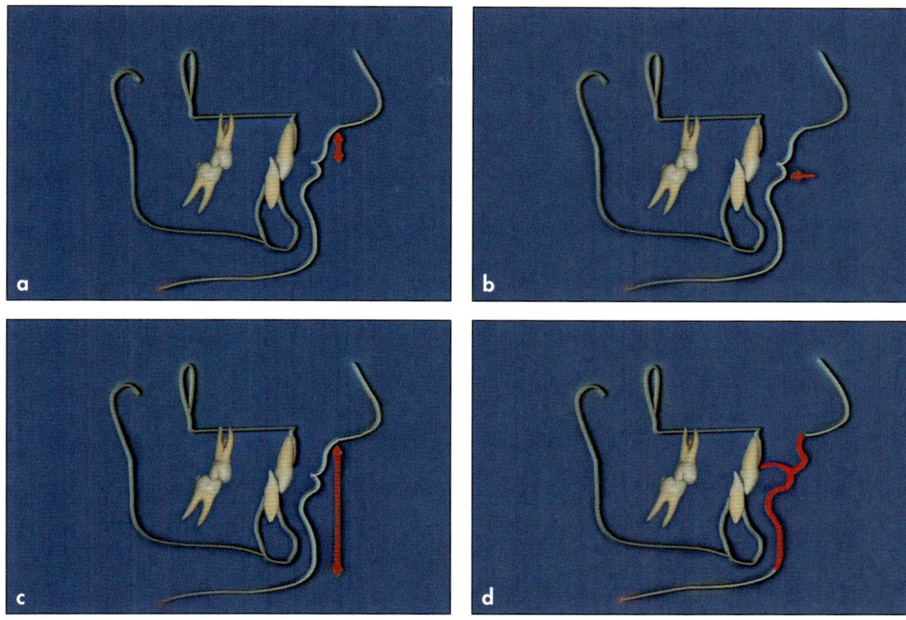

Fig 12-3 Predisposing characteristics for the development of a Class II, division 2 malocclusion. *(a and b)* A short upper lip. *(c)* A reduced anterior lower facial height with a horizontally oriented mandibular lower border and a small gonial angle. *(d)* An excess of labial soft tissues.

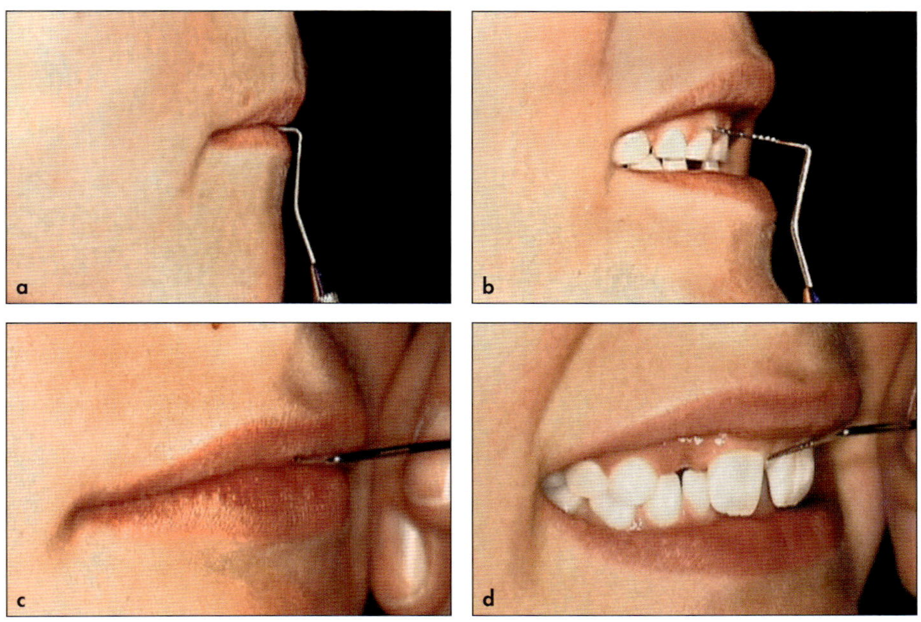

Fig 12-4 The height of stomion in a developing Class II, division 2 malocclusion. *(a and b)* In the deciduous dentition, the lower lip covers the maxillary incisors. *(c and d)* After the transition, the lower lip covers an excessive amount of the maxillary permanent incisors.

Initially, Class II, division 2 malocclusions develop as Class II, division 1 malocclusions. In both malocclusions, the mandibular dental arch is positioned too far to the posterior in relation to the maxillary dental arch, ie, there is a distoclusion. The essential difference between the two in the deciduous dentition phase is the height of stomion, which is situated in Class II, division 2 malocclusions at the cervical border of the maxillary central deciduous incisors (Fig 12-4). In Class II, division 1 malocclusions, the lip line is located near the incisal edges of the maxillary deciduous incisors. Through the high position of stomion and the force exerted by the lower lip on the maxillary permanent incisors, two or more of them gradually tip palatally[3–8] (Figs 12-5 and 12-6). When the palatally tipped maxillary central incisors start to contact the mandibular central incisors, the latter will tip to the lingual. In a Class I malocclusion with symptoms of a Class II, division 2 malocclusion, this happens at an earlier stage and to a larger extent (Fig 12-7).

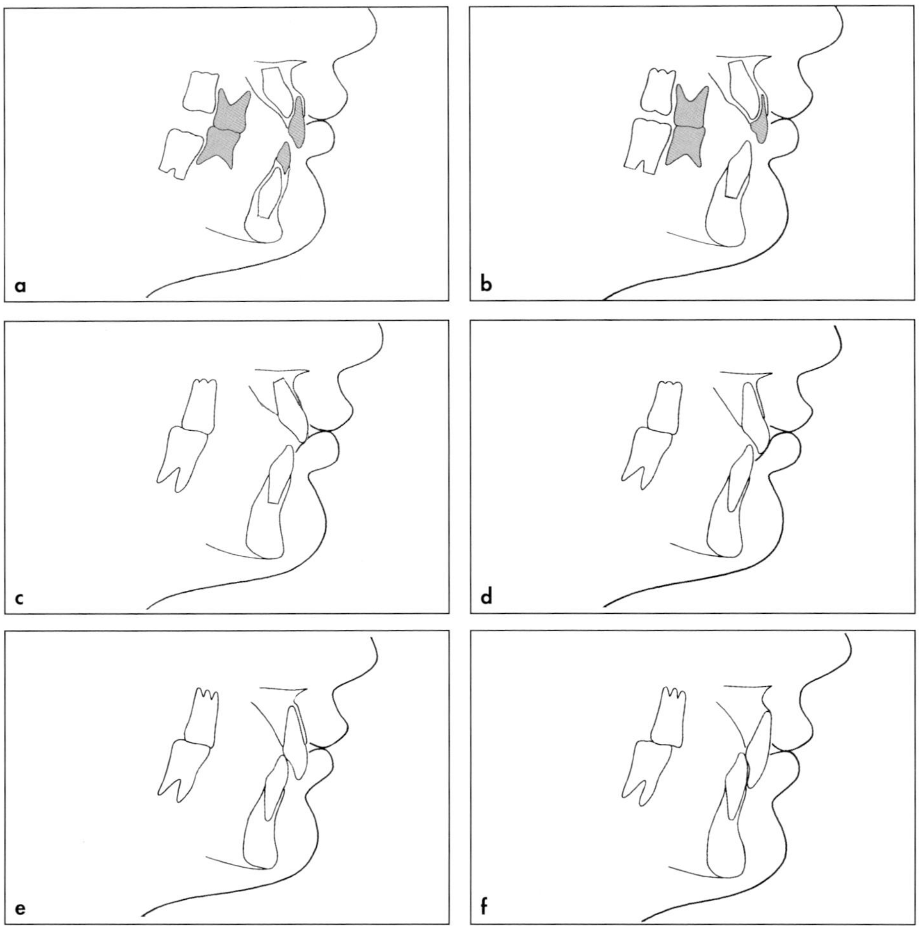

Fig 12-5 Development of a Class II, division 2 malocclusion (compare with Figs 3-4 and 11-5). *(a)* Stomion is situated near the cervical border of the maxillary deciduous incisors. The overjet is large. *(b)* The mandibular central permanent incisors emerge normally. The maxillary central permanent incisors start to tip palatally prior to their emergence.[9] *(c)* Due to its high position, the upper lip has only a limited effect on the erupting maxillary central incisors. *(d)* The latter become more and more influenced by the lower lip, leading to progressive palatal tipping. *(e)* After sagittal incisal contact is established, the pressure of the lower lip is transferred through the maxillary incisors to the mandibular incisors, which also start to tip lingually. The lower lip covers the maxillary incisors completely. *(f)* The incisors overerupt in the mandible until they touch the palate and in the maxilla until the gingiva labial to the mandibular incisors is reached.

The difference between a normal transition and the one in a Class II, division 2 malocclusion is demonstrated in Figs 12-8 and 12-9 with longitudinally collected cephalometric radiographs of two children.

The obvious difference between the two is the extent that the lower lip covers the crowns of the maxillary deciduous and permanent incisors. In addition, there is a marked difference in lower anterior facial height and in the amount of lip material. Longitudinal investigations have demonstrated that, in normal development, the inclination of erupting maxillary central incisors changes little before and after emergence. In Class II, division 1 malocclusions, the labial inclination increases after emergence. In Class II, division 2 malocclusions, the inclination alters when the crown of the maxillary central permanent incisor has perforated the occlusal surface of the bone but not the gingiva. This continues after emergence; the maxillary incisors gradually become more palatally inclined.[9]

It is not clear why in some cases the forming part of the maxillary central incisors does not become displaced, and in other cases it moves labially. If the forming part stays in place, a curved root will develop, and the alveolar process at the apical level will not advance anteriorly (see Fig 12-9d). An angle between the crown and root is a typical feature of some patients with a total complete overbite.

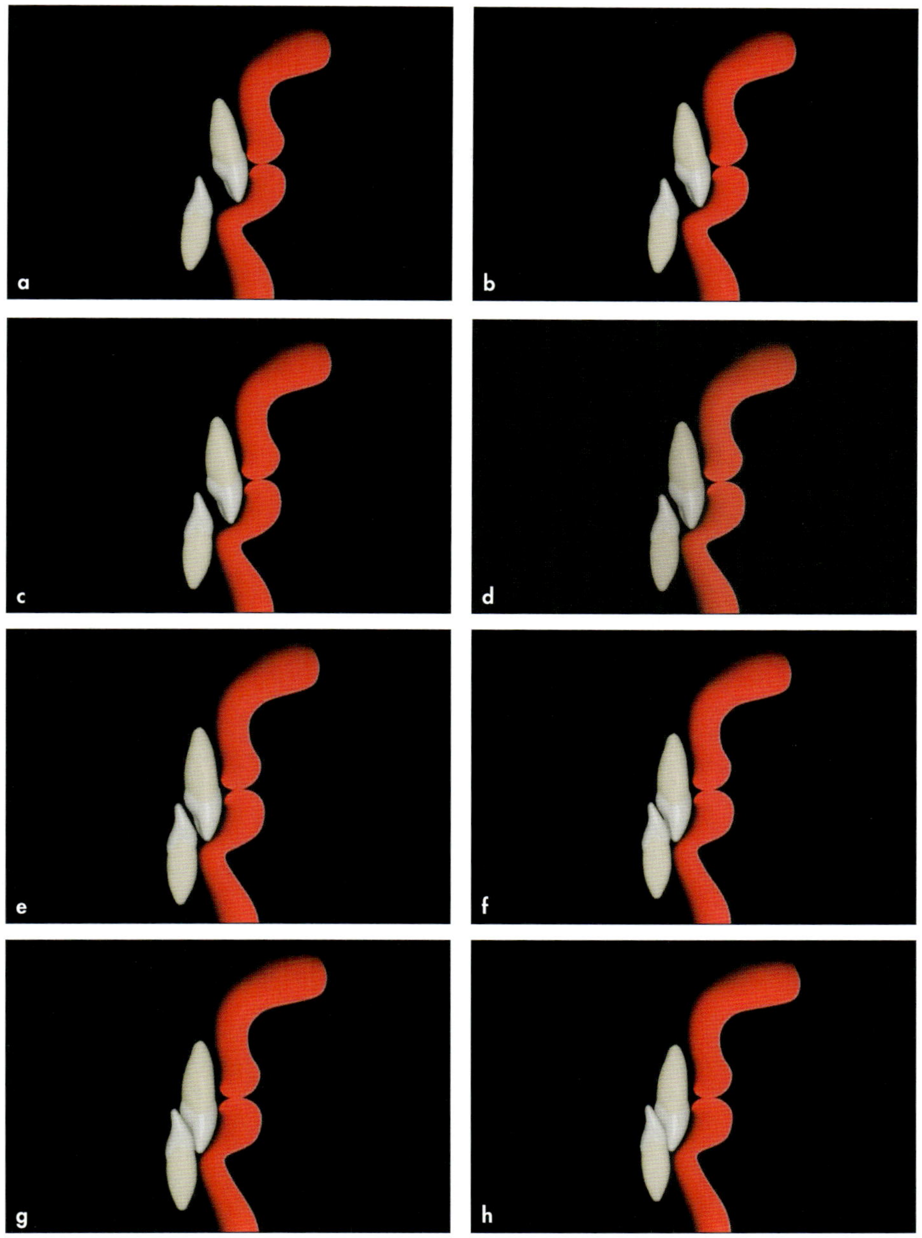

Fig 12-6 Alterations of central permanent incisors in relation to the lips in a Class II, division 2 malocclusion. *(a)* The mandibular incisors erupt normally. The maxillary incisors have tipped palatally prior to emergence. *(b and c)* Thereafter, they continue to tip palatally and overerupt. *(d to h)* When contact is established, the mandibular incisors also start to tip lingually. See video clip 34. (Printed from Van der Linden et al[10] with permission.)

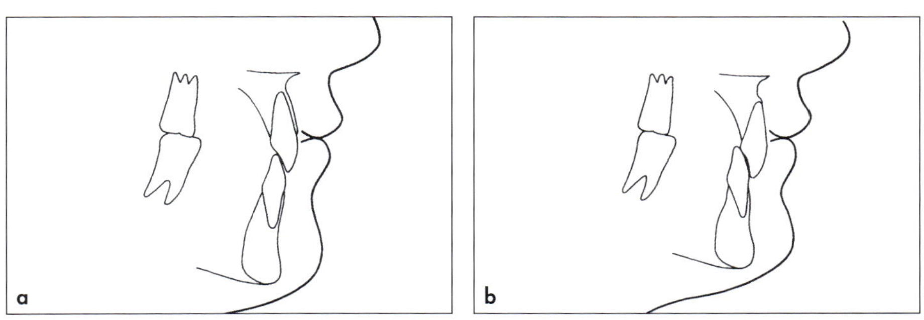

Fig 12-7 Changes in a neutroclusion with symptoms of a Class II, division 2 malocclusion. *(a)* In a neutroclusion, contact between the incisors is established earlier. *(b)* The mandibular incisors start to tip lingually sooner; the occurrence and increase of crowding in the mandibular arch also occurs earlier.

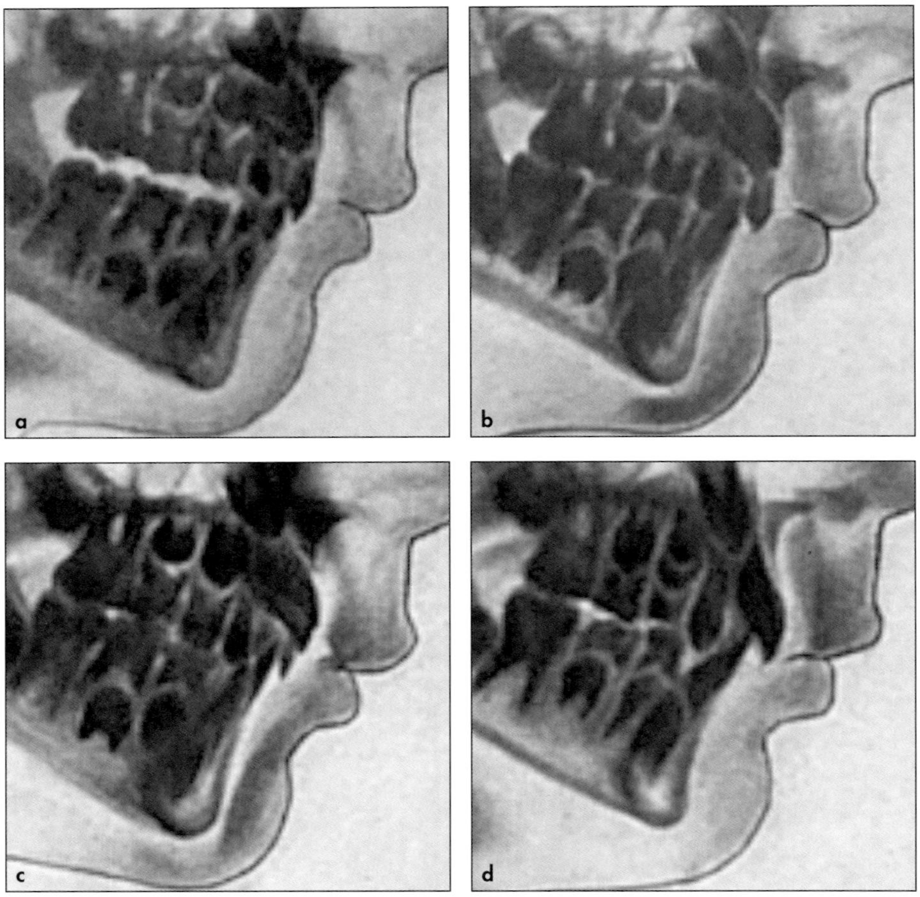

Fig 12-8 Radiographs of normal development in the anterior region. *(a)* In a normal situation, the maxillary central permanent incisors are formed within the jaw in a labially inclined position. *(b)* Six months later, the maxillary central permanent incisors have erupted further, and the bone at their labial side has become thinner. *(c)* Seven months thereafter, their predecessors are still present, and the unemerged permanent incisors have erupted further, without an alteration in angulation, while the bone at the labial side has been resorbed. *(d)* Eighteen months later, the maxillary central permanent incisors as well as the mandibular incisors have erupted completely and reached occlusal contact. The lower lip lies against the incisal edges of the maxillary incisors and covers only a small portion of their labial surfaces. The inclination of the maxillary central incisors has exhibited little or no change during the whole eruption process. The developing part of roots of the incisors remained at the same location. (Reprinted from Falck and Fränkel[3] with permission.)

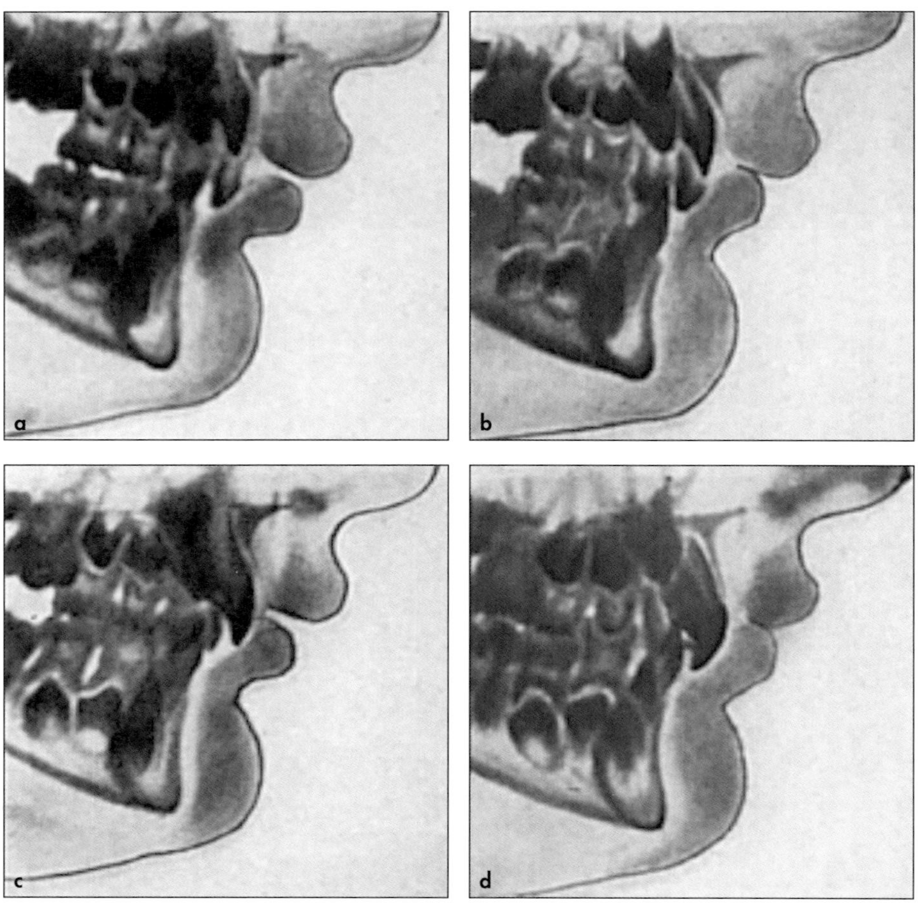

Fig 12-9 Radiographs of development in the anterior region in a Class II, division 2 malocclusion. *(a)* In a developing total complete overbite, an excessive amount of the maxillary deciduous incisors is covered by the lower lip. Prior to emergence, the maxillary permanent incisors are in a more upright position than normal. *(b)* Seven months later, the maxillary permanent incisors are more labially and occlusally positioned, and their predecessors are ready to exfoliate. *(c)* Six months thereafter, the maxillary central permanent incisors have emerged, and about half their crown height is covered by the lower lip. *(d)* Eighteen months later, occlusal contact has been established, and the lower lip completely covers the crowns of the maxillary central permanent incisors. These sections from lateral cephalometric radiographs demonstrate that the initially somewhat steeply inclined maxillary central incisors first move labially but tip palatally after emergence. Furthermore, in this individual, a bend developed between the long axis of the crown and the long axis of the root—the so-called collum angle of Andresen. (Reprinted from Falck and Fränkel[3] with permission.)

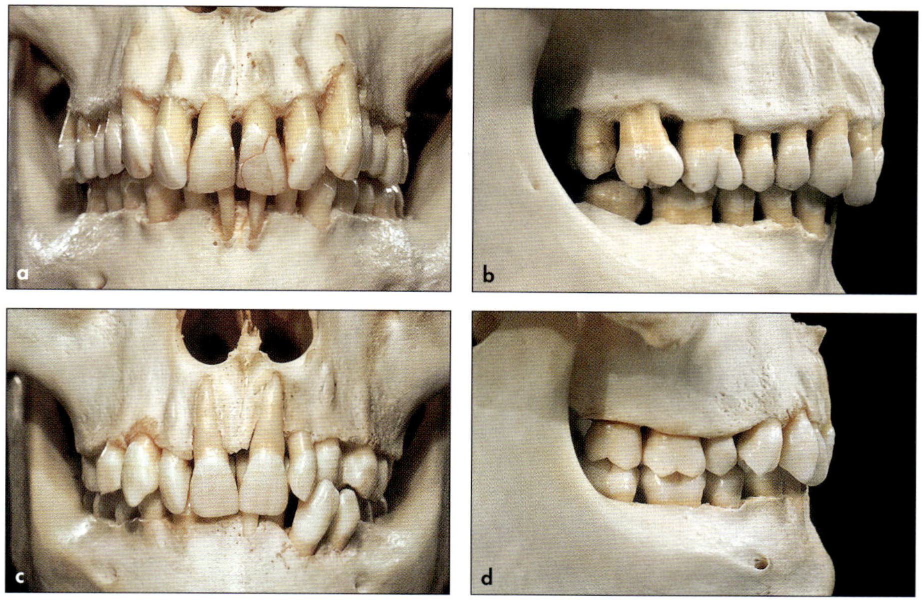

Fig 12-10 Changes in the alveolar processes in total complete overbites. *(a and b)* In total complete overbites, mostly the crowns of the maxillary incisors become palatally displaced, with the apices moving labially. Bone is deposited anteriorly at the alveolar process to maintain root coverage, and the concavity at the level of the apices disappears. *(c and d)* The potential to deposit bone at the labial surfaces is limited and insufficient if the roots move far outside their normal boundaries. The labial surfaces of the roots can become denuded of bone.

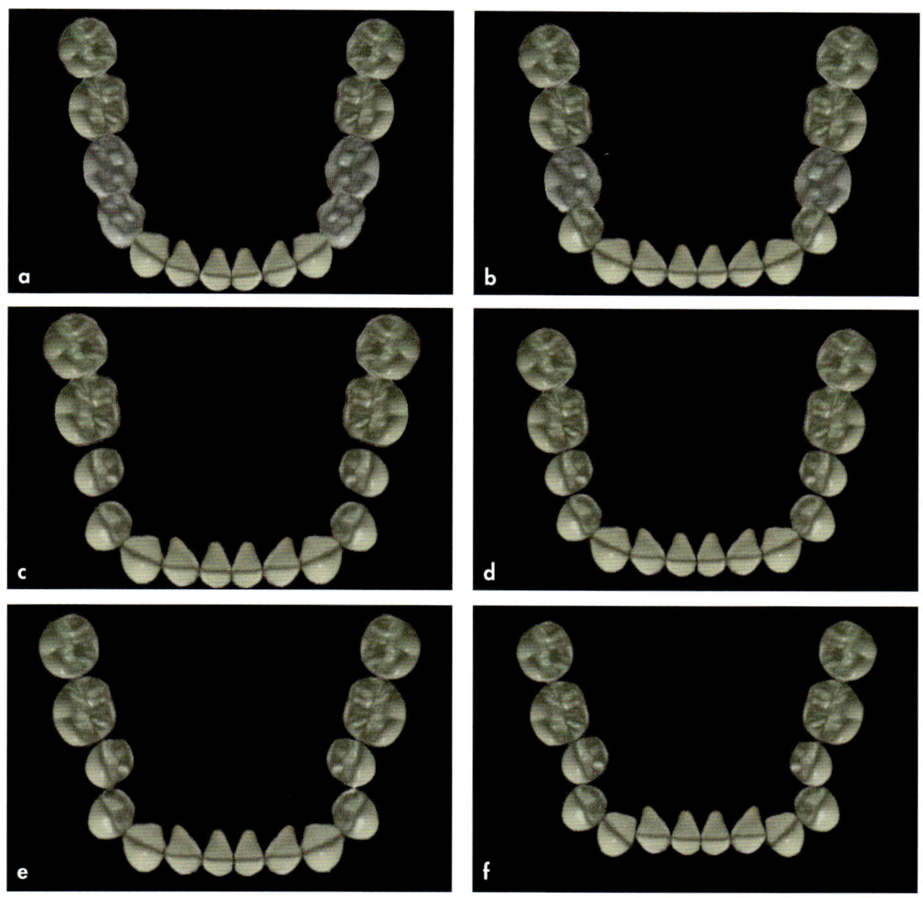

Fig 12-11 Development of mandibular crowding in total complete overbites. *(a)* Initially, there is enough space in the mandibular dental arch. *(b and c)* That changes when the mandibular incisors tip lingually. *(d)* Crowding develops. *(e and f)* Canines can be forced outside the dental arch and second premolars inside the dental arch through pressure exerted at the anterior teeth.

If the forming part moves labially, no curving of the root will occur, but the alveolar process will be built out too anteriorly. In excessive displacements, the bone coverage at the labial side of the roots can be lost (Fig 12-10). When palatally tipped maxillary incisors contact mandibular incisors, crowding in the mandibular dental arch develops or increases (Fig 12-11).

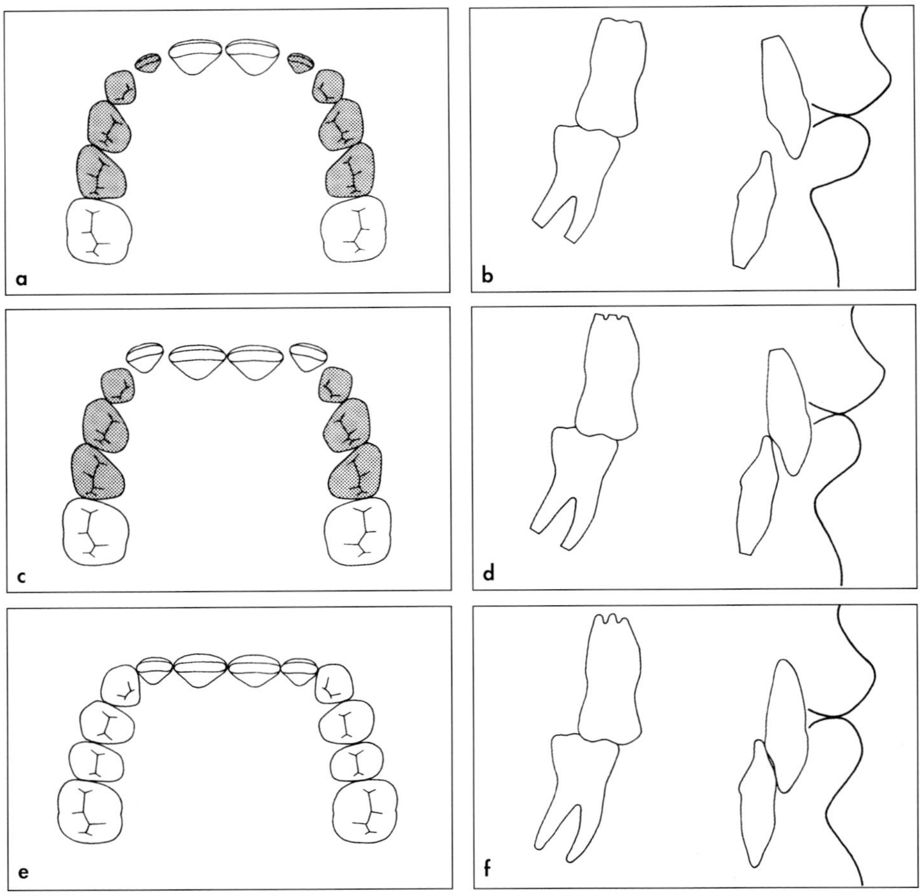

Fig 12-12 Development of a Class II, division 2, Type A malocclusion: more than sufficient space in the maxillary dental arch. *(a and b)* The maxillary permanent incisors are palatally tipped, and more than half of their crown height is covered by the lower lip. *(c and d)* There is sufficient space in the dental arch for the maxillary lateral incisors even after further palatal tipping of the central incisors. The lateral incisors also are covered by the lower lip and tip palatally. After contact is established, the mandibular incisors begin to tip lingually. *(e and f)* The maxillary lateral incisors tip farther palatally, and their incisal edges are arranged in a straight line with those of the central incisors. Sufficient space remains in the dental arch for the maxillary permanent canines. The maxillary and mandibular incisors are oriented perpendicular to the occlusal plane and do not support each other vertically.

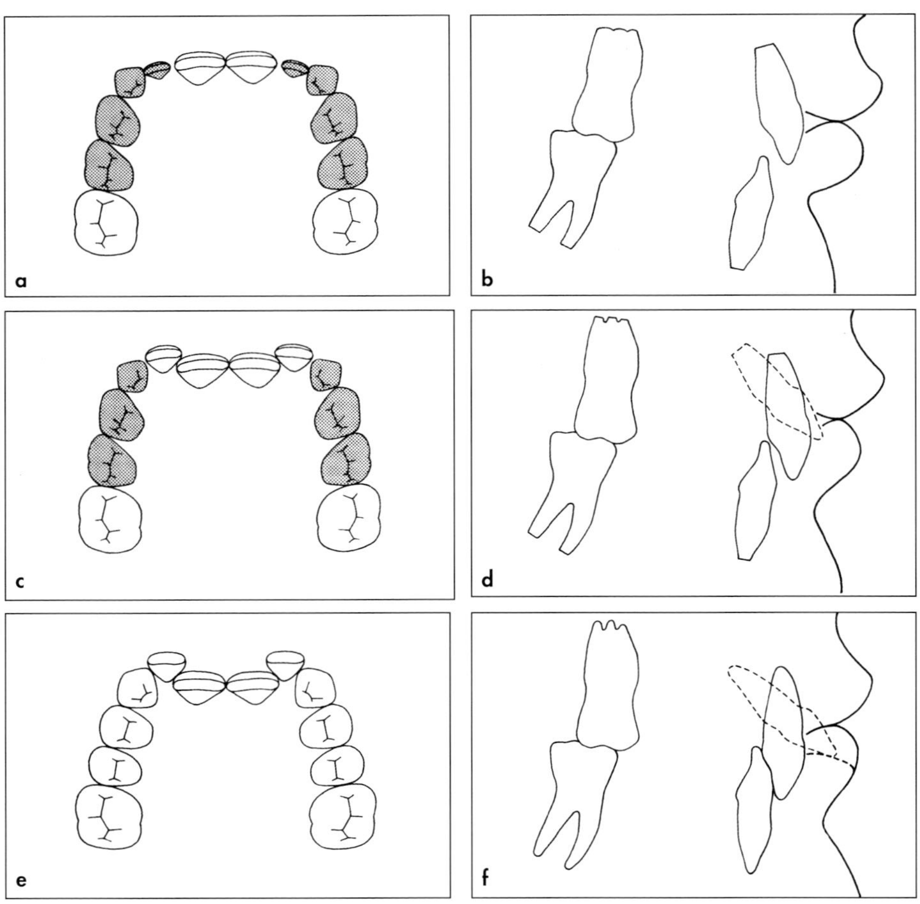

Fig 12-13 Development of a Class II, division 2, Type B malocclusion: no or little crowding in the maxillary dental arch. *(a and b)* The maxillary central incisors have emerged and tipped palatally. *(c and d)* The little space that remains for the maxillary lateral incisors is reduced further as the central incisors continue to tip palatally. The erupting lateral incisors diverge labially. *(e and f)* The lower lip becomes positioned behind their palatal surfaces, which increases their labial tipping. The lower lip covers the crowns of the maxillary central incisors completely. In some cases, only one lateral incisor diverges labially, and the other one tips palatally.

Fig 12-14 Development of a Class II, division 2, Type C malocclusion: severe crowding in the maxillary dental arch. *(a and b)* There is not enough space in the maxillary dental arch for the emergence of the lateral permanent incisors. The space is further reduced by the palatal tipping of the maxillary central incisors. *(c and d)* With the eruption of the lateral permanent incisors, not only their predecessors but also the neighboring deciduous canines are exfoliated. This provides extra space for the emergence of the lateral incisors, which will tip palatally through the pressure exerted by the lower lip. *(e and f)* Too little space is left for the maxillary canines, which will emerge buccally, outside the dental arch. Crowding in the maxillary dental arch is usually associated with crowding in the mandibular dental arch, which increases as the incisors tip lingually. If the shortage of space is concentrated on one side, only the canine on that side will become positioned outside the dental arch.

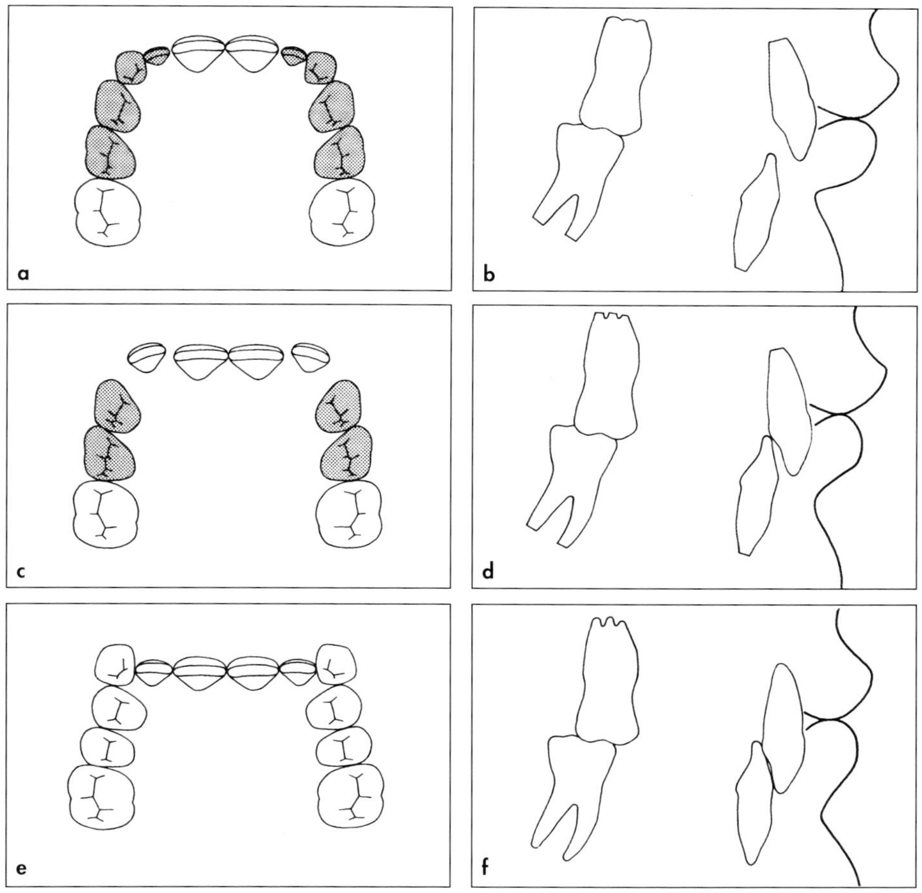

Spatial Conditions in the Maxilla

The three differentiated types of Class II, division 2 malocclusions can be traced back to differences in spatial conditions in the maxillary dental arch. With excess space, all four incisors can tip palatally without the occurrence of crowding—Type A (Fig 12-12). If the space available in the dental arch is limited, palatal tipping of the central incisors will reduce the space further. The lateral incisors will diverge labially—Type B (Fig 12-13). Their palatal surfaces will rest on top of the lower lip, which increases their labial inclination further (see Fig 12-13f). The labial divergence may also occur on one side only, with the other lateral tipped palatally. In severe crowding, the eruption of the maxillary lateral incisors coincides with the resorption and loss not only of their predecessors but also of the adjacent deciduous canines. Then space becomes available for the lateral incisors to tip palatally. Subsequently, not enough space remains for the permanent canines. They emerge buccally, outside the dental arch—Type C (Fig 12-14). If there is asymmetry in the maxillary anterior region, one canine may emerge within and the other outside the dental arch.

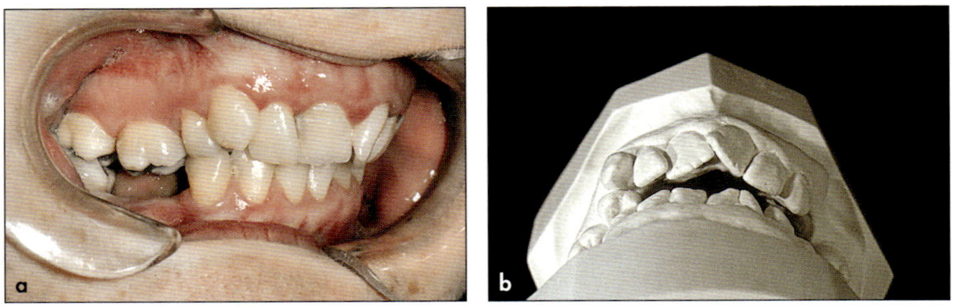

Fig 12-15 *(a and b)* Severely palatally tipped maxillary incisors combined with anterior nonocclusion. If in a total complete overbite the resting position of the tongue is between the mandibular anterior teeth and the palate, vertical contact is not achieved.

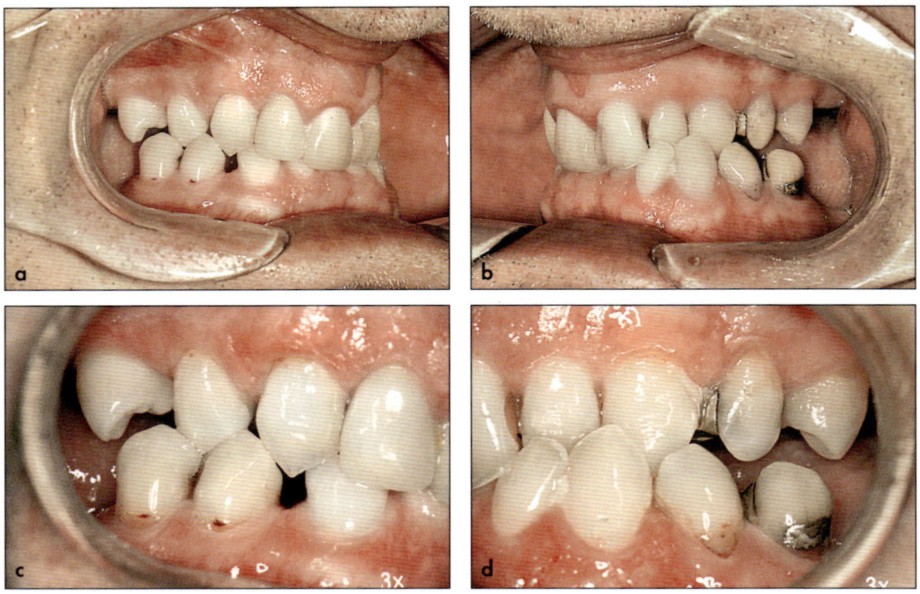

Fig 12-16 Total complete overbite combined with a partial negative overjet and a lateral open bite. A 60-year-old man had agenesis of the maxillary right lateral incisor and all permanent molars, a total complete overbite of the maxillary central incisors, and negative overjet of the left lateral incisor and canine. There is an open bite of second premolars on the right side *(a and c)* and all premolars on the left side *(b and d)*. The combination of short dental arches, total complete overbite, and reverse overjet have not led to any functional disturbances in speech or chewing or to temporomandibular joint complaints.

Development of Class I Neutroclusion with Symptoms of Class II, Division 2 Malocclusion

As explained previously, the phenomenon of a high position of the lip also occurs in neutroclusions. The development of such a malocclusion is comparable to that of Class II, division 2 malocclusion, albeit with normal intercuspation of premolars and molars and a more lingual tipping of the mandibular incisors. Total complete overbites occur in combination with other malocclusions, even with nonocclusion in the anterior region and with a partial negative overjet (Figs 12-15 and 12-16).

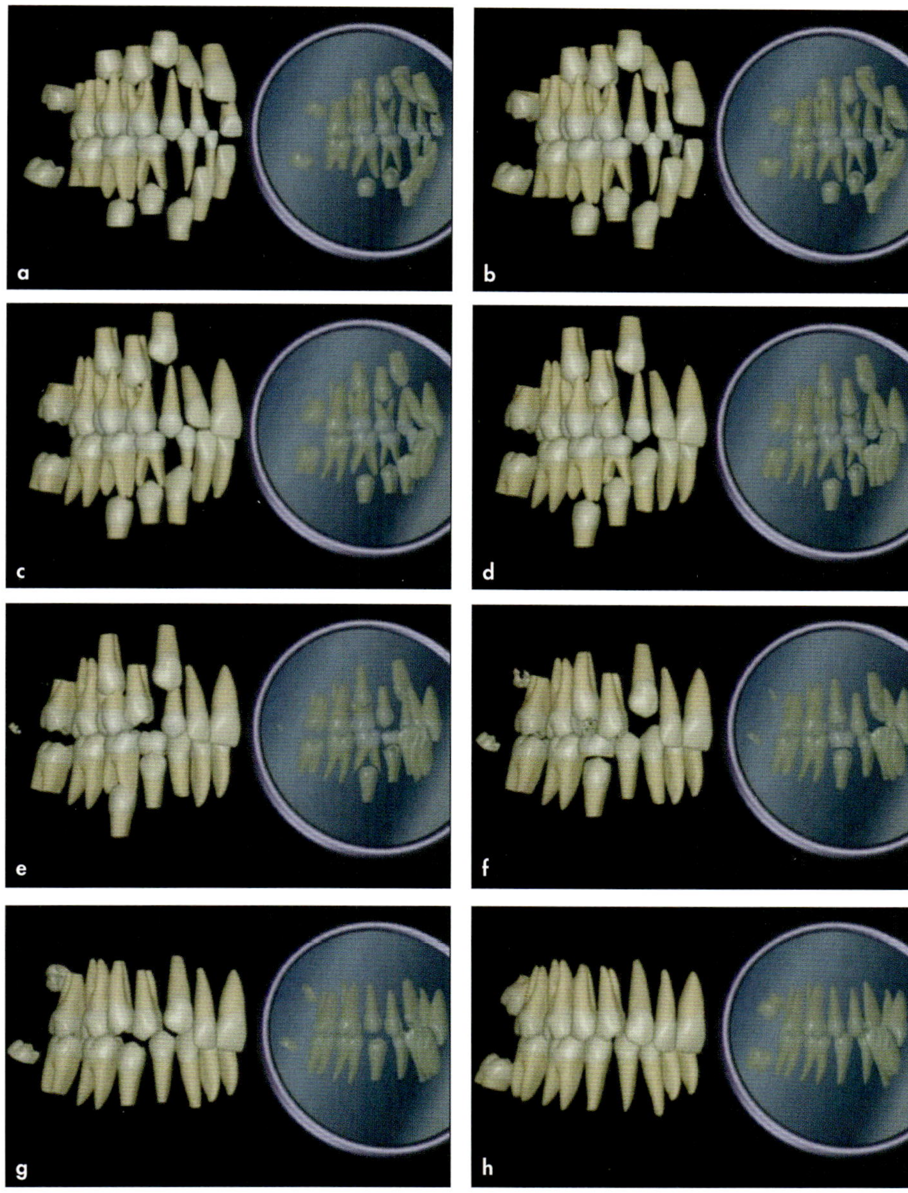

Fig 12-17 Development of a Class I occlusion with symptoms of a Class II, division 2, Type A malocclusion. *(a)* There is a neutroclusion. *(b and c)* Soon after emergence of the central permanent incisors, contact is reached in the anterior region. *(d and e)* With further palatal tipping of the maxillary incisors, the mandibular incisors are pushed lingually. *(f and g)* The transition of the canines and deciduous molars/premolars is not affected. *(h)* The four maxillary incisors are in a steep position, and their incisal edges are arranged in a straight line. The mandibular incisors are significantly lingually inclined. The maxillary canines emerge without space problems and become well positioned in the dental arch. See video clip 35. (Printed from Van der Linden et al[10] with permission.)

In Fig 12-17, the development of a Class I occlusion with symptoms of a Class II, division 2, Type A malocclusion is shown. In Fig 12-18, a Class II, division 2, Type C malocclusion is shown. In addition, some other aspects of the development of Class II, division 2 malocclusions, especially Type B, are shown in video clips 34 and 36 to 40.

As with Class II, division 1 malocclusions, the development of Class II, division 2 malocclusions is mainly presented in severe forms. However, Class II, division 2 malocclusions also occur in less severe forms. The extent of the distoclusion and in the degree of lingual tipping of maxillary and mandibular incisors varies. The severity of a Class II, division 2 malocclusion depends mainly on the extent to which the lower lip overlaps the maxillary incisors. If more than one-third of the labial surface of the maxillary central incisors is covered, they will be tipped palatally.

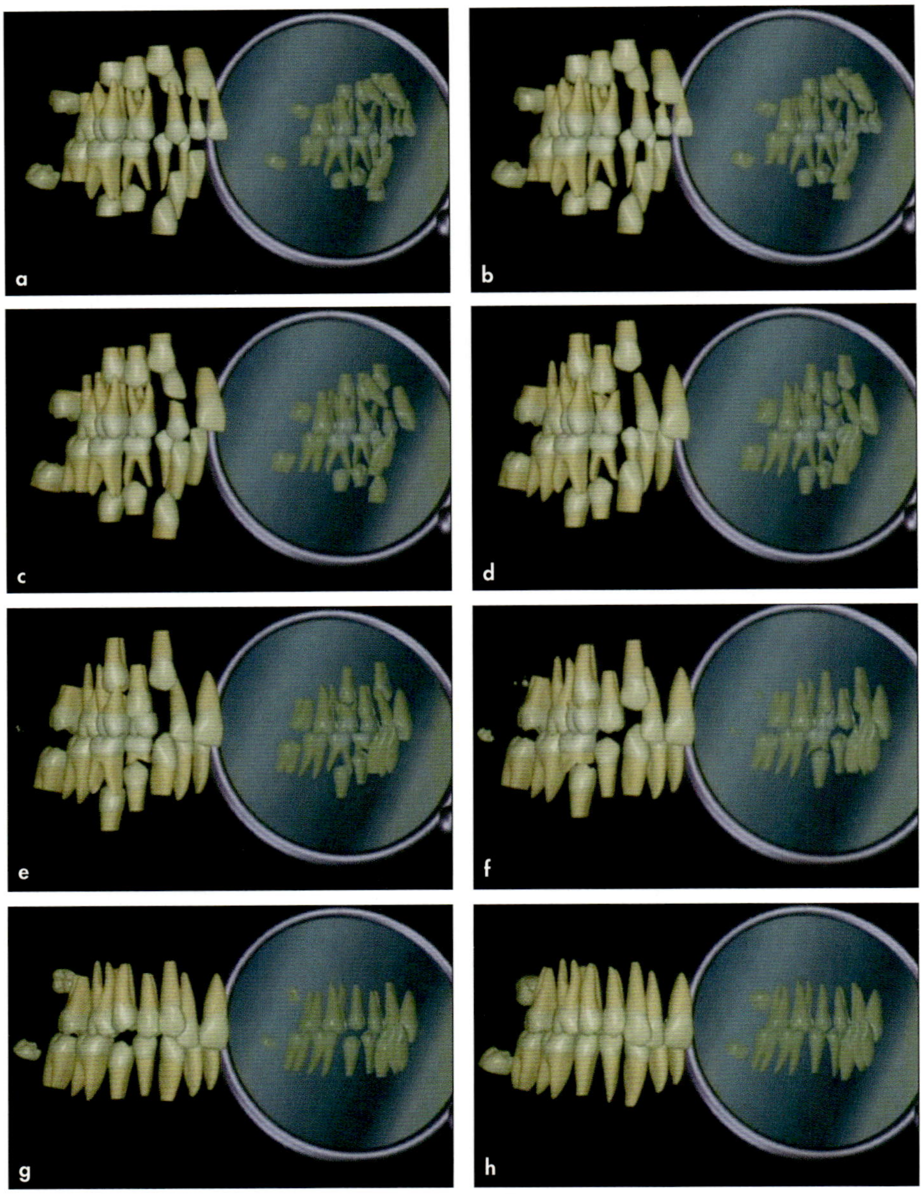

FIG 12-18 Development of a Class II, division 2, Type C malocclusion. *(a to c)* With the eruption of the maxillary central incisors, not only their predecessors but also the adjacent lateral deciduous incisors are lost. *(d)* Prior to the emergence of the maxillary lateral permanent incisors, the roots of the adjacent deciduous canines are resorbed and the crowns exfoliated. *(e)* Too little space remains for the maxillary permanent canines. *(f and g)* They emerge buccally outside the dental arch. *(h)* The mandibular incisors are tipped lingually. See video clip 41. Note that in Fig 12-14, the development of a Class II, division 2, Type C malocclusion was illustrated without premature loss of the lateral deciduous incisors. There, the lateral deciduous incisors and canines were lost simultaneously shortly prior to the emergence of the lateral permanent incisors. Both modes of transition occur in the development of Class II, division 2, Type C malocclusions and in Class I malocclusions with a total complete overbite. (Printed from Van der Linden et al[10] with permission.)

In addition, a total complete overbite can develop subsequent to an orthodontic treatment that is concluded with an excessive overlap of the maxillary incisors by the lower lip. This can happen with inadequate correction of a Class II, division 1 malocclusion with overerupted maxillary incisors (Fig 12-19).

The esthetic perception of Class II, division 2 malocclusions varies by type. Type A, with flattened aligned incisors and well-positioned canines, rarely causes concern. Type B, with severely proclined lateral incisors, is experienced as unesthetic and distracting. This also applies to the buccally positioned canines in Type C. Their mesial surfaces are visible, and the sharp cusp tips protrude.

FIG 12-19 Development of a total complete overbite after inadequate treatment of a Class II, division 1 malocclusion with overerupted maxillary incisors. *(a and b)* A boy aged 10 years 4 months had a Class II, division 1 malocclusion with a distoclusion of one premolar crown width. His lower lip was positioned palatal to the maxillary incisors, which were overerupted. The mandibular incisors were tipped lingually. *(c and d)* After problematic treatment for 2 years with cervical headgear, a maxillary plate, a lip bumper in the mandible, and finally an activator, a seemingly acceptable result with a neutroclusion was obtained. However, the maxillary incisors were too upright and the bite too deep. Continuation of the treatment with fixed appliances was not an option. *(e and f)* The treatment was not followed by a retention period. After 1 year, the maxillary central incisors were more palatally inclined, and the overbite had increased. *(g and h)* At that time, the excessive coverage of the maxillary incisors by the lower lip was verified. *(i and j)* Photographs taken 2 years 6 months later revealed that the maxillary incisors, except the right lateral incisor, had tipped more palatally and the overbite had increased further. Concomitantly, the mandibular incisors had tipped lingually, and crowding had developed in the mandibular anterior region. However, the solid intercuspation in neutroclusion was maintained. *(k and l)* Three years later, at the age of 18 years 10 months, the situation had worsened.[11] (Printed from Van der Linden[11] with permission.)

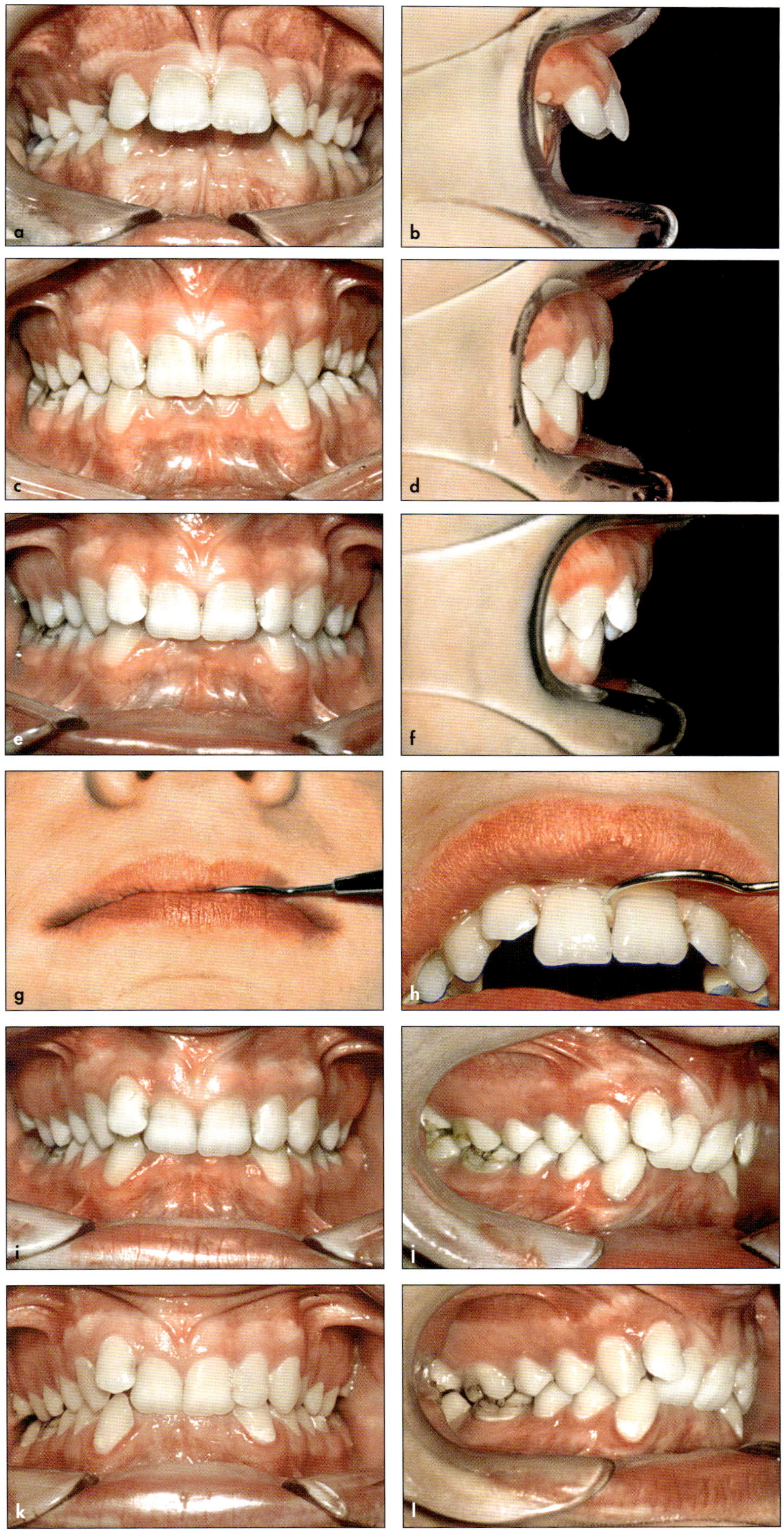

References

1. Daskalogianakis J. Glossary of Orthodontic Terms. Chicago: Quintessence, 2000.
2. Posen AL. The influence of maximum perioral and tongue forces on the incisor teeth. Angle Orthod 1972;42:285–309.
3. Falck F, Fränkel R. Die labiale Alveolenwand unter dem Einfluss des durchbrechenden Schneidezahnes. Fortschr Kieferorthop 1973;34:37–47.
4. Fränkel R, Falck F. Zahndurchbruch und Vererbang beim Deckbiss. Fortschr Kieferorthop 1967;28:175–182.
5. Fletcher GGT. The retroclined upper incisor. Br J Orthod 1975;2:207–216.
6. Kolf J. Anterior hypertonic syndrome in cases of Class II div. 2 [in French]. Rev Orthop Dento Faciale 1976;10:149–161.
7. Mills JRE. The problem of overbite in Class II, division 2 malocclusion. Br J Orthod 1973;1:34–48.
8. Nicol WA. The lower lip and the upper incisor teeth in Angle's Class II, division 2 malocclusion. Dent Pract (Bristol) 1963;14:179–182.
9. Leighton BC, Adams CP. Incisor inclination in Class 2 division 2 malocclusions. Eur J Orthod 1986;8:98–105.
10. Van der Linden FPGM, Radlanski RJ, McNamara JA Jr. Dynamics of Orthodontics: Malocclusions and Interventions [DVD 3B]. Berlin: Quintessence, 2000.
11. Van der Linden FPGM. Orthodontic Concepts and Strategies. Chicago: Quintessence, 2004.

13

Class III Malocclusions

Characteristics of Class III Malocclusions

In Class III malocclusions, the mandibular dental arch is positioned anterior to the maxillary dental arch. This leads to mesioclusion and a negative overjet. In occlusion, the edges of the mandibular incisors are anterior to the maxillary incisors. As mentioned previously, the Angle classification does not specify if the malocclusion is caused by an abnormality in the mandible, the maxilla, or a combination of the two.

Between 1% to 2% of the Western population and 5% to 10% of the Asian population have a Class III malocclusion.[1–3] The primary factor in Class III malocclusions is the mesial relationship of the jaws. Secondary aspects are the negative overjet and, in severe cases, the tipping of the maxillary incisors to the labial and the mandibular incisors to the lingual.

The development of Class III malocclusions cannot be explained using a normal mandibular dental arch as a starting point, as was done for the Class II, division 1 malocclusion. As described previously, in Class II, division 1 malocclusions, the overjet and overbite enlarge gradually with the increase of the distoclusion. The form of the mandibular dental arch, as seen from the occlusal, is unchanged or only slightly affected. In Class III malocclusions, however, the increase in mesioclusion leads to a reverse sagittal contact of the incisors with specific deviations in tooth positions in both jaws.

Class III malocclusion is shown for the deciduous dentition in Fig 13-1, the intertransitional period in Fig 13-2, and the permanent dentition in Fig 13-3. In addition, the malocclusion is illustrated with clinical photographs in Fig 13-4. This is followed by the presentation of the transition of the incisors and the emergence of the first permanent molars in Fig 13-5.

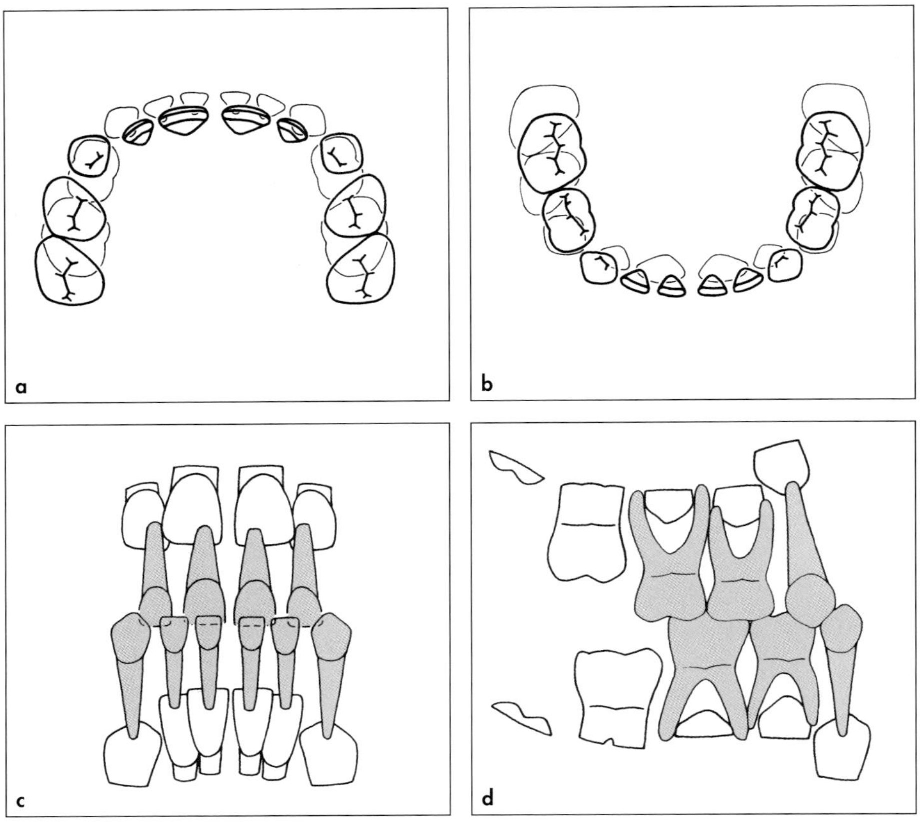

Fig 13-1 Class III malocclusion in the deciduous dentition (compare with Fig 2-26). *(a and b)* The mandibular dental arch is too anterior in relation to the maxillary dental arch. The deciduous molars occlude adequately in the transverse direction. There is a negative overjet at the incisors and canines. *(c)* There is a slight overbite. *(d)* The occlusion of the mandibular deciduous molars with the maxillary deciduous molars is too mesial. The terminal plane has an abnormally large mesial step.

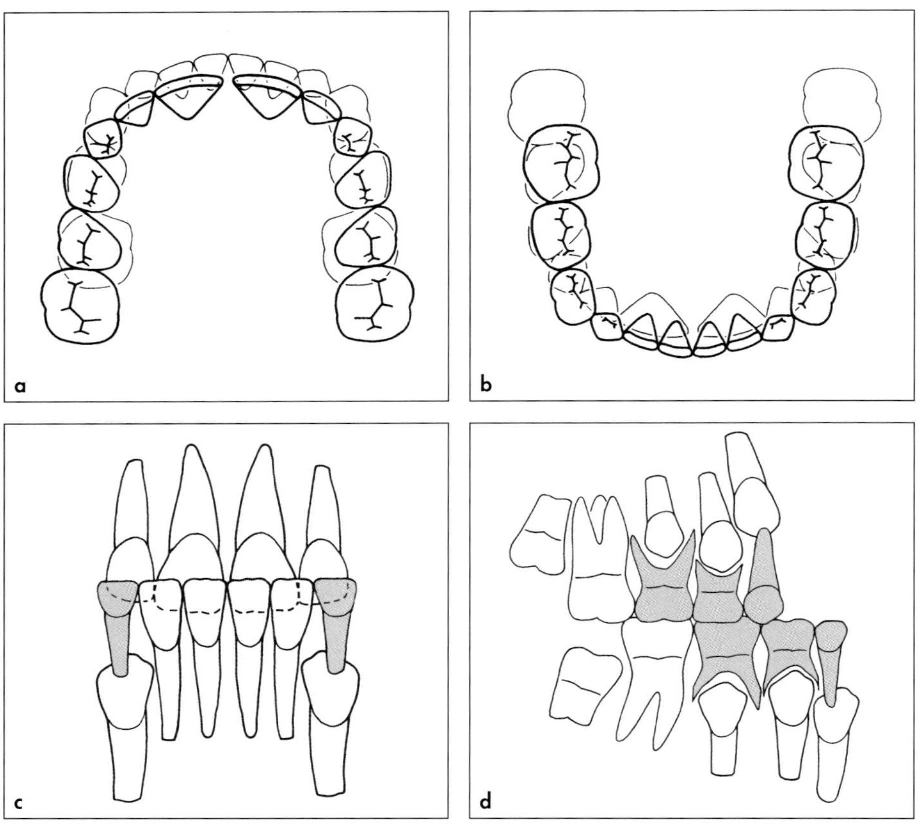

Fig 13-2 Class III malocclusion in the intertransitional period (compare with Fig 4-1). *(a and b)* The mandibular dental arch is too anterior in relation to the maxillary dental arch. There is a negative overjet. The positions of the individual teeth are adapted to the occlusion, which crosses at the canine region. The mandibular incisors overlap the maxillary incisors. *(c)* The edges of the maxillary incisors are in contact with the lingual surfaces of the mandibular incisors. *(d)* The mandibular first permanent molar occludes too mesially, making only slight contact with the maxillary first permanent molar.

FIG 13-3 Class III malocclusion in the permanent dentition (compare with Fig 7-1). *(a and b)* The mandibular dental arch is too anterior in relation to the maxillary dental arch. There is a negative overjet. *(c)* The mandibular canines are located labial to the maxillary lateral incisors. *(d)* All posterior teeth occlude one premolar crown width too far to the mesial.

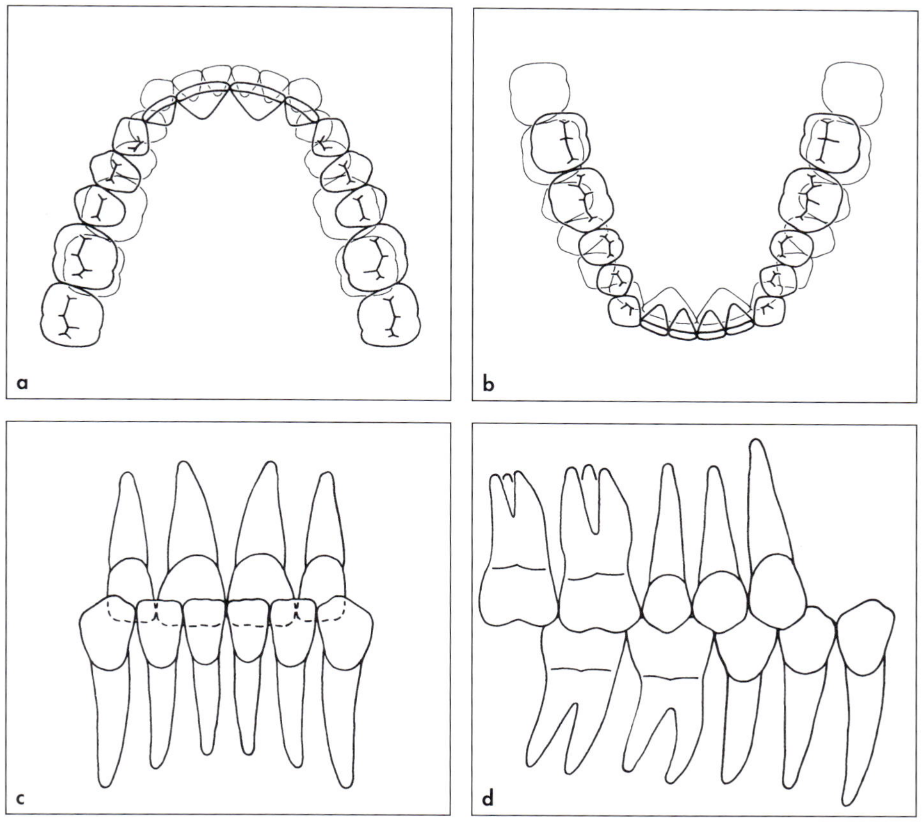

FIG 13-4 Class III malocclusion. *(a)* The midface recedes, the mandible dominates, and the lower lip protrudes. *(b to d)* The mandibular incisors are tipped lingually and occlude anterior to the maxillary incisors. There is mesioclusion on both sides.

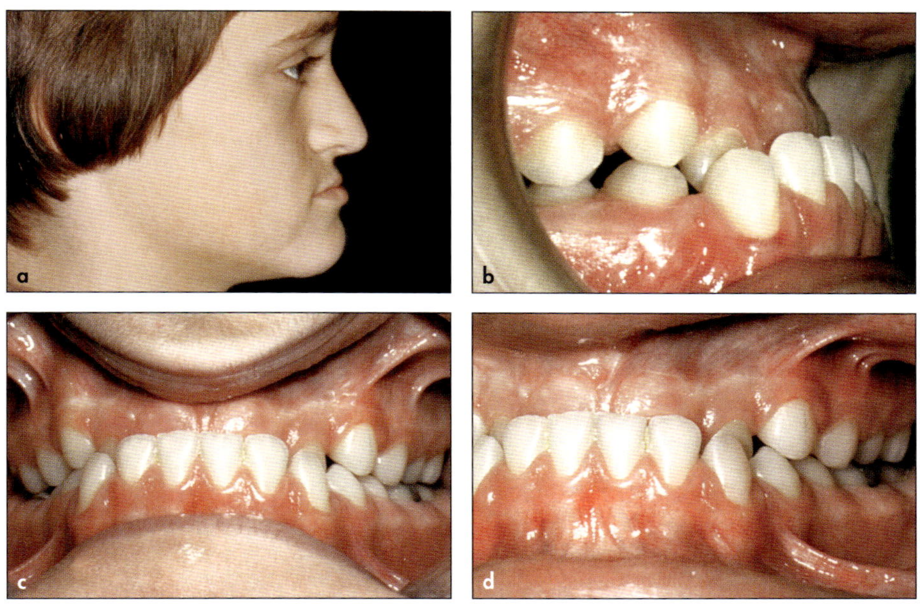

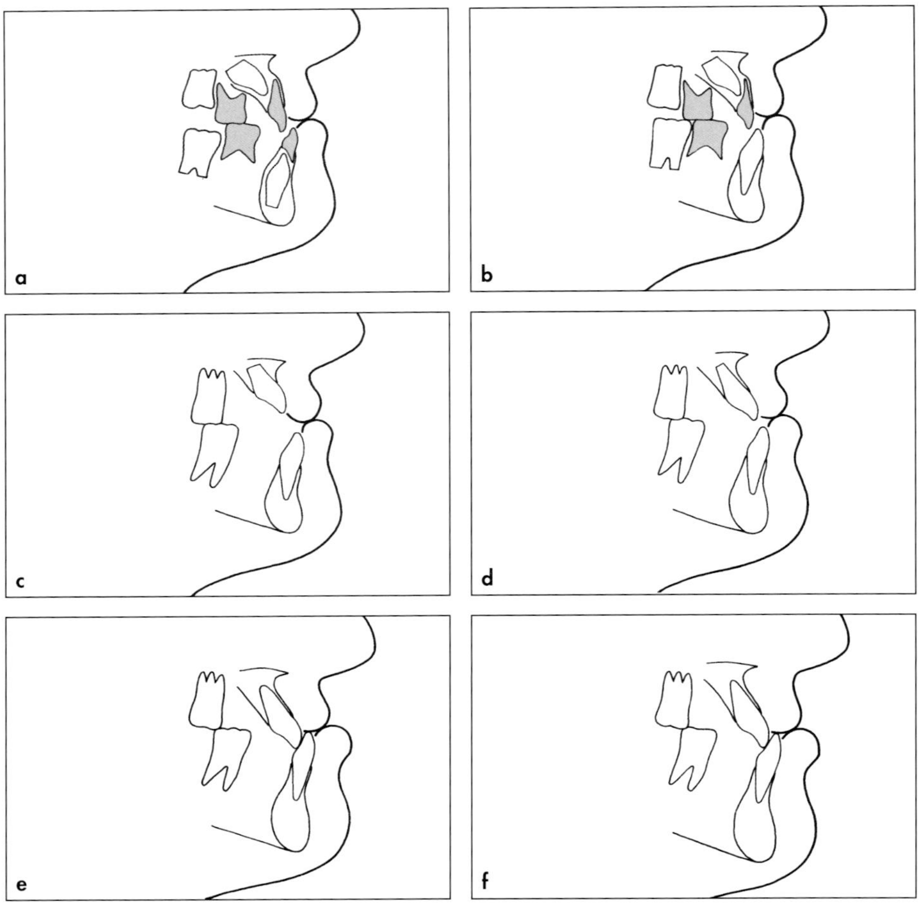

FIG 13-5 Development of a Class III malocclusion (compare with Fig 3-4). *(a)* There is already a negative overjet in the deciduous dentition. The position and inclination of the permanent incisors within the jaws is normal. The lower lip is more anteriorly located than the upper lip. *(b)* The mandibular central permanent incisors erupt and emerge normally. The lower lip does not touch the maxillary central deciduous incisors. *(c)* The first permanent molars have emerged in mesioclusion. The mandibular central incisors erupt further. The maxillary central incisors erupt from the position they occupied in the jaw. *(d)* The lower lip does not touch the maxillary central incisors and does not affect their inclination. The maxillary central incisors are not vertically supported by the lower lip. *(e)* Their labial incisal edges contact the lingual surface of the mandibular incisors. *(f)* The prominence of the chin has increased.

In Class III malocclusions, the lower lip is clearly positioned more anteriorly than the upper lip. Together with the dominant chin, it causes the characteristic appearance and profile of a Class III malocclusion (Fig 13-6). The negative overjet leads to a specific relationship between the lips and incisors and affects the sagittal and vertical support of the incisors.

The development of Class III malocclusion presented shows a mesioclusion of the width of one premolar crown. However, most Class III malocclusions are not so severe, and some are more severe. In Class II malocclusions, the scale from a neutroclusion to a severe malocclusion is gradual. In Class III malocclusions, on the other hand, the transition from a normal to a negative overjet is abrupt; in between are increasing levels of mesioclusion resulting in distinguishable degrees of anterior forced bites.

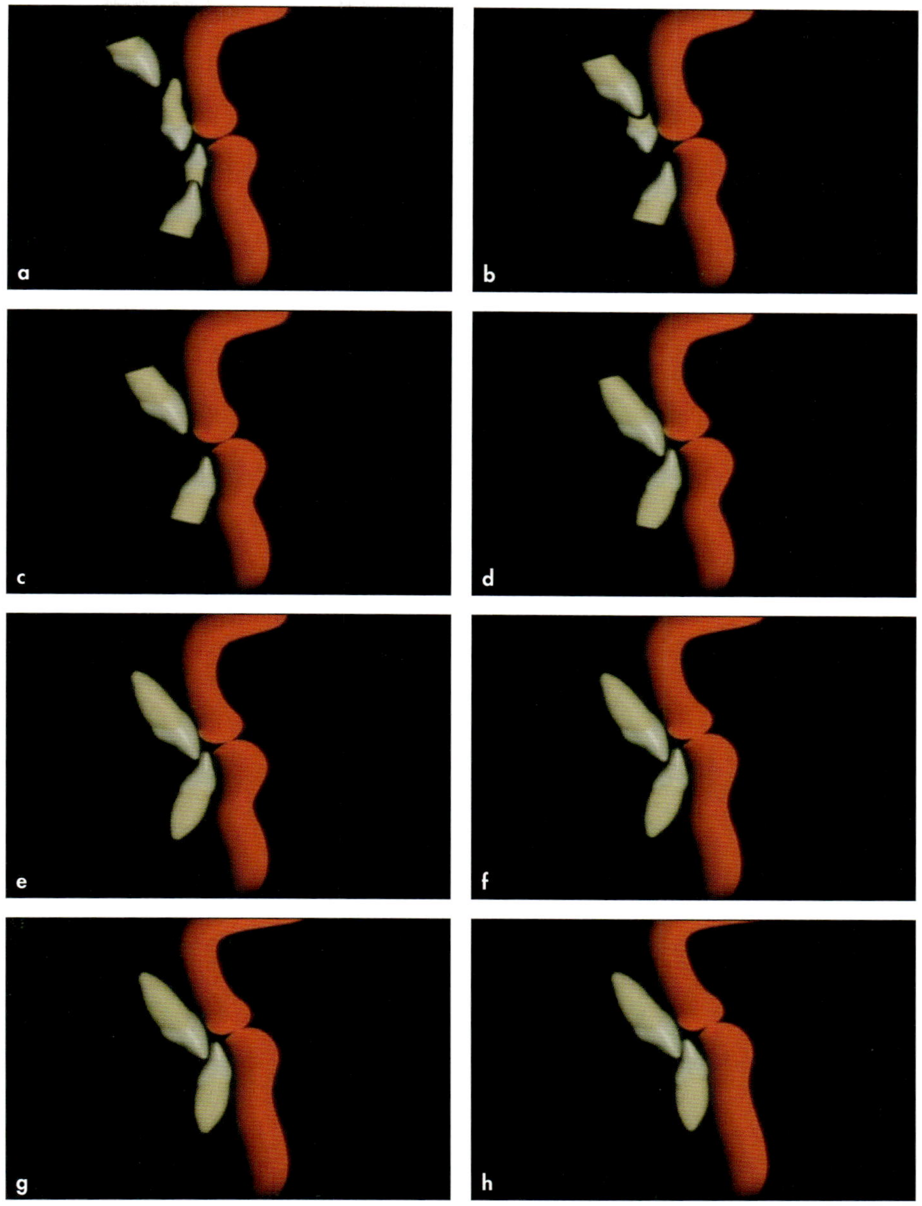

FIG 13-6 Influence of tongue and lips on the incisors in a Class III malocclusion. The amount of negative overjet and the extent to which the teeth overlap vertically depend on the sagittal occlusion and the local conditions in the dental arches. Furthermore, the tongue and lips play an essential role. *(a to d)* In extreme Class III malocclusions, the maxillary incisors become tipped labially, and the mandibular incisors become tipped lingually. This tipping increases as the mesioclusion advances. *(e to h)* The maxillary and mandibular incisors support each other vertically. The degree of vertical support and the associated amount of overbite vary. With growth to adulthood, the typical profile that characterizes the Class III malocclusion intensifies. The lower lip protrudes more, and the dominance of the chin increases. See video clip 42. (Printed from Van der Linden et al[4] with permission.)

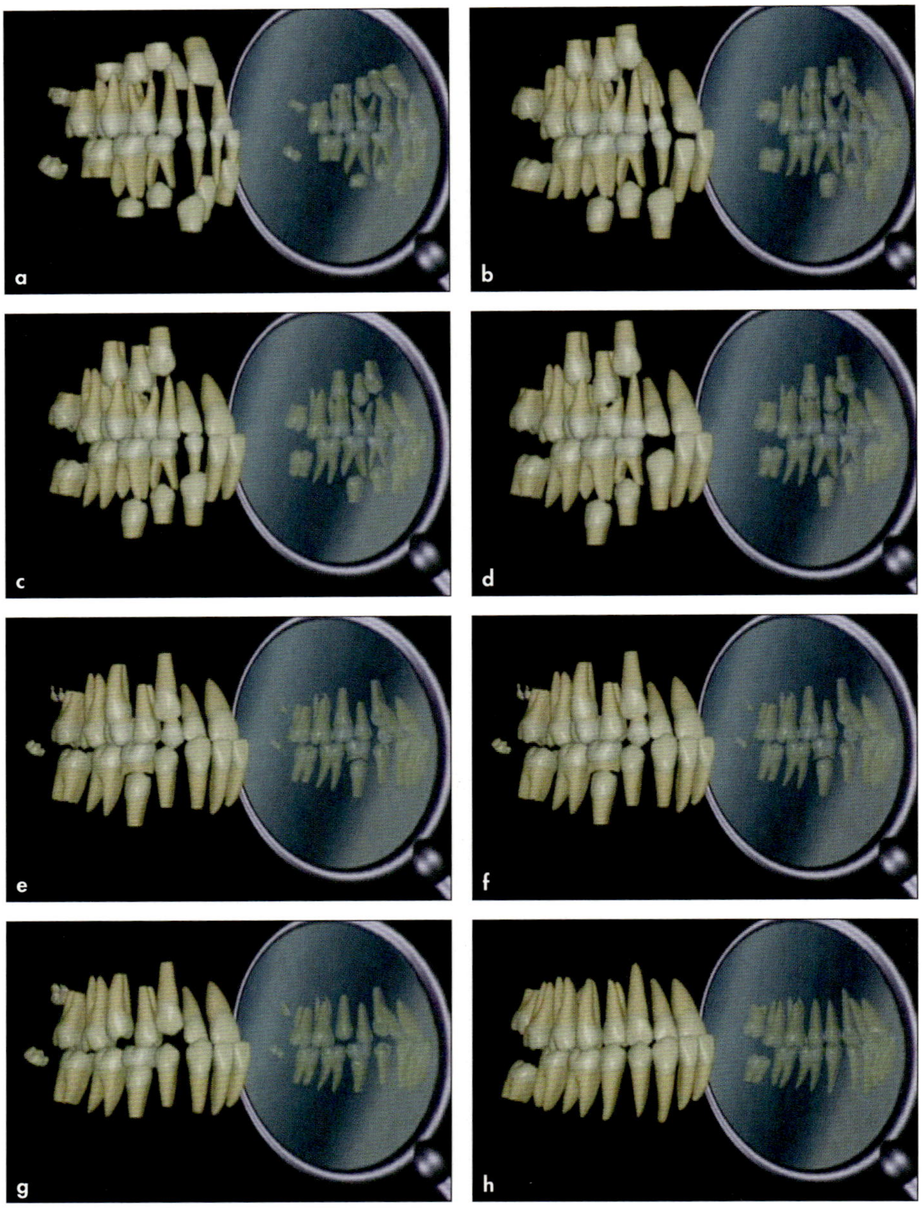

Fig 13-7 Development of a mild Class III malocclusion. *(a and b)* After emergence, the permanent incisors are in a negative overjet. *(c and d)* The transition of the canines and deciduous molars/premolars proceeds normally, albeit in mesioclusion. *(e and f)* In a mild Class III malocclusion, the mesioclusion is about half the width of a premolar crown. *(g and h)* In such cases, the incisors do not tip or tip only slightly. See video clip 43. (Printed from Van der Linden et al[4] with permission.)

In the deciduous dentition, there is end-to-end occlusion of the incisors or a slight negative overjet. The negative overjet usually arises after the transition of the incisors. The mesioclusion can increase by excessive anterior growth of the mandible, insufficient anterior development of the maxilla, or a combination of both.

In most cases, the anterior growth of the mandible is not progressive, and as a result, the Class III malocclusion does not become extreme (Fig 13-7). However, sometimes mandibular growth is excessive and continues even after the adolescent growth spurt is concluded (Figs 13-8 and 13-9). In such cases, the mesioclusion may exceed one premolar crown width. (See video clip 44.)

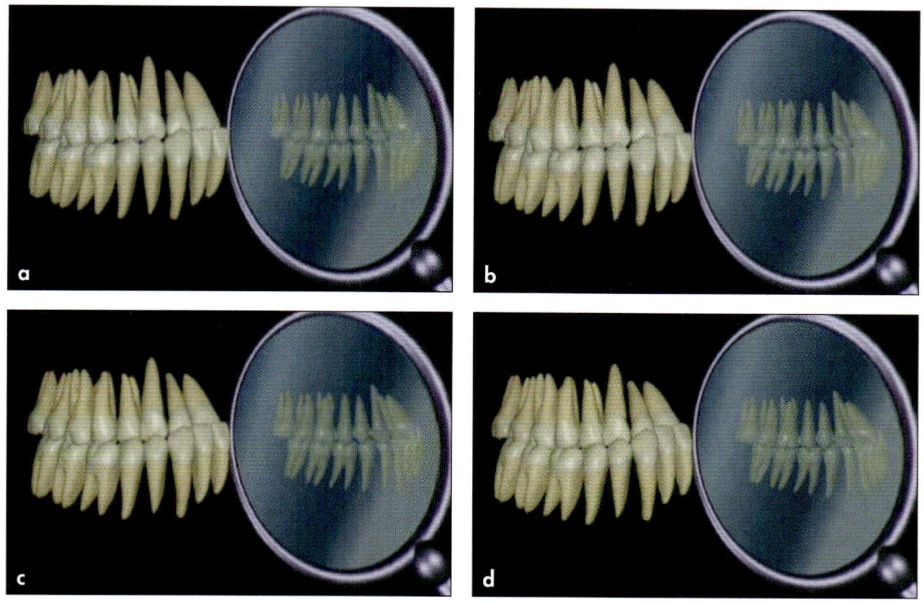

FIG 13-8 Increase in severity of Class III malocclusions. The range of variations in Class III malocclusions is large, exceeding the width of a premolar crown. The greater the mesioclusion, the more the incisors tip. See video clip 45. (Printed from Van der Linden et al[4] with permission.)

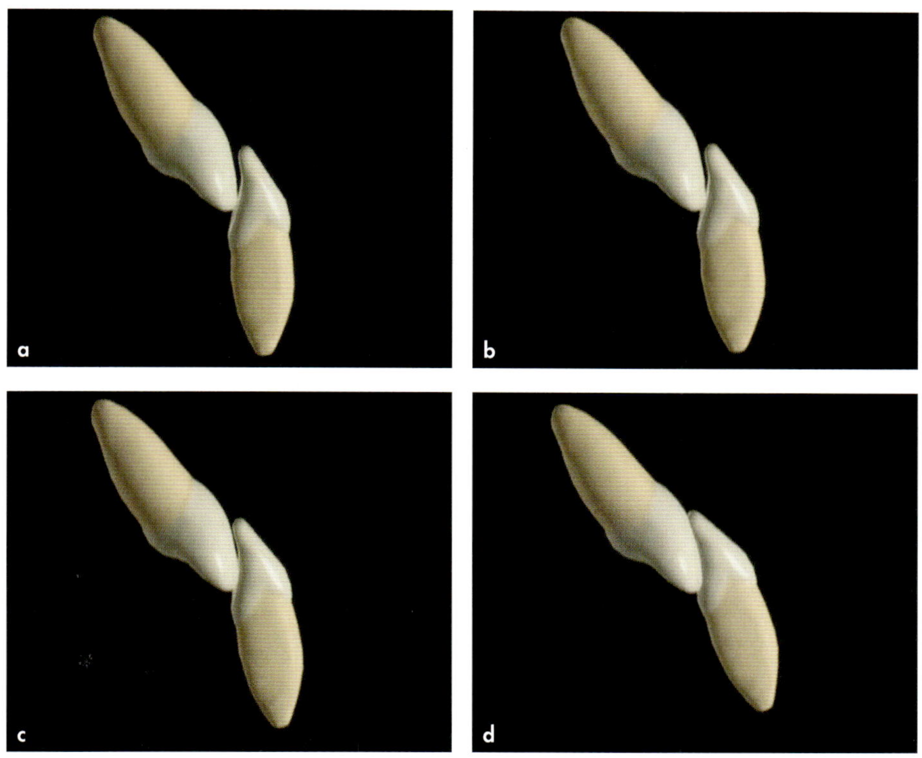

FIG 13-9 Tipping of incisors in Class III malocclusions. The larger the sagittal discrepancy, the greater the labial tip of the maxillary incisors and the lingual tip of the mandibular incisors. See video clip 46. (Printed from Van der Linden et al[4] with permission.)

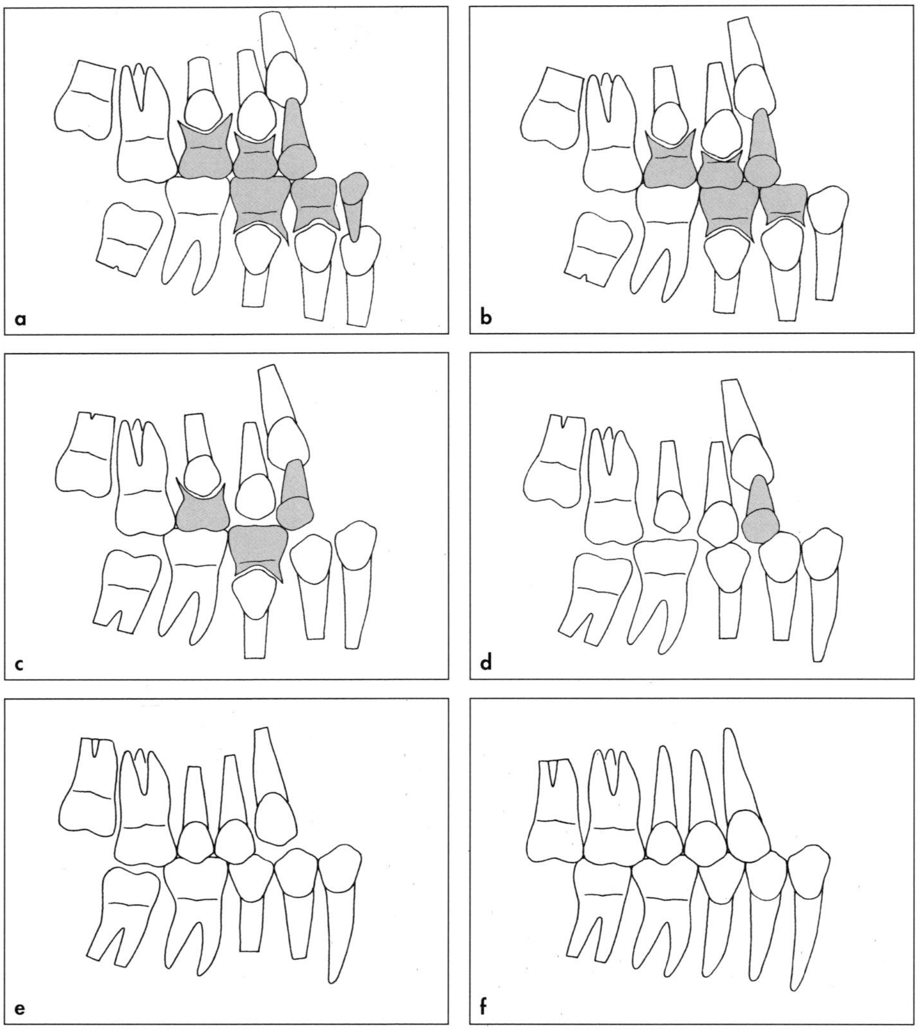

Fig 13-10 Transition of the canines and deciduous molars/premolars and emergence of the first permanent molars in a Class III malocclusion of the width of a premolar crown that did not progress further (compare with Fig 5-1). *(a)* The mandibular posterior teeth occlude mesial to the maxillary ones. The position of the second permanent molars within the jaws is consistent with the mesioclusion. *(b)* The resorption of the deciduous teeth and the eruption of the permanent teeth proceed normally. *(c and d)* With the emergence of the premolars, the mesioclusion is consolidated. *(e)* The maxillary permanent canine will occlude distal to the mandibular first premolar. *(f)* The occlusal contact between the first and newly emerged second permanent molars is limited.

Adequate transverse contact of the posterior teeth can be present in mesioclusions (Fig 13-10). In severe Class III malocclusions, however, the maxillary premolars and molars may arrive in crossbite, and the mandibular dental arch will be wider than the maxillary dental arch.

The position of the individual teeth depends on the occlusal contacts. In mild Class III malocclusions and anterior forced bites, the maxillary incisors are inclined palatally, and the mandibular incisors are inclined labially (Fig 13-11). In severe Class III malocclusions, the maxillary incisors are inclined labially, and the mandibular incisors are inclined lingually. The tipping of the incisors increases with greater mesioclusion. With this adaption in inclination, the sagittal discrepancy is partly compensated. Severe Class III malocclusions have a typical facial appearance (Fig 13-12).

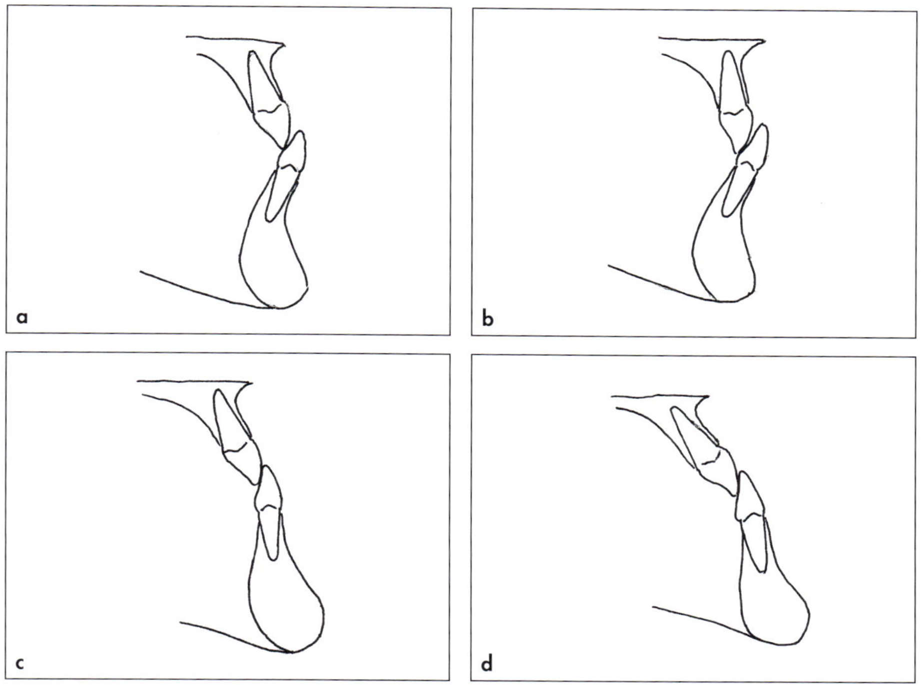

Fig 13-11 Variations in inclination of incisors in Class III malocclusions. *(a)* In an anterior forced bite the mandibular incisors can be tipped labially and the maxillary incisors palatally. *(b)* In a slight mesioclusion, the inclination will be normal or deviate only slightly. *(c and d)* In severe Class III malocclusions, the maxillary incisors tip labially, and the mandibular incisors lingually.

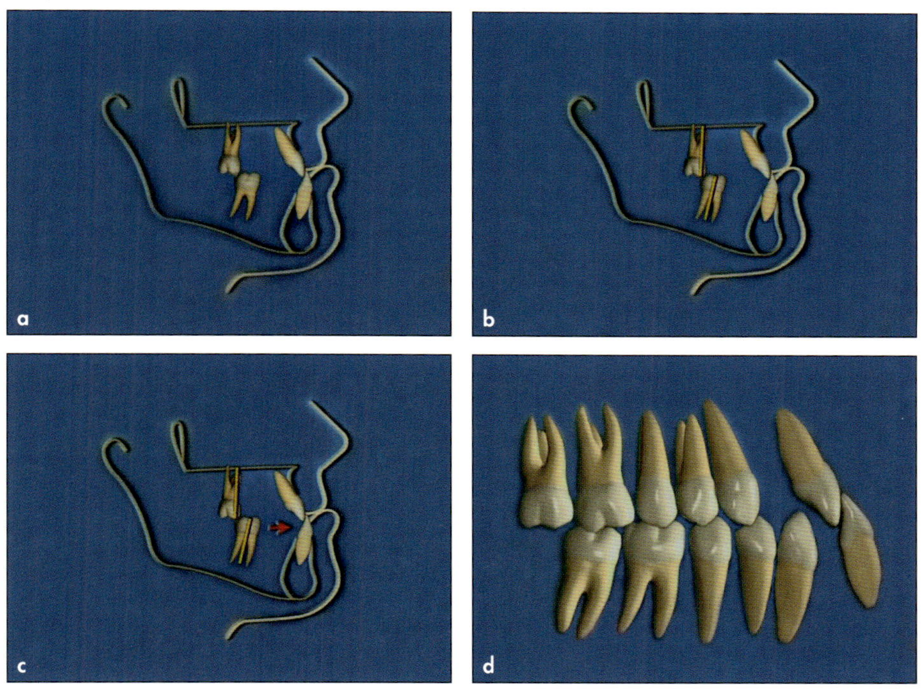

Fig 13-12 Characteristics of a Class III malocclusion. *(a)* The increased anteroposterior step between the upper and lower lip and the chin dominance are typical. *(b)* The first permanent molars are in mesioclusion. *(c)* The tongue and lips play an essential role in the tipping of the incisors. *(d)* There is a negative overjet and, as is often the case, an adequate transverse occlusion in the posterior region.

Forced Bite

The habitual occlusion is affected by the initial contact reached in centric relation. If premature contact is made, closing will proceed with a slide in the anterior and/or lateral direction. This phenomenon is called forced bite. Anterior forced bites occur in moderate mesioclusion (see video clip 47). In these cases, with the mandible in the most retruded position, contact is made with the incisors (Fig 13-13). In spontaneous closure, premature contact followed by a slide to habitual occlusion does not occur. Individuals with forced bites move directly to the habitual occlusion.[5]

Mild Class III malocclusions are associated with anterior forced bites, which are sometimes referred to as pseudo Class III malocclusions. The size of the forced bite is measured by the difference between the most retruded position of the mandible and its position in habitual occlusion. This is accomplished by manually moving the mandible from habitual occlusion to its most retruded position (Fig 13-14). Forced bites are discussed further in chapter 15 (see video clip 48).

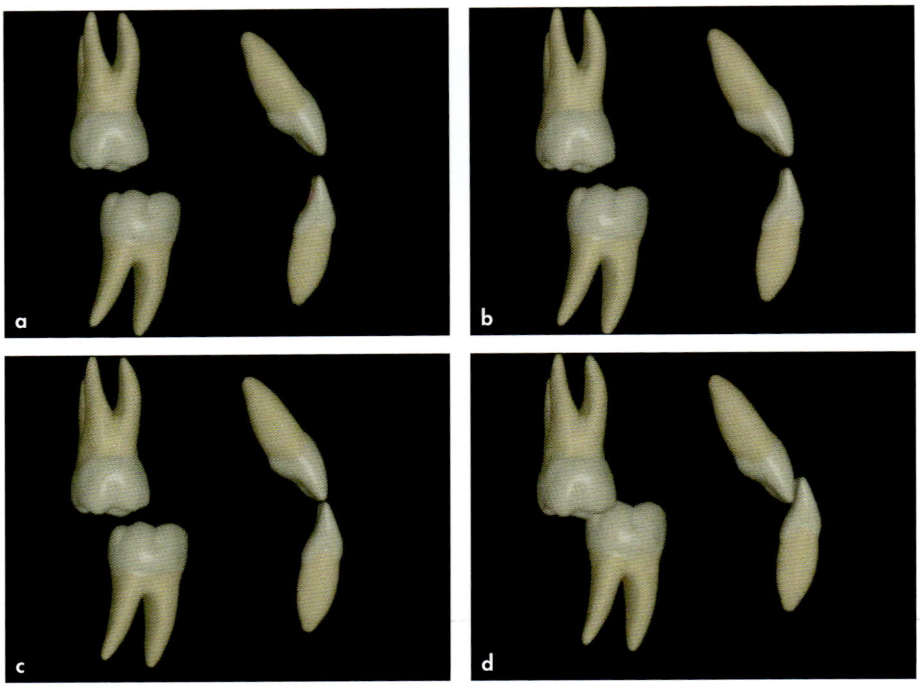

FIG 13-13 Closing in an anterior forced bite. *(a)* With the mandible in the most retruded position, the central incisors are in end-to-end position. *(b and c)* The posterior teeth can occlude only after a diversion is made to the anterior. *(d)* The result is a negative overjet. In spontaneous closing, patients with an anterior forced bite avoid premature contact and move directly to the final position. See video clip 47. (Printed from Van der Linden et al[4] with permission.)

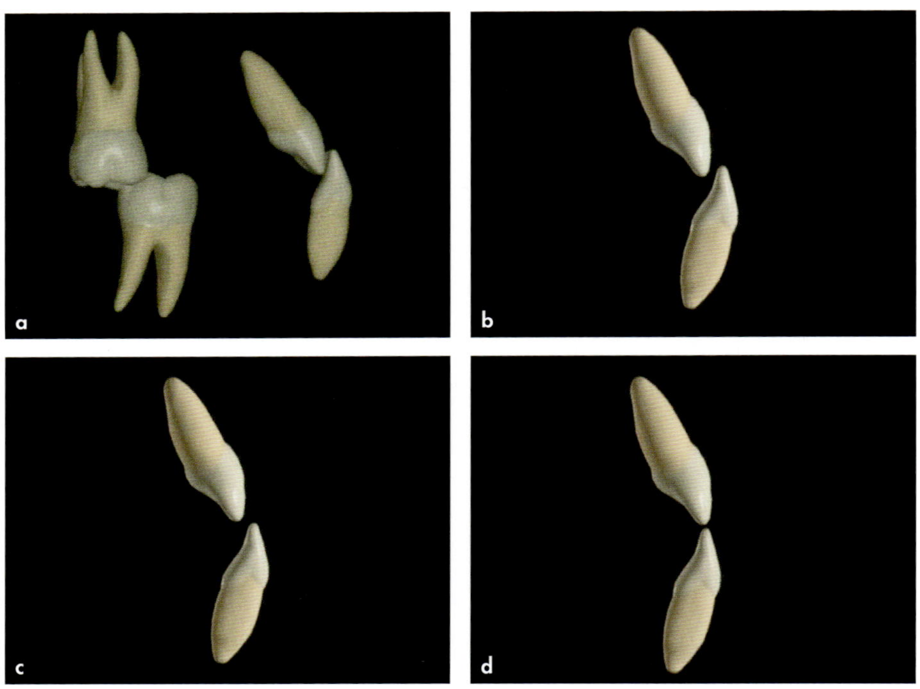

FIG 13-14 Assessing the extent of an anterior forced bite. *(a)* The negative overjet is the result of the diverging movement. *(b)* With a small anterior forced bite, the mandible can only make a slight movement to the posterior in habitual occlusion. *(c)* In a moderate forced bite, the mandible can make a larger posterior movement. *(d)* At most, an end-to-end occlusion can be reached. See video clip 27. (Printed from Van der Linden et al[4] with permission.

References

1. Kitai N, Takada K, Yasuda Y, et al. Prevalence of malocclusions and demand for orthodontic treatment among students at a woman's high school [in Japanese]. Osaka Daigaku Shigaku Zasshi 1990;35:321–327.
2. Lin JJ. Prevalence of malocclusion in Chinese children age 9-15. Clin Dent (Taiwan) 1985;5:57–65.
3. Proffit WR, Rields HW, Moray LS. Prevalence of malocclusion and orthodontic treatment need in the United States: Estimates from the NHANES-III survey. Int Adult Orthod Orthognath Surg 1998;13:97–106.
4. Van der Linden FPGM, Radlanski RJ, McNamara JA Jr. Dynamics of Orthodontics: Malocclusions and Interventions [DVD 3B]. Berlin: Quintessence, 2000.
5. Hamerling J. Mandibular Movement Patterns [thesis]. Amsterdam: University of Amsterdam, 1983.

14

Open Bites and Nonocclusion

In dentistry, the prevailing standard is that teeth should be in maximal contact with a solid intercuspation of the posterior teeth in habitual occlusion. However, that is not the reality. Open bites (Fig 14-1), characterized by a lack of overlap of opposing teeth, are not uncommon. Even more prevalent is nonocclusion (Fig 14-2), in which opposing teeth overlap or make no or only limited contact and no optimal occlusal contacts exist.

Causes of Open Bites and Nonocclusion

Open bites and nonocclusion are usually caused by factors that inhibit and stop eruption and occasionally by a disturbance in the eruption mechanism, eg, ankylosis and primary failure of eruption.

Anterior open bites are fairly common in the deciduous dentition and are mostly caused by digit sucking or pacifier use. The size and location of the open bite depends on the position of the objects in the mouth. If the open bite is caused exclusively by digit sucking or pacifier use, it will disappear spontaneously when the habit is stopped if this occurs prior to or during the transition of the incisors and if the tongue is not positioned at rest in the open space.[1–4] The induced protrusion, labial inclination, and asymmetric position of anterior teeth will also dissipate. If the habit is stopped later, improvements, if not full resolution of the problems, still can occur.

In adolescents and adults, tongue interposition is usually the cause of open bites and nonocclusion. The size of the open bite or nonocclusion in the anterior region depends on the extent to which the tongue is held between the mandibular and maxillary anterior teeth or between the mandibular teeth and the palate. If this is limited and the tongue is kept inside the maxillary dental arch, a nonocclusion will result. When a significant portion of the tongue is held between the opposing anterior teeth, then an open bite will be produced.

The tongue position is primarily genetically determined. The attainment of another position during growth and maturation of the face can be traced back to changes in the size and relations of the various structures involved. However, age-related, genetically encoded alterations in tongue position also play a role. A tongue that initially appears to be large can become less dominant with continued growth of the face. In addition, neuromuscular aspects can change and result in another tongue position. Unfortunately, it is difficult to predict if open bites and nonocclusion will be maintained or disappear spontaneously.

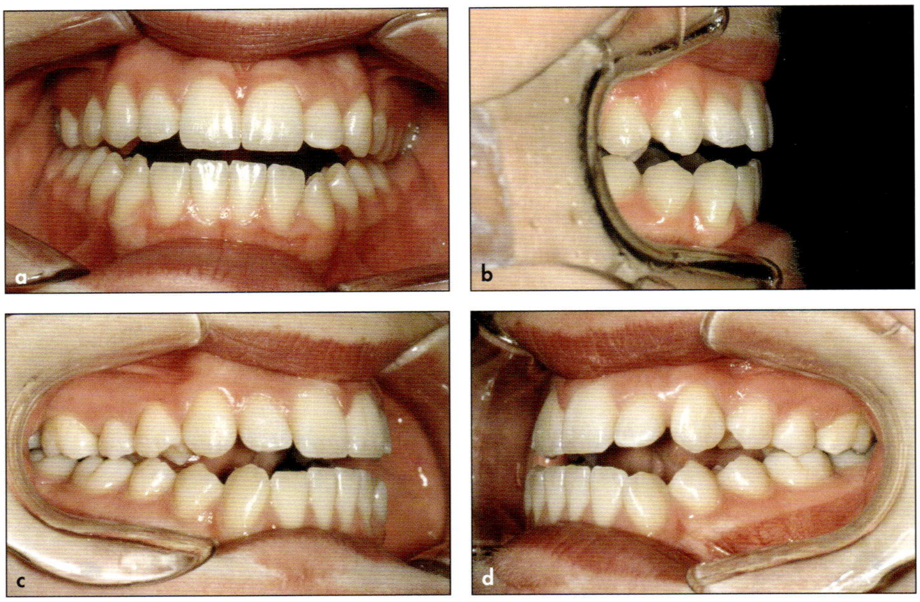

FIG 14-1 Open bite. *(a to d)* A large anterior open bite extending to the second premolars in a 14-year-old girl.

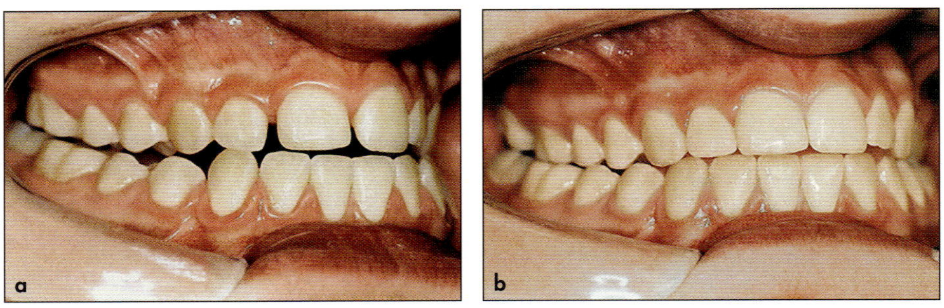

FIG 14-2 Nonocclusion in daughter and mother. *(a)* The 13-year-old daughter has complete nonocclusion and an open bite at the maxillary central incisors. *(b)* The 35-year-old mother has nonocclusion in the anterior, premolar, and molar regions.

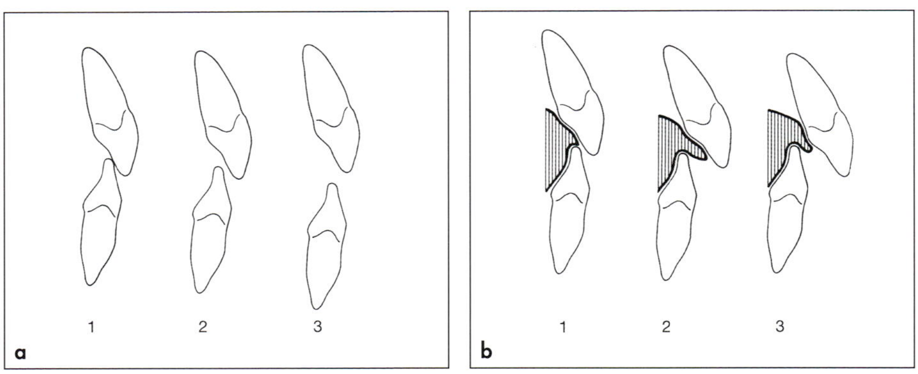

FIG 14-3 Variations in open bites and nonocclusion. *(a)* The change-over where nonocclusion becomes open bite (2 and 3) is somewhat arbitrary. *(b)* Slight nonocclusion with a small overjet (1), large nonocclusion with a large overjet (2), and large nonocclusion with a very large overjet and overbite (3). Note the differences in vertical overlap of the incisors.

Forms of Open Bites and Nonocclusion

The distinction between an open bite and nonocclusion is somewhat arbitrary but based on whether or not there is vertical overlap of opposing teeth[5] (Figs 14-3 to 14-5). Open bites and nonocclusion, whether they occur in the anterior or posterior regions, can be partial or complete and can occur unilaterally or bilaterally (Fig 14-6). The most extreme form is the total open bite or nonocclusion, in which no teeth have optimal vertical contact during swallowing (see Fig 14-2). The tongue is held between all opposing teeth at rest and during swallowing.

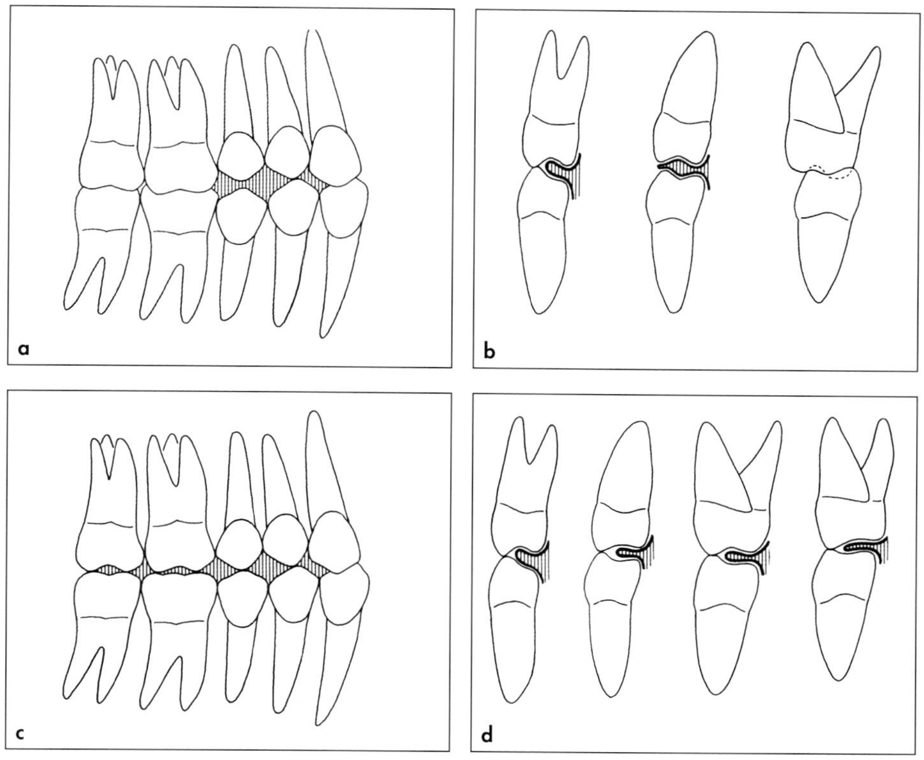

Fig 14-4 Open bites and nonocclusion in the posterior regions. *(a and b)* Local open bite at the second premolars and nonocclusion at the first premolars. The molars intercuspate adequately. *(c)* Nonocclusion along the entire length of the right posterior region. There is incomplete contact between the opposing teeth. *(d)* The teeth are not adjusted in the transverse direction. In many cases of nonocclusion in the posterior regions, the tongue lies only between the lingual cusps, while the buccal cusps touch each other.

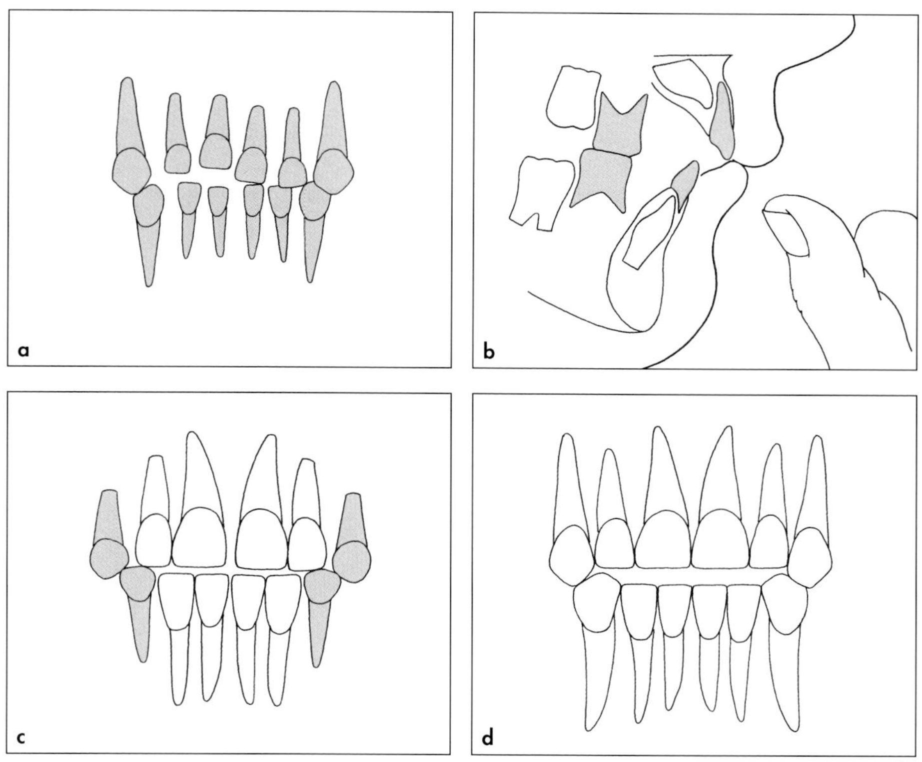

Fig 14-5 Anterior open bites. *(a and b)* An asymmetric open bite caused by digit sucking is quite common in the deciduous dentition. An open bite caused by pacifier use is symmetric in shape. If the habit is not stopped in due time, the permanent incisors will have a similar position. *(c and d)* Open bites caused by tongue interposition can vary in extent.

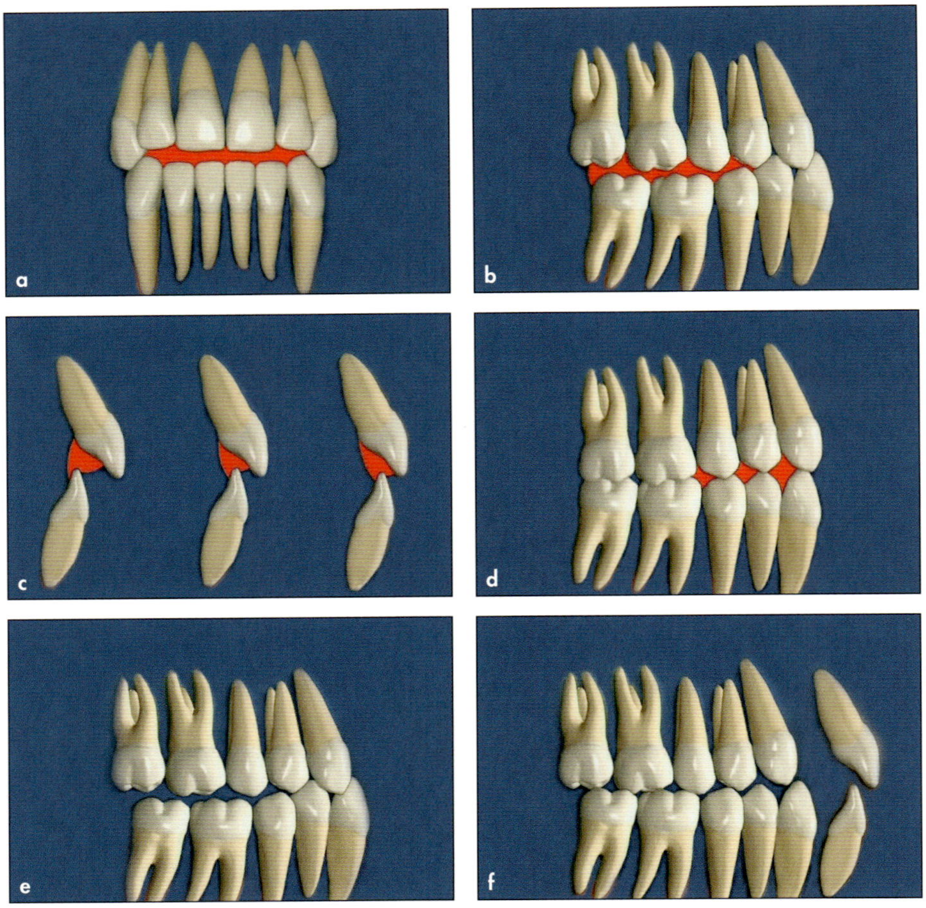

Fig 14-6 Open bites and nonocclusion. *(a)* Anterior open bites due to tongue interposition are usually shaped symmetrically. *(b)* Open bites can also develop in the posterior regions, unilaterally or bilaterally. *(c)* In the anterior region, the prevalence of nonocclusion is much higher than that of open bites. *(d)* This also holds true in the posterior regions, where in nonocclusion the buccal cusp tips usually contact each other. *(e)* Open bite in the premolar and molar regions, not at the canines. *(f)* Total nonocclusion.

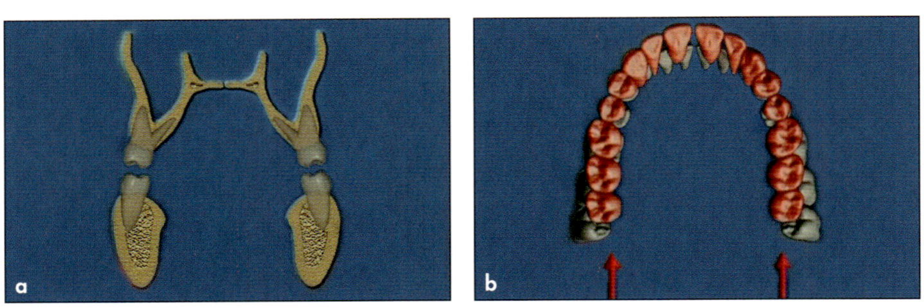

Fig 14-7 Effects of open bites and nonocclusion on the posterior regions. *(a)* The tongue interposition interferes with guidance to optimal occlusion through the cone-funnel mechanism. *(b)* In addition, the rail mechanism cannot function; as a result, the maxillary dental arch does not widen.

Nonocclusion in the anterior region occurs quite often in Class II, division 1 malocclusions. It is not troublesome as long as the teeth are well aligned. Observers and the individual with nonocclusion usually do not know that there is any abnormality. In addition, from a functional standpoint, nonocclusion in the anterior region is seldom a source of complaints.

Open bites and nonocclusion in the posterior region vary in size and in the number of teeth involved. They are often associated with a narrow maxillary dental arch and a broad mandibular dental arch. That is partly due to the absence of the cone-funnel mechanism and the lack of adaptation of the inclination of opposing teeth. Also, the rail mechanism does not function with tongue interposition (Fig 14-7). An overly narrow maxillary dental arch and posterior teeth positioned on top of each other transversely (ie, end-to-end occlusion) are caused mostly by tongue interposition.

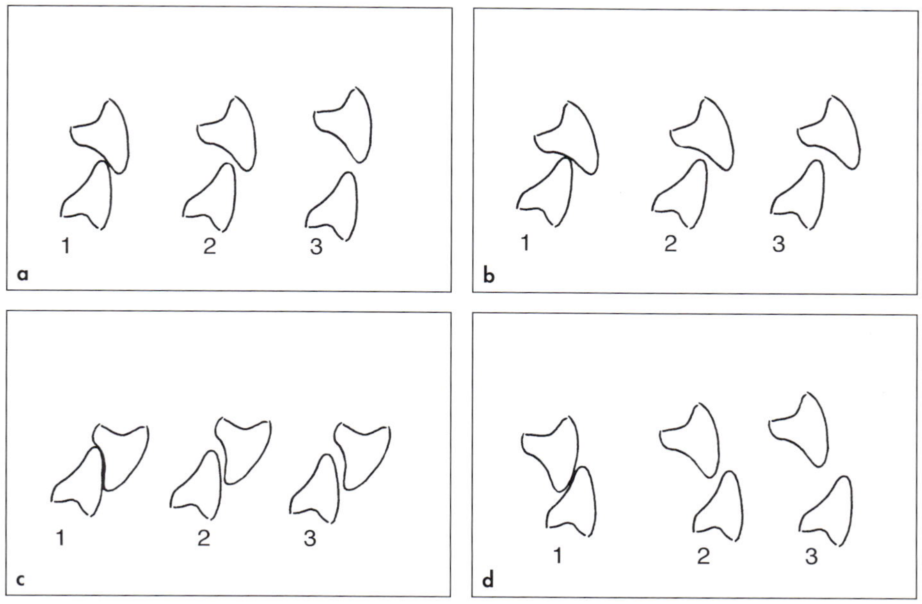

FIG 14-8 Variations in relationships between opposing incisors. *(a)* In a Class I situation (1), the incisors overlap each other with contact in the anterior region. In nonocclusion (2), the anterior teeth overlap but do not contact each other; there is some space between them. Only when there is no overlap (3) is the term *open bite* used. *(b)* In a Class II, division 1 malocclusion, antagonists can be separated by a large space while still overlapping each other (3), ie, nonocclusion. *(c)* The same applies to Class II, division 2 malocclusions (2 and 3). *(d)* In Class III malocclusions, anterior nonocclusion (2) seldom occurs, and open bites (3) sometimes occur.

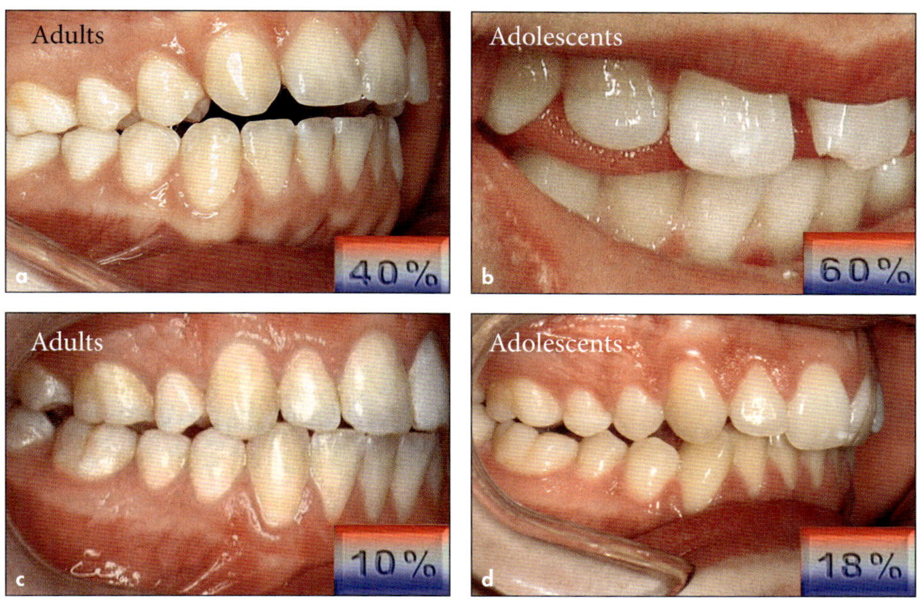

FIG 14-9 Prevalence of open bites and nonocclusion. *(a)* A national epidemiologic survey carried out in the Netherlands in the 1980s revealed that in 40% of 2,273 individuals between 15 and 70 years of age, the mandibular incisors contacted neither the maxillary incisors nor the palate.[8] *(b)* Of the 525 adolescents (between 15 and 20 years of age), 60% had no anterior contact. *(c and d)* For the posterior regions, the prevalence of open bites and nonocclusion combined was 10% and 18%, respectively.[7]

Incidence of Open Bites and Nonocclusion

Open bites and nonocclusion occur in all types of malocclusions and incisor relationships (Fig 14-8), even in total compete overbites (see chapter 12, Figs 12-15 and 12-16). They are quite common in the Netherlands but also occur in other countries.[6] A large population study in the Netherlands revealed that open bites and nonocclusion occur less frequently in adults than in adolescents[7] (Fig 14-9). Based on the results of other investigations, the conclusion can be reached that half of the open bites and nonocclusion in children between 8 and 15 years of age disappear spontaneously, in adolescents one-third.[9,10] These late changes are associated with the growth and maturation of the face, which sometimes eliminates the tongue interposition.

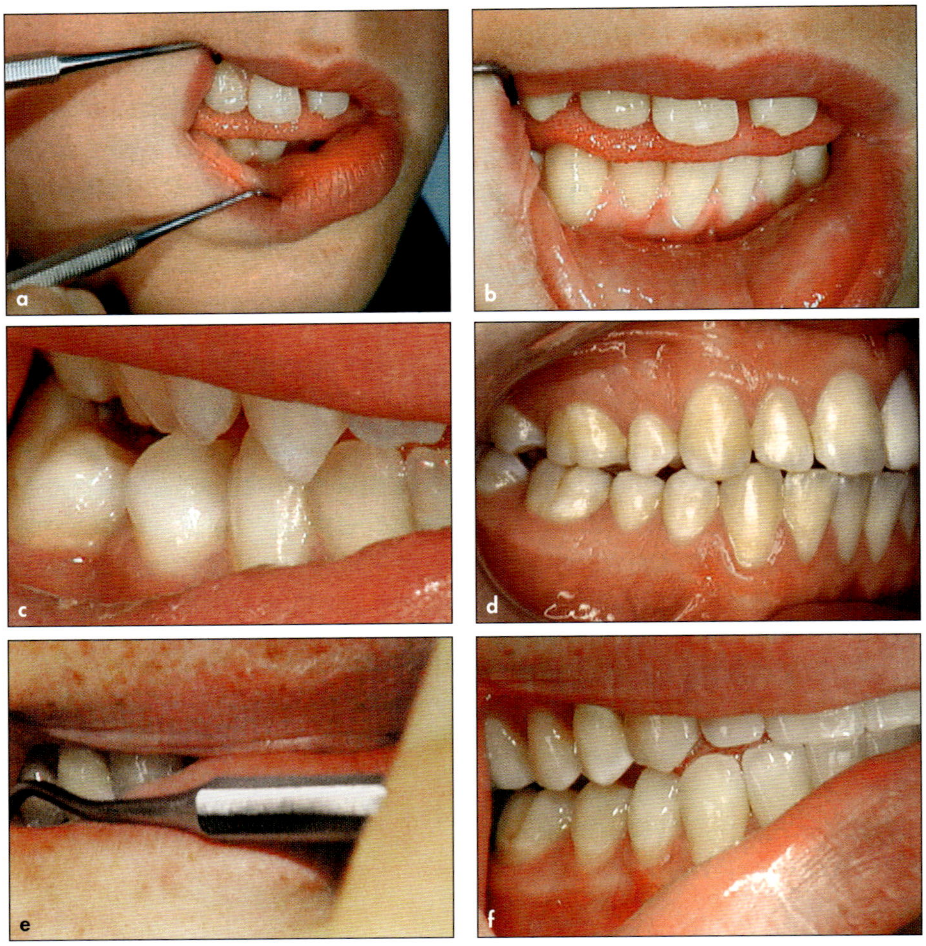

FIG 14-10 Detection of open bites and nonocclusion. *(a and b)* In an anterior open bite, the tongue interposition becomes visible when the lips are quickly moved apart. Anterior nonocclusion is difficult to detect by inspection, particularly when the distance between the mandibular and maxillary incisors is small. However, biting on a cellophane strip or a soft piece of wax can provide evidence. *(c and d)* Similarly, posterior open bites are easy to detect, but nonocclusion can be difficult to ascertain. *(e and f)* Posterior tongue interpositions are difficult to detect because patients tend to withdraw the tongue when the lips are touched. However, a tongue interposition can usually be observed when the lips are carefully separated with two blunt instruments at the corner of the mouth. See video clip 49.

Assessing Open Bites and Nonocclusions

Open bites in the anterior and posterior regions are easy to detect clinically; however, nonocclusions in the posterior region are not. It is difficult to assess the tongue position at rest unless the mouth is kept open, which often happens in individuals with an anterior open bite but not in those with nonocclusion (Fig 14-10). However, nonocclusions are easy to detect on dental casts. Looking at the occlusion from every labial/buccal and palatal/lingual perspective, it can be determined if the teeth are in optimal occlusion. If that is not the case, tongue interposition is the most likely cause. As mentioned previously, tongue interposition is also the most likely reason for a maxillary dental arch that is too narrow in relation to the mandibular dental arch. Cephalometric radiographs taken in habitual occlusion offer the ability to assess if an open bite or nonocclusion exists in the posterior regions (Fig 14-11).

Individuals with an open bite and nonocclusion in the anterior region exhibit a different type of tongue movement when swallowing than those whose incisors make contact. They move the tongue anteriorly when swallowing to close off the space between the opposing teeth. It is incorrect to consider this tongue movement that is typical in swallowing (tongue thrust) as a cause of an open bite. As stated before, the tongue movement adapts to the existing morphologic situation, not vice versa. Indeed, the position of the tongue at rest determines to a large extent the position of the teeth. Even if one swallows many times a day, the total time that the tongue exerts a force during swallowing is not more than 15 to 20 minutes a day. That is far too little time to affect the position of teeth.

Dental and Skeletal Open Bites

The open bites discussed above are caused by local factors (ie, dental open bites; Fig 14-12). In addition, there are open bites that are associated with a deviating skeletal configuration (ie, skeletal open bites; Fig 14-13). In dental open bites there is no excessive increase in the lower anterior facial height; in skeletal open bites there is. It is assumed that in the latter the dominance of internal over external functional components leads to excessive vertical growth of the lower face (see chapter 9).

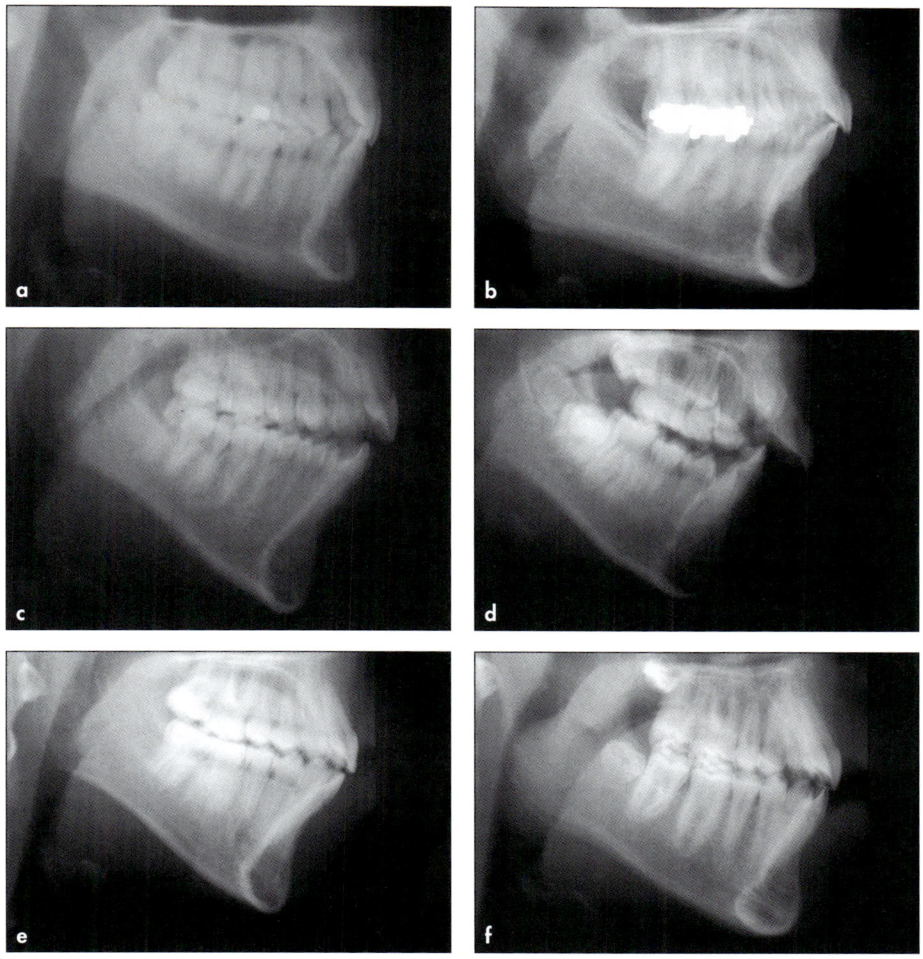

Fig 14-11 Open bites and nonocclusion on lateral cephalometric radiographs. *(a)* Lateral cephalometric radiographs made with the patient in habitual occlusion can provide insight into the overlapping of posterior teeth. In a symmetric situation, the corresponding teeth will be projected on top of each other, and the enamel of the intercuspating teeth will be visible as a light gray zone. *(b)* In an asymmetric lower face, the light gray zone will not be even. However, in this case, radiopaque restorations interfere with diagnosis. *(c)* Large anterior open bites can be easily seen. *(d)* The same applies to posterior open bites. *(e)* Total nonocclusion is projected as a small, dark strip. *(f)* In bilateral posterior nonocclusion in an asymmetric lower face, two small, dark strips appear.

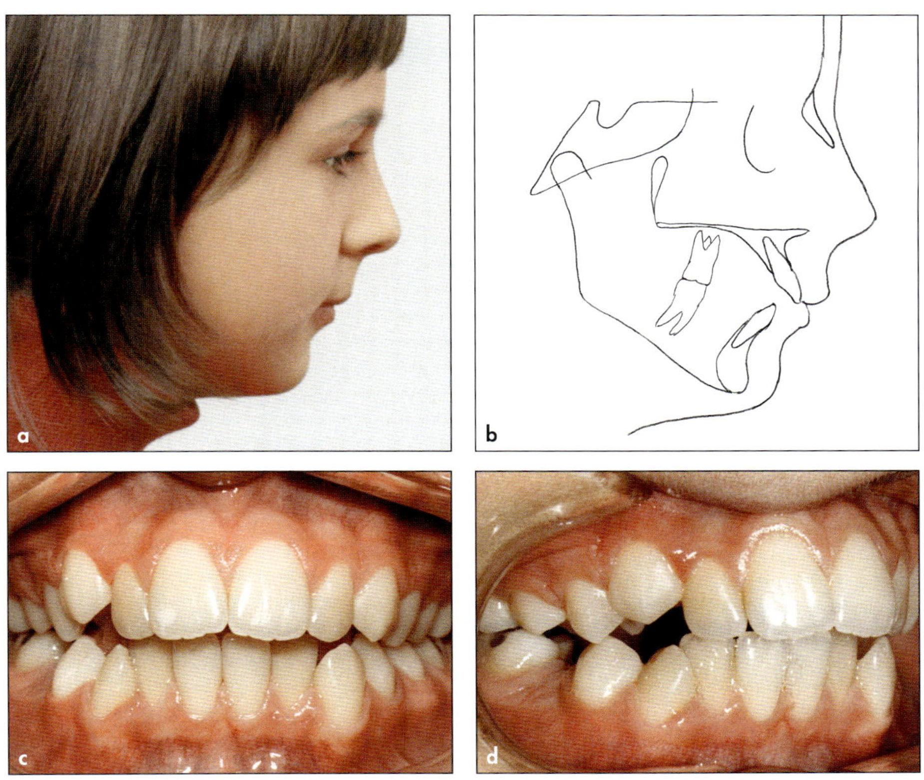

Fig 14-12 Dental open bite. *(a and b)* This 11-year-old girl has a borderline anterior open bite/nonocclusion. The lower face has not grown significantly in the inferior direction. The chin recedes slightly. *(c and d)* There is solid intercuspation on the left side and partial nonocclusion on the right side.

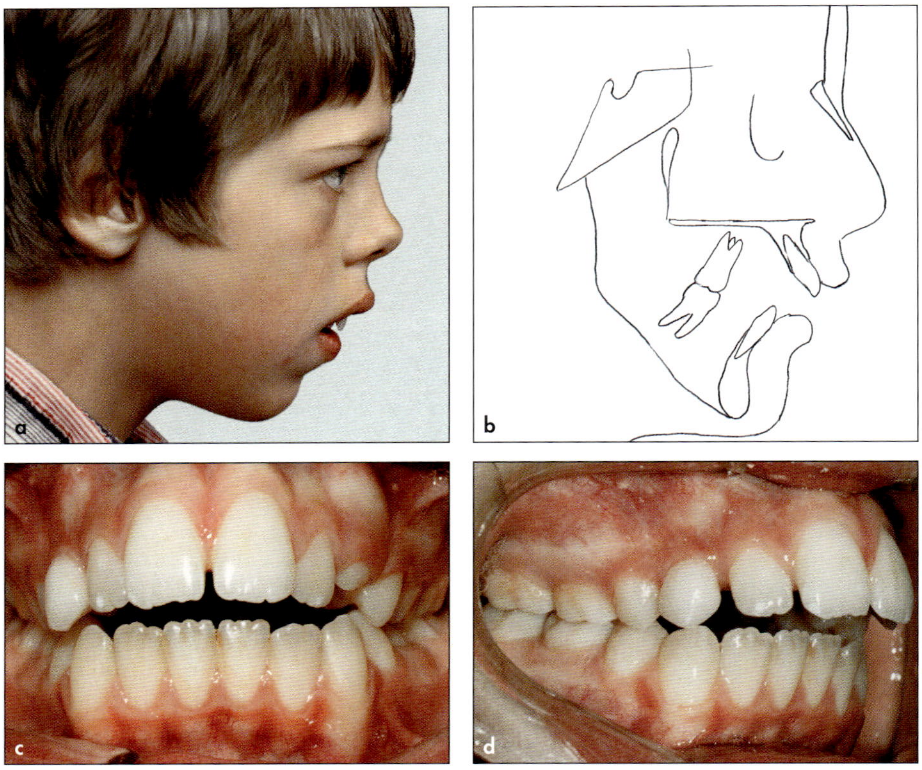

FIG 14-13 Skeletal open bite. *(a and b)* In this 12-year-old boy, the dominance of the internal over the external functional components presumably has resulted in an excessive vertical development of the lower face and a receding chin. *(c and d)* There is a large open bite; the posterior teeth occlude well.

References

1. Kjellgren B. Fingersugningsvana hos barn fran dentalortopedisk synpunkt. Nord Med 1939;3:2918.
2. Larsson E. Dummy- and finger-sucking habits with special attention to their significance for facial growth and occlusion. 5. Improvement of malocclusion after termination of the habit. Sven Tandlak Tidskr 1972;65:635–642.
3. Popovich F, Thompson GW. Thumb- and finger-sucking: Its relation to malocclusion. Am J Orthod 1973;63:148–155.
4. Van Hillegondsberg AJ. Over de betekenis van enkele postnatale factoren voor het ontstaan van dentomaxillaire afwijkingen in het temporaire gebit [thesis]. Utrecht: Utrecht University, 1959.
5. Moyers RE. Handbook of Orthodontics, ed 4. Chicago: Year Book, 1988.
6. Sarita PTN, Kreulen CM, Witter DJ, van 't Hof M, Creugers NHJ. A study on occlusal stability in shortened dental arches. Int J Prosthodont 2003;16:375–380.
7. Frankenmolen FWA. Orale gezondheid en zelfzorg van Nederlandse adolescenten [thesis]. Nijmegen: University of Nijmegen, 1990.
8. De Kanter RJAM. Prevalence and etiology of craniomandibular dysfunction [thesis]. Nijmegen: University of Nijmegen, 1990.
9. Goldstein MS, Stanton FL. Various types of occlusion and amounts of overbite in normal and abnormal occlusion between two and twelve years. Int J Orthod 1936;22:549–569.
10. Helm S. Prevalence of malocclusion in relation to development of the dentition. An epidemiological study of Danish school children. Acta Odontol Scand 1970;28(suppl 58).

15

Asymmetries, Transverse Deviations, and Forced Bites

Asymmetries

Asymmetry in the dentition can be caused by a difference between the left and right sides in terms of facial skeletal configuration or position of teeth within the jaws or by a combination of both. Small asymmetries of the skull and face, as well as misalignment of the midlines of the dental arches, occur frequently and are rarely troublesome.[1–3] Asymmetries in facial configuration can be traced to genetic factors, trauma, or pathological processes. Deviating facial growth can cause and/or exacerbate asymmetries. Asymmetries in tooth position may be caused by differences in the location where corresponding teeth are formed, premature loss or extraction of deciduous teeth followed by migration, or agenesis or extraction of permanent teeth.

Angle added subdivisions to his classification to account for asymmetries. A Class II subdivision has distoclusion on one side and neutroclusion on the other side. An analogous condition exists in a Class III subdivision, in which mesioclusion is present on one side and neutroclusion on the other side. According to Angle, it is not possible to have distoclusion on one side and mesioclusion on the other side.[4] In untreated Class II subdivisions, the assymetric occlusion will persist.[5]

Asymmetries in the occlusion caused by the facial skeletal configuration are usually caused by a deviation in the mandible (Fig 15-1). There are various types of asymmetries caused by deviant locations of tooth formation sites[7,8] (Fig 15-2).

As indicated, asymmetry in the dental arches can arise secondary to or become aggravated by premature loss of deciduous teeth (Fig 15-3) and agenesis or extraction of permanent teeth. This occurs because teeth tend to migrate in the direction where a tooth is missing (Fig 15-4).

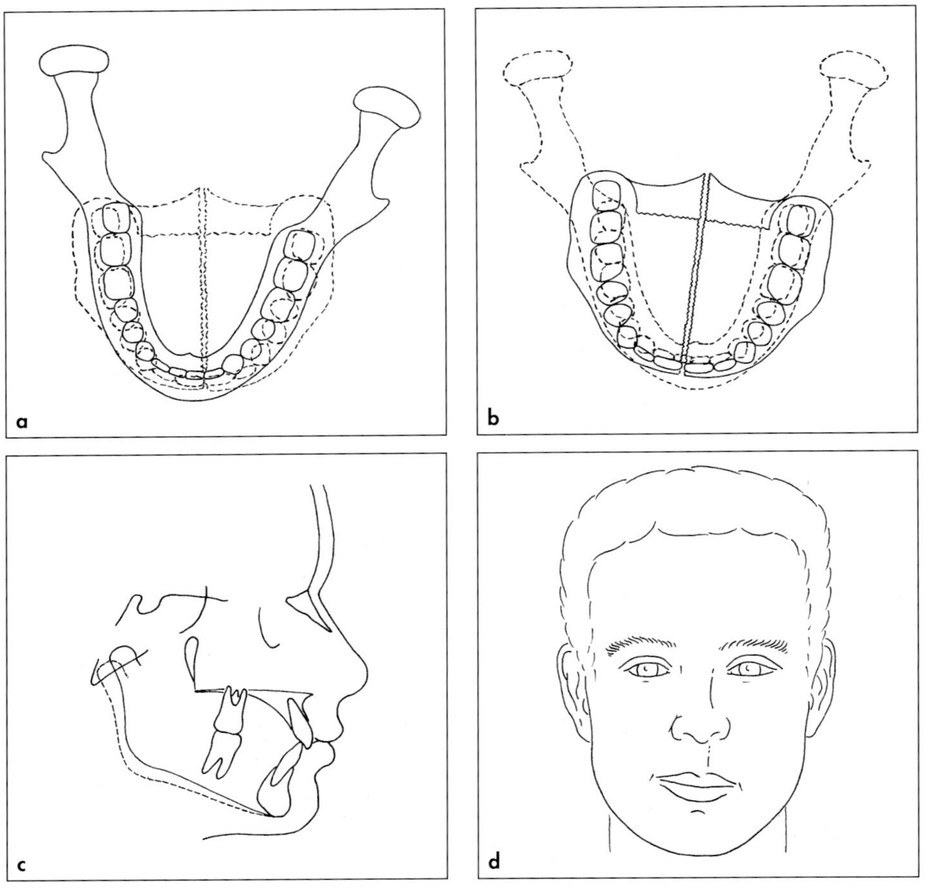

FIG 15-1 Asymmetry in facial configuration. In most humans, the facial skeleton is slightly asymmetric.[6] Also, muscles and other soft tissues often differ between the left and right sides. The mandible can be positioned asymmetrically because the locations of the temporal fossae do not correspond. *(a)* In addition, the mandible itself can be asymmetric. *(b)* Asymmetry of the face and the maxilla is usually associated with some asymmetry of the mandible. *(c)* In asymmetry of the lower part of the face, both the size and the shape of the two sides of the mandible are usually different. *(d)* A small asymmetry in the face is not noticed; a large one is. The positions of the teeth adjust to the asymmetry of the facial skeleton. The dentoalveolar compensatory mechanism plays an essential role in this adjustment.

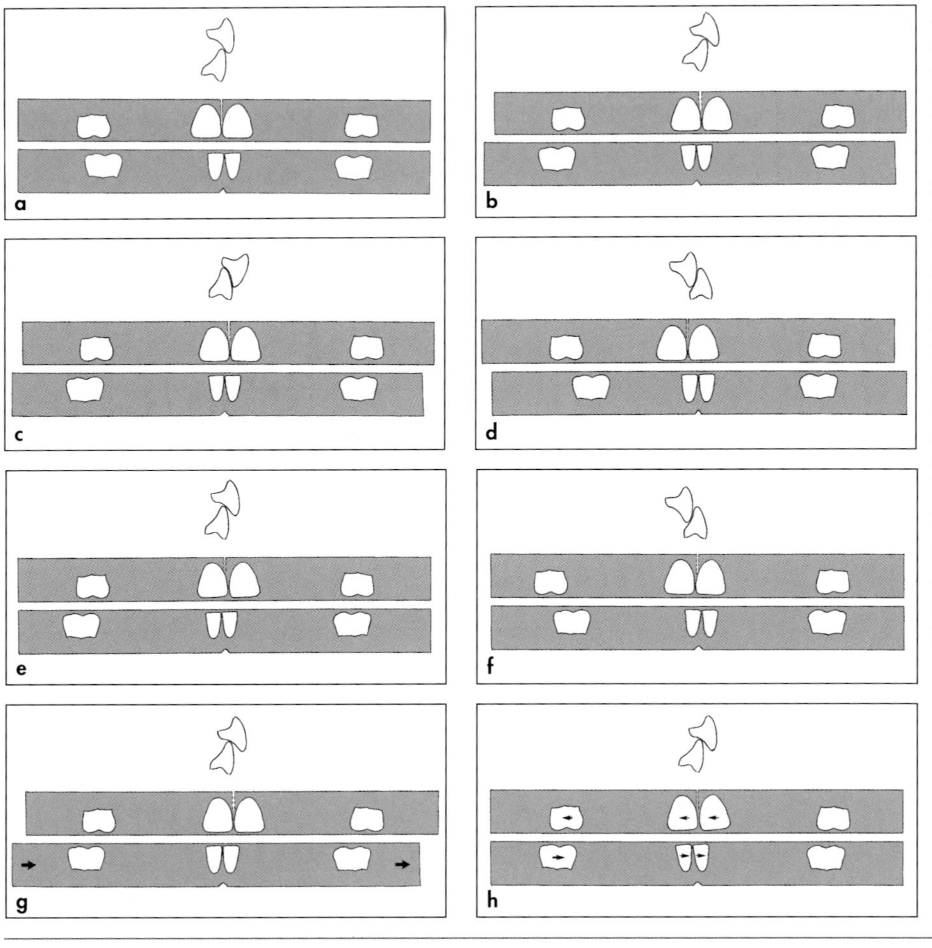

FIG 15-2 Asymmetry in occlusion. *(a)* Schematic presentation of an ideal situation. An asymmetry in jaw size or position can lead to deviations in the occlusion, such as a Class II, division 1 subdivision *(b)*, Class II, division 2 subdivision *(c)*, or a Class III subdivision *(d)*. The midlines of the two dental arches also can deviate without asymmetry of the jaws or the posterior occlusion. Such an asymmetry can result from a deviating position of the mandibular or maxillary anterior teeth, or from a combination of both. If the molars are also positioned asymmetrically, a Class II subdivision *(e)* or a Class III subdivision *(f)* will result. *(g)* The asymmetry can also be caused by an anomaly in the mandible and result in a Class II subdivision. *(h)* Asymmetries in the dental arches may simply be the result of abnormal tooth positions.

FIG 15-3 Asymmetry after premature loss of deciduous teeth. Premature loss of deciduous anterior teeth is usually a sign of crowding. *(a)* A maxillary lateral deciduous incisor may resorb when the central permanent incisor erupts. *(b)* A deciduous canine may resorb when the lateral permanent incisor erupts. *(c)* The latter occurs more often in the mandible than in the maxilla.[9] *(d)* Premature loss of deciduous molars—mostly due to tooth decay—can lead to tooth migration and result in asymmetry of the occlusion.

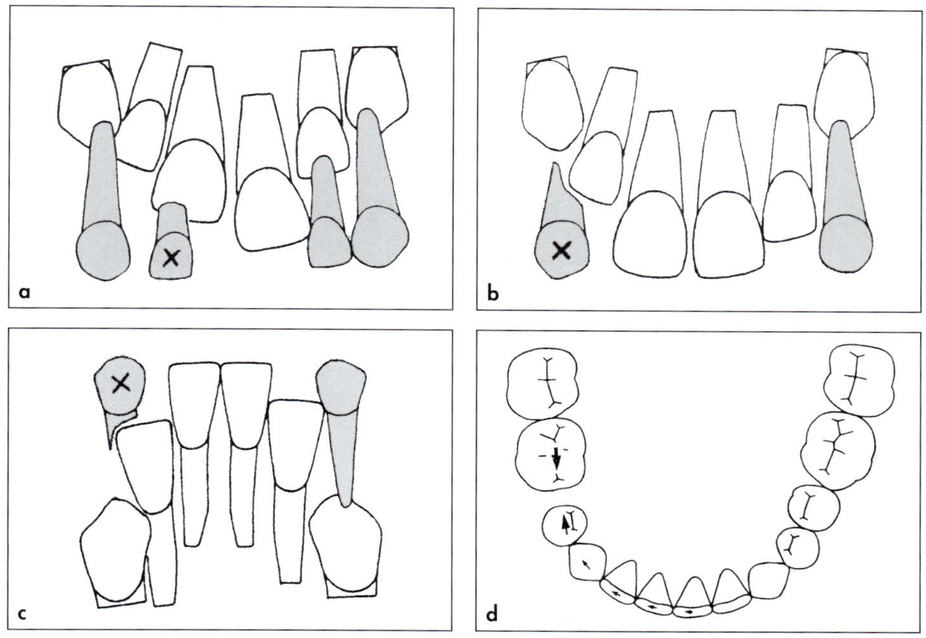

FIG 15-4 Asymmetry due to agenesis or extraction of a permanent tooth. *(a)* A missing maxillary right lateral permanent incisor will result in tipping of the other three incisors to the right side, but the roots will not pass the median suture. *(b)* However, there is no structure in the mandible that prevents the migration of an incisor through the median plane when one incisor is missing. *(c)* Agenesis of a mandibular second premolar leads to migration on both sides. *(d)* Agenesis of a maxillary right lateral permanent incisor and of a mandibular left second premolar have a cumulative effect on the deviation of the midlines of the dental arches.

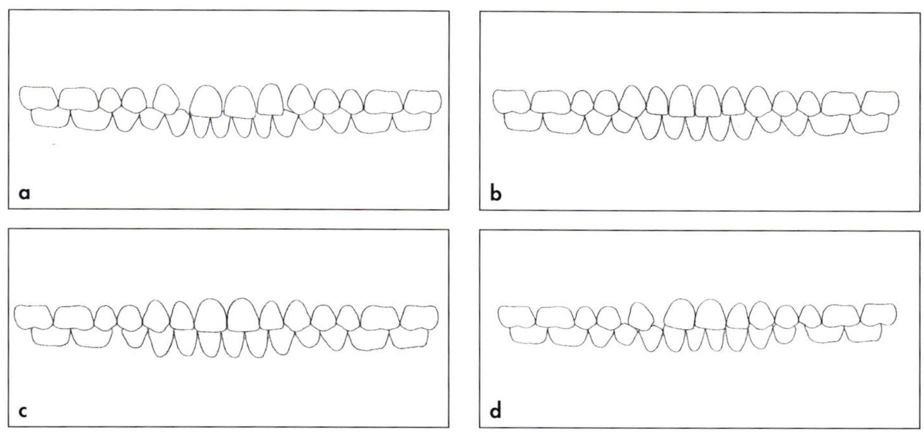

Transverse Deviations

There is a large variation in asymmetries and transverse deviations of the dentition in children and adults. Differences between the left and right side in sagittal occlusion of the posterior region (ie, subdivisions) are associated with deviations of the midlines of the dental arches (Figs 15-5 to 15-7). Sometimes the transverse occlusion deviates only on one side (Fig 15-8). The transverse occlusion can also deviate on both sides, as in a telescoping bite, ie, complete maxillary buccal crossbite (Figs 15-9 and 15-10). A complete maxillary palatal crossbite is very rare but may occur in an extreme Class III malocclusion. Bilateral posterior maxillary palatal crossbites are not uncommon (Fig 15-11).

Forced Bites

In asymmetries in facial configuration and location and occlusion of teeth, centric relation and habitual occlusion sometimes do not coincide. This condition is associated with forced bites. In forced bites, closing in centric relation leads to contact at one or more points that prevents completion of the closing movement in the initial direction. The neuromuscular system adapts to that condition, and premature contact is avoided in closing as the mandible moves directly into habitual occlusion.[10]

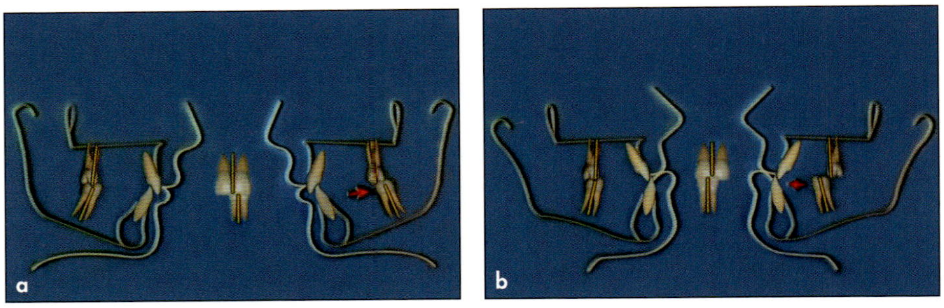

FIG 15-5 Subdivisions. *(a)* Class II subdivisions can be caused by asymmetry in the skeletal configuration or the position of the teeth. *(b)* The same applies to Class III subdivisions.

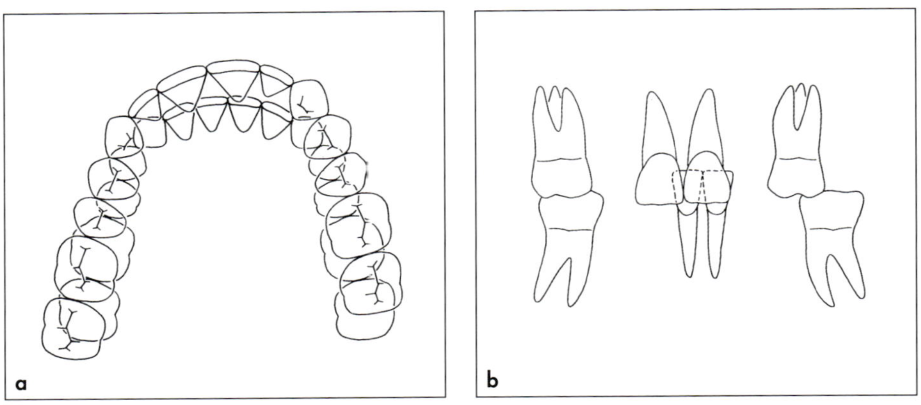

FIG 15-6 Class II, division 1 subdivision. *(a)* The posterior teeth are in an adequate transverse occlusion. On the left side is a distoclusion, on the right side a neutroclusion. There is a large overjet and overbite. *(b)* The midlines of the dental arches do not match.

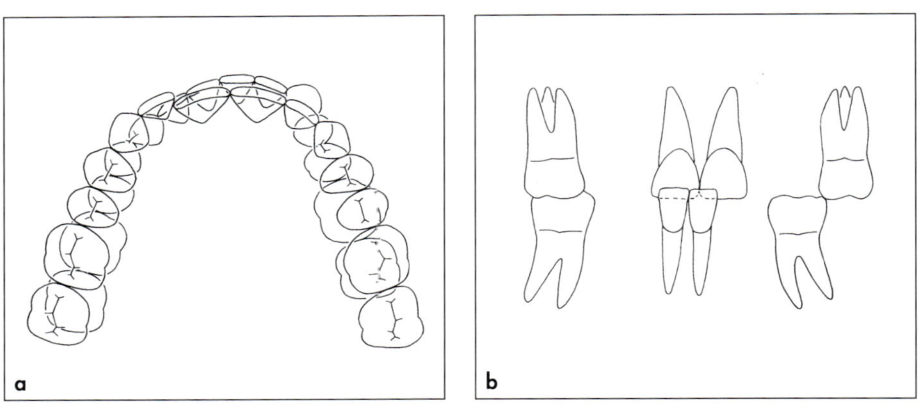

FIG 15-7 Class III subdivision. *(a)* There is a mesioclusion on the left side and a neutroclusion on the right side. There is a negative overjet (anterior crossbite) of the majority of the incisors and the mandibular left canine. *(b)* The midlines of the dental arches do not match.

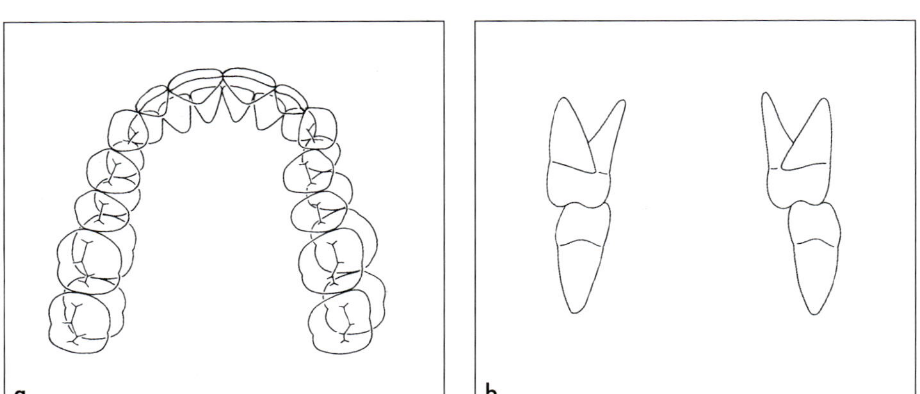

FIG 15-8 Unilateral posterior maxillary palatal crossbite without forced bite. *(a)* The maxillary dental arch crosses the mandibular dental arch distal to the maxillary left canine. *(b)* There is adequate transverse occlusion on the right side and a posterior maxillary palatal crossbite on the left side.

FIG 15-9 *(a to f)* Clinical views of Class II, division 1 malocclusion with complete maxillary buccal crossbite, also called *telescoping bite* or *Brodie syndrome*. The mandibular posterior teeth are tipped lingually; the maxillary posterior teeth are tipped buccally. The mandibular dental arch is abnormally narrow; the maxillary dental arch is abnormally broad.

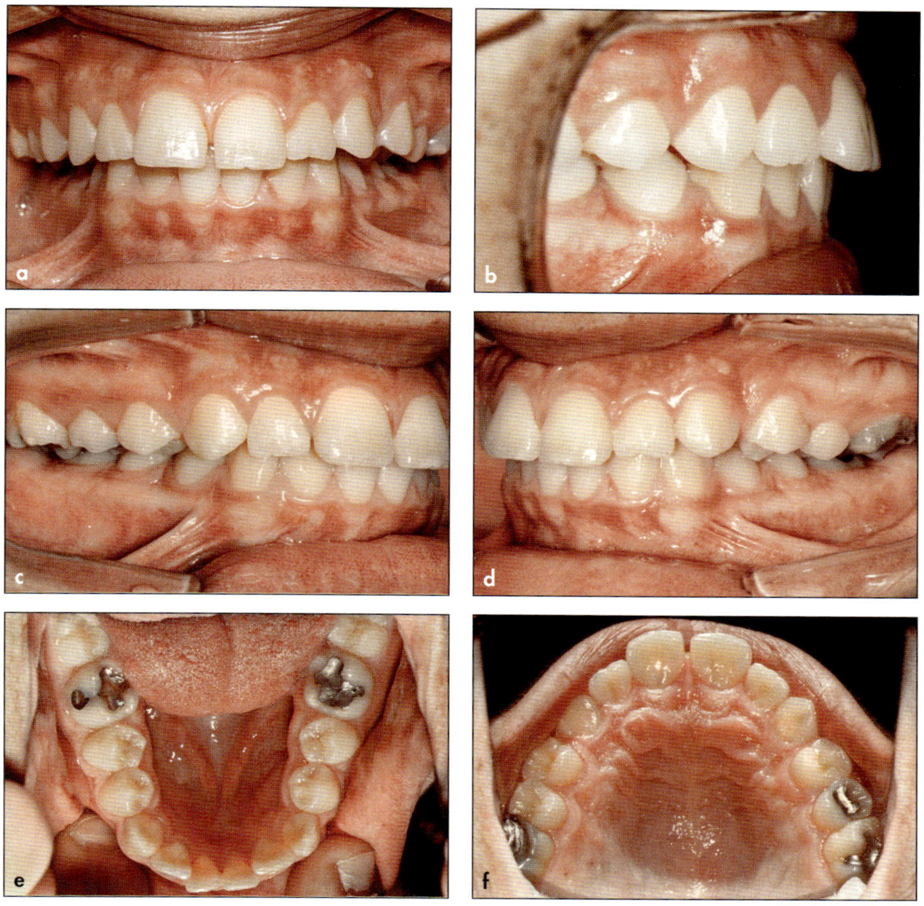

FIG 15-10 Class II, division 1 malocclusion with complete maxillary buccal crossbite. *(a)* The occlusal surfaces of the opposing posterior regions do not make contact. All maxillary teeth are positioned buccal to the mandibular teeth. *(b)* The maxillary posterior teeth are tipped buccally; the mandibular posterior teeth are tipped lingually.

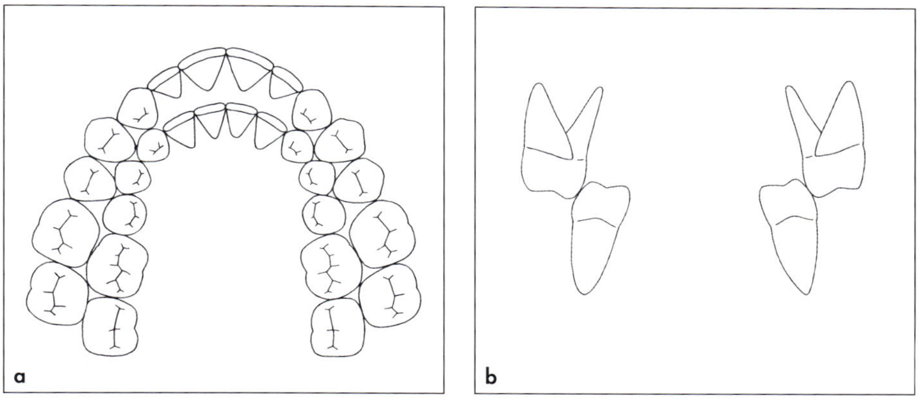

FIG 15-11 Bilateral posterior maxillary palatal crossbite. *(a)* The maxillary posterior teeth interdigitate with their buccal cusps instead of their palatal cusps. *(b)* There is a posterior maxillary palatal crossbite on both sides.

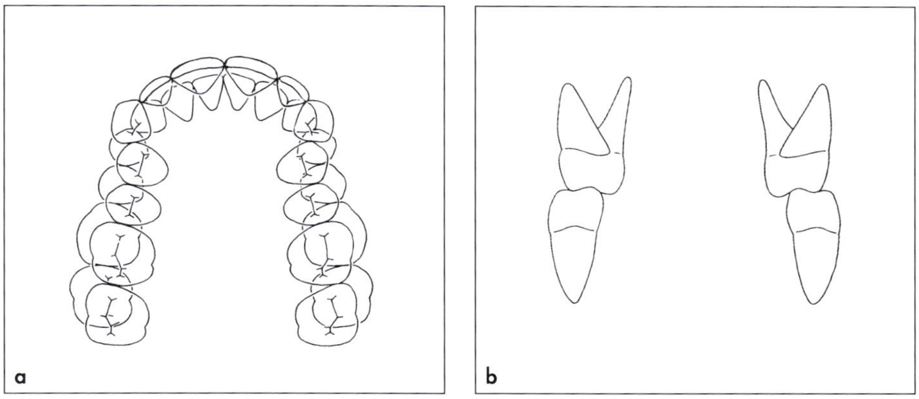

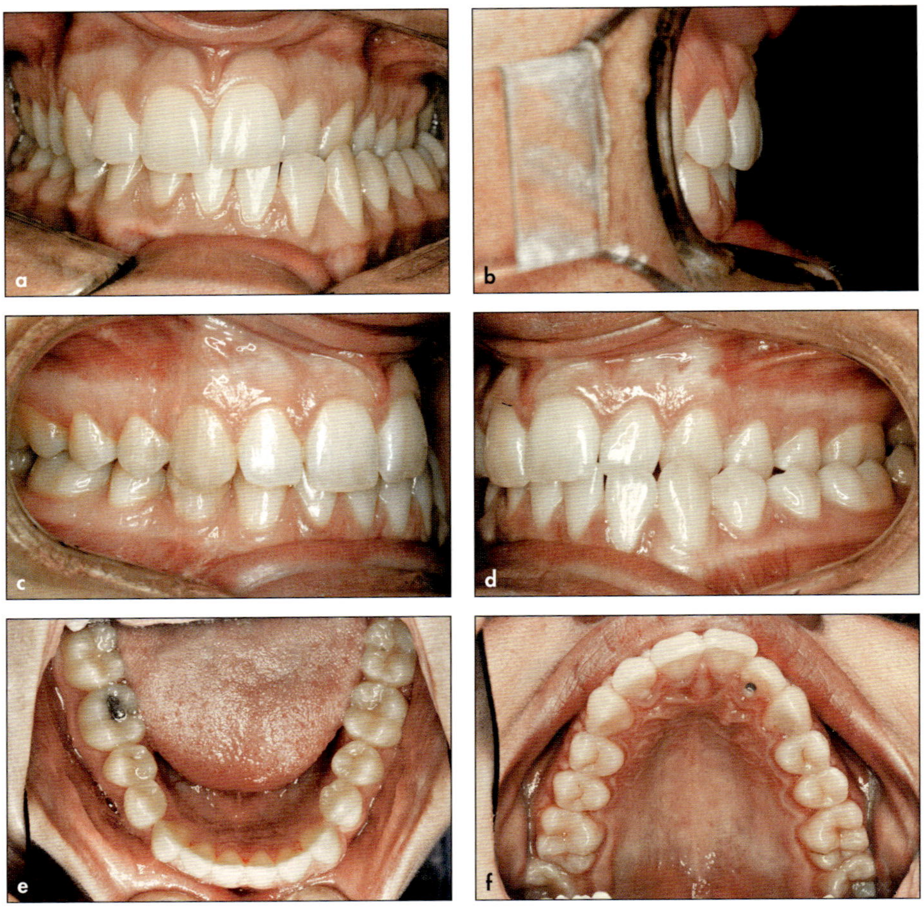

Fig 15-12 *(a to f)* Clinical views of a lateral forced bite. A crossbite of all teeth, except the central incisor, on the left side is combined with a lateral forced bite of 3 mm to the left. The most retruded position of the mandible is 1 mm posterior to the habitual occlusion. The premolars and molars are in neutroclusion, albeit in crossbite on the left side. On the left side, solid intercuspation has led to buccal tipping of the mandibular posterior teeth and palatal tipping of the maxillary posterior teeth.

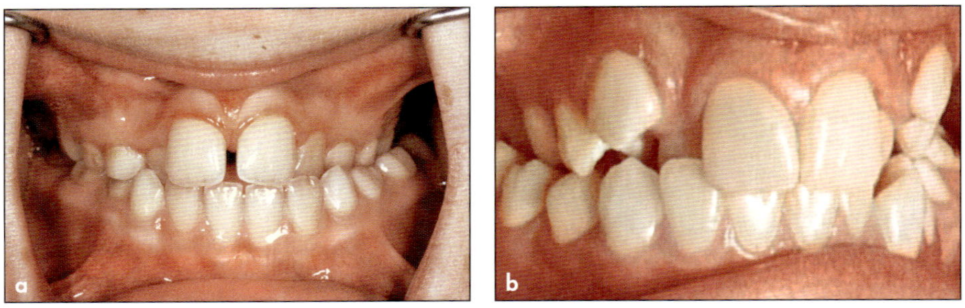

Fig 15-13 Clinical views of a lateral forced bite. *(a)* The maxillary dental arch is narrow. In closing, it is diverged to the right. There is a crossbite on the left side. *(b)* Lateral forced bite with an anterior component through palatal positioning of the maxillary lateral incisors. There is a maxillary posterior crossbite on both sides.

Forced bites occur in all stages of development of the dentition. They are differentiated into lateral and anterior forced bites and combinations of both. In lateral forced bites, the first contact in closing in centric relation is mostly at the canines, and the maxillary dental arch is often too narrow in relation to the mandibular dental arch. In habitual occlusion, a crossbite on one side results, and the midlines of the dental arches do not match (Figs 15-12 and 15-13a). The transverse occlusion can also deviate on both sides (Fig 15-13b). In lateral forced bites, the mandible must shift to one side to arrive in habitual occlusion (Figs 15-14 and 15-15).

In anterior forced bites, the first contact in closing in centric relation is at the incisors. The habitual occlusion is more anterior. This leads to a negative overjet (Figs 15-16 and 15-17). An anterior forced bite can also come about in a Class II malocclusion with crowding in the maxillary anterior region if a maxillary lateral deciduous incisor is lost with the emergence of the adjacent central permanent incisor, and the maxillary lateral permanent incisor emerges too far palatally. When the latter attains contact with the lingual aspect of the mandibular teeth, further palatal displacement will result. The occlusion adapts to the new situation. During closure in habitual occlusion, it appears that there is a neutroclusion or a slight distoclusion. However, with careful, manually guided closure in the most retruded position, the palatally positioned maxillary lateral incisor will be touched first. A slide to the anterior is needed to reach habitual occlusion (Figs 15-18 and 15-19). This type of forced bite is easily overlooked. An anterior forced bite can also be caused by unfavorable contact of the posterior teeth.

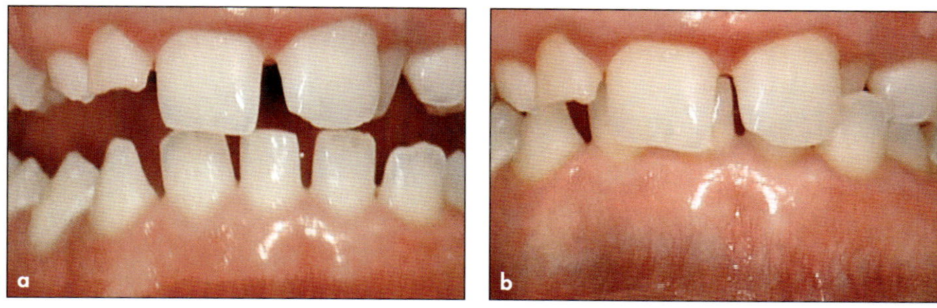

FIG 15-14 Clinical views of a lateral forced bite. *(a)* In closure in centric relation, the maxillary central incisors make end-to-end contact with the mandibular incisors. *(b)* To achieve habitual occlusion, divergence of the mandible to the right side is needed.

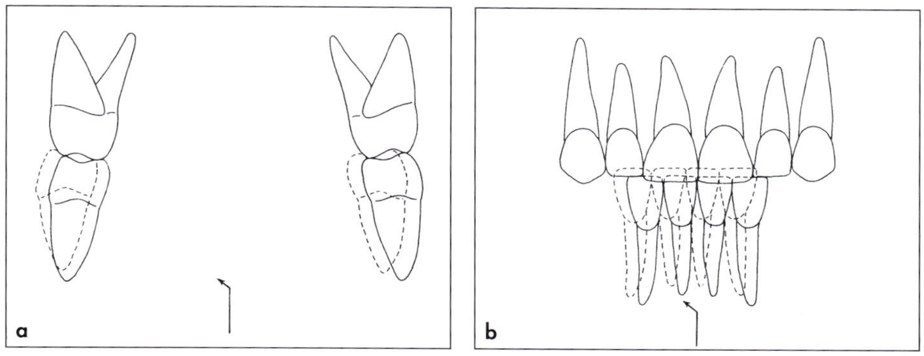

FIG 15-15 Lateral forced bite. *(a)* In closure in centric relation, partial contact is made in the posterior regions *(solid lines)*. Habitual occlusion requires a mandibular shift to the right, through which more extensive contact is attained at both sides *(dotted lines)*. At the right side is a posterior crossbite. *(b)* The midlines of the two dental arches deviate accordingly.

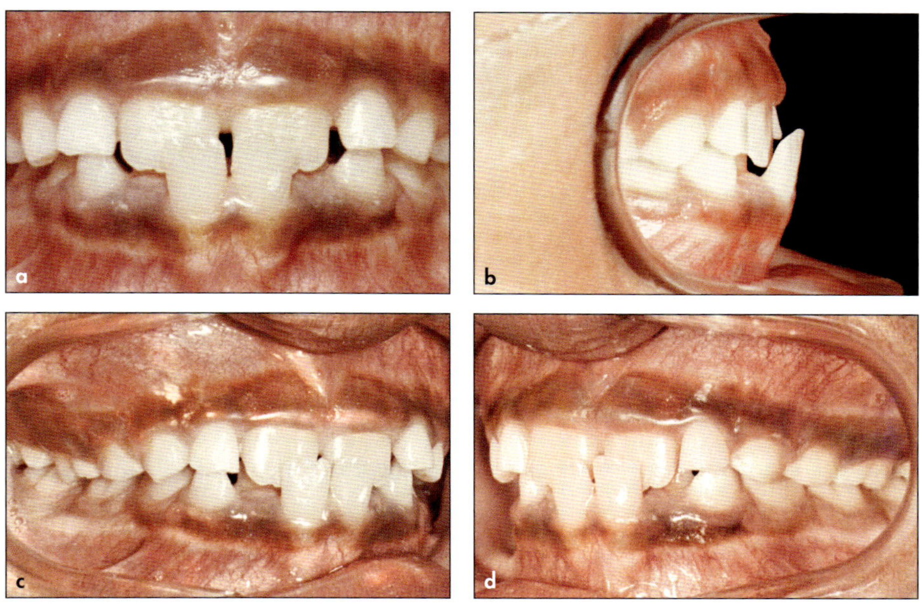

FIG 15-16 *(a to d)* Clinical views of anterior forced bite (pseudo Class III malocclusion). The mandible can be moved posteriorly into end-to-end occlusion of the central incisors. In closure, the mandible moves directly to the anterior, without a slide to achieve habitual occlusion.

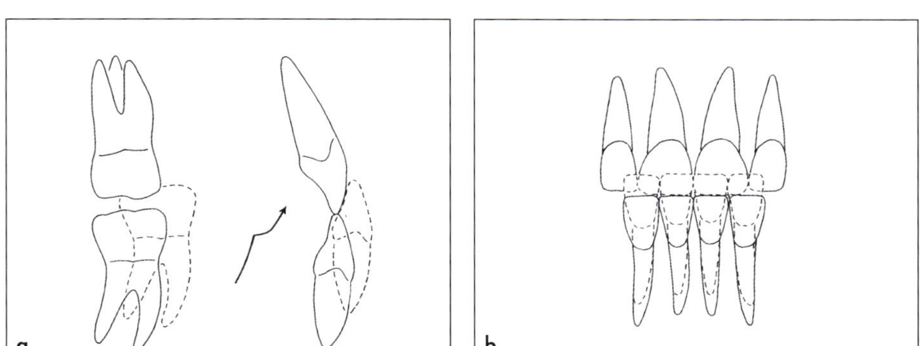

FIG 15-17 Anterior forced bite. *(a)* In closure in centric relation, initial contact is made at the incisal edges, with the central incisors in end-to-end occlusion *(solid lines)*. For habitual occlusion the mandible must slide anteriorly *(dotted lines)*. *(b)* Frontal view of contact in centric relation *(solid lines)* and in habitual occlusion *(dotted lines)*.

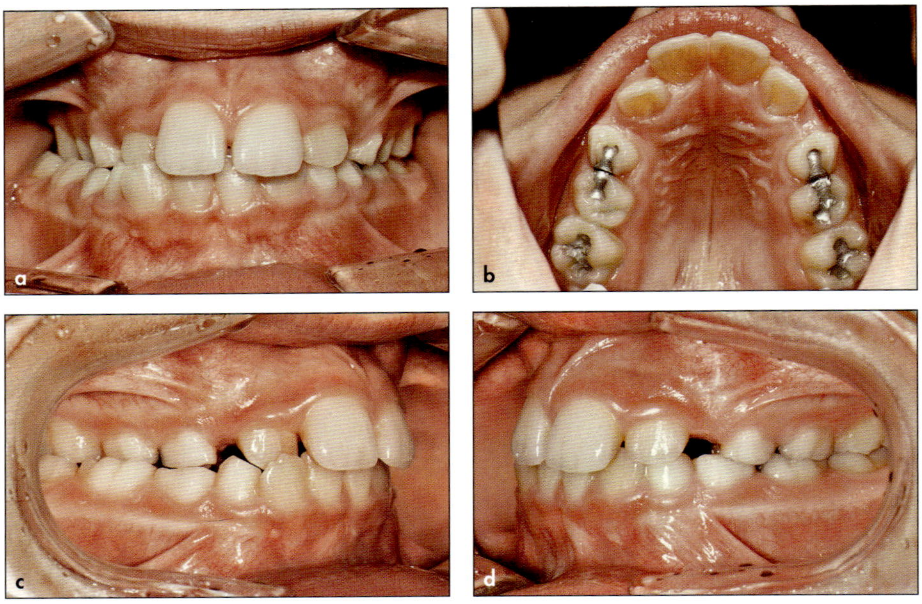

Fig 15-18 *(a to d)* Clinical views of a Class II, division 1 malocclusion with anterior and lateral forced bite. The maxillary right lateral incisor has emerged palatally. It is impossible for the mandibular teeth to close behind that tooth. The habitual occlusion in forced bite is 4 mm anterior and 2 mm left of centric relation. There is a crossbite on the right side and adequate transverse occlusion on the left side. In the most retruded position of the mandible, the incisal edges of the opposing right lateral incisors are in end-to-end occlusion. That also applies to the posterior teeth in transverse direction. The position of the teeth is adapted to habitual occlusion.

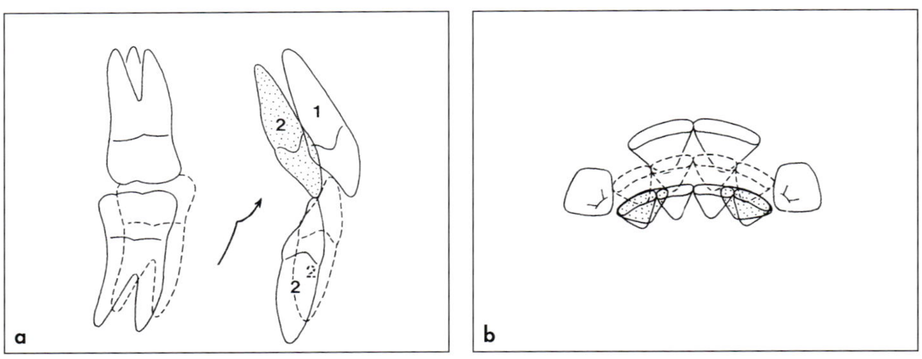

Fig 15-19 Anterior forced bite in a Class II, division 1 malocclusion. *(a)* In closure in centric relation *(solid lines)*, the opposing lateral incisors (2) contact each other. The habitual occlusion *(dotted lines)* is more anterior, with the mandibular lateral incisors (2) caught between the maxillary lateral incisors (2) and central incisors (1). The molars are then in neutroclusion. *(b)* Initial contact of the mandibular lateral incisors in centric relation *(solid lines)* and in habitual occlusion *(dotted lines)*. As in *a*, the maxillary incisors are completely dotted.

Many forced bites are a combination of the anterior and the lateral type. In forced bites, the position of the individual teeth adapts to the deviant habitual occlusion.

References

1. Beyer JW, Lindauer SJ. Evaluation of dental midline position. Semin Orthod 1998;4:146–152.
2. Miller EL, Bodden WR Jr, Jamison HC. A study of the relationship of the dental midline to the facial median line. J Prosthet Dent 1979;41:657–660.
3. Zachrisson BU. Dental to facial midline positions. World J Orthod 2001;2:362–364.
4. Angle EH. Classification of malocclusion. Dent Cosmos 1899;41:248–264,350–357.
5. Veli I, Yuksel B, Uysal T. Longitudinal evaluation of dental arch asymmetry in Class II subdivision malocclusion with 3-dimensional digital models. Am J Orthod Dentofac Orthop 2014;145:763–770.
6. Rossi M, Ribeiro E, Smith R. Craniofacial asymmetry in development. An anatomical study. Angle Orthod 2003;73:381–385.
7. Bishara SE, Burkey PS, Kharouf JG. Dental and facial asymmetries: A review. Angle Orthod 1994;64:89–98.
8. Janson GRP, Metaxas A, Woodside DG, De Freitas MR, Pinzan A. Three-dimensional evaluation of skeletal and dental asymmetries in Class II subdivision malocclusions. Am J Orthod Dentofacial Orthop 2001;119:406–418.
9. Helm S, Siersbæk-Nielsen S. Crowding in the permanent dentition after early loss of deciduous molars or canines. Trans Eur Orthod Soc 1973;137–149.
10. Hamerling J. Mandibular Movement Patterns: A Methodological and Clinical Investigation of Children with a Lateral Forced Bite [thesis]. Amsterdam: University of Amsterdam, 1983.

16

Premature Loss of Deciduous Teeth

Causes of Premature Loss of Deciduous Teeth

Deciduous teeth can be lost early because of premature resorption of their roots, trauma, or decay (caries) followed by extraction. Loss by premature resorption and trauma happens only in the anterior region. Untimely loss due to caries and extraction mainly affects the deciduous molars.

Premature resorption of the roots of deciduous incisors and canines is a symptom of crowding. In addition, the distal root of maxillary second deciduous molars can resorb prematurely if the first permanent molar erupts too far to the mesial. However, the deciduous molar will not exfoliate, and the eruption of the permanent molar will be blocked.[1,2] Premature loss of deciduous molars can lead to migration of adjacent teeth and to shortage of space for their successors.

Premature loss of deciduous molars due to caries happens twice as often in the mandible than in the maxilla.[3–7] Deciduous canines are somewhat resistant to decay, as are deciduous incisors, which are present in the mouth only a relatively short period of time. Decayed deciduous molars can lose part or all of their crowns. Complaints of pain are often the reason for their removal. Infections are an indication for extraction, especially because they can affect succeeding teeth. Deciduous teeth with a nonvital pulp can cause large purulent periapical infections. In contrast with permanent teeth, no fibrous encapsulation of the abscess takes place in deciduous teeth. Hence successors can be damaged, and abnormal shapes, hypocalcifications, and caries lesions can result.[8–10]

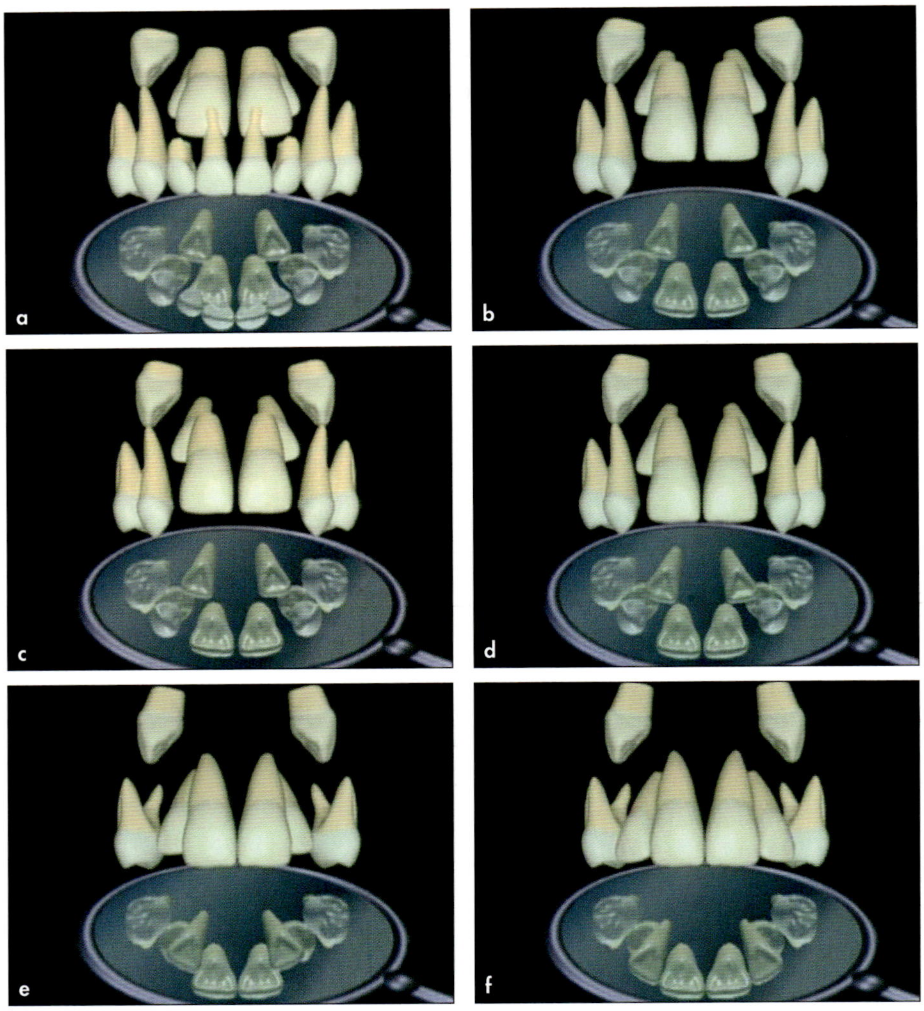

Fig 16-1 Premature loss of deciduous incisors and canines. *(a and b)* With crowding in the maxilla, the lateral deciduous incisors can be shed prematurely during the eruption of the central permanent incisors. *(c and d)* Too little space remains for the lateral permanent incisors. *(e)* Their eruption can lead to premature resorption and loss of the deciduous canines. *(f)* Subsequently, the lateral permanent incisors move labially and occupy their positions in the dental arch. Too little space remains for the permanent canines. Sometimes in such cases the deciduous canines are not lost prematurely; instead, the lateral permanent incisors emerge palatally (see Fig 15-18). See video clip 14.

Effects of Premature Loss of Deciduous Teeth

The effects of premature loss of deciduous teeth are predictable and can be well estimated. The occurrence of migrations after premature loss of deciduous teeth depends on which tooth is lost as well as on the occlusion.[3,11–14] These migrations are greater and happen more quickly in the maxilla than in the mandible.[3,15,16] Furthermore, migrations in the maxilla are mainly limited to mesial movement and rotation of the first permanent molar. In the mandible, teeth mesial to the lost tooth have a greater tendency to move distally.[15]

In addition, the spatial conditions in the dental arches are important.[12,17,18] In general, premature loss of deciduous teeth in dental arches with excess space has no or only little effect on the development of the dentition. In the absence of excess space, complications might appear; in cases of crowding, complications are a certainty.

Tongue and buccal musculature also play an essential role,[3,5] and the timing of the loss is relevant.[12,17] Loss long before the time of emergence of the successor leads to its delayed emergence; loss shortly before emergence has an accelerating effect.[19] Moreover, loss of deciduous teeth at an early age has more negative sequelae than loss occurring later. Migrations of adjacent teeth take place mainly in the first 6 months after the premature loss.[18]

It is important to emphasize that the loss of space is often limited and of little relevance for the development of the dentition.[11–14,20–22] In addition, in the mandible some of the lost space can be regained at the end of the second transitional period.[23]

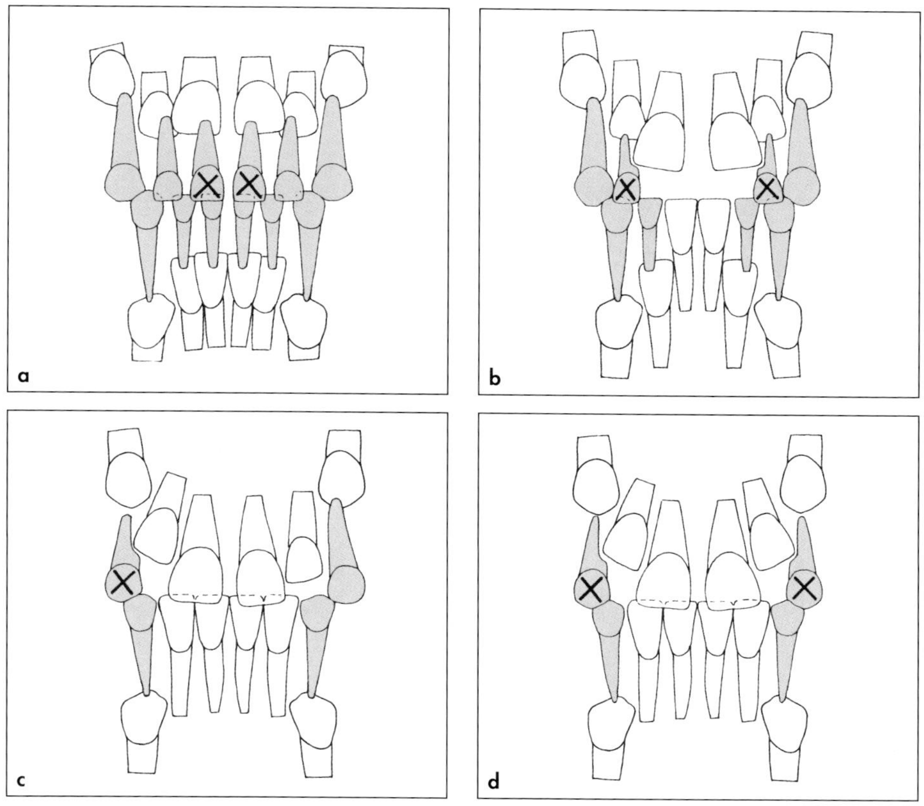

Fig 16-2 Effect of premature loss of deciduous anterior teeth. *(a)* Trauma of maxillary deciduous incisors can disturb the formation and eruption of their successors. Premature loss of central deciduous incisors in most cases has no effect on the development of the dentition. *(b)* In situations with severe crowding, the lateral deciduous incisors can be lost prematurely. Consequently, the displacement of the deciduous canines associated with the eruption of the central permanent incisors will not take place. *(c)* With unilateral premature loss of a maxillary deciduous canine, the incisors will migrate in that direction, and the midlines of the dental arches will no longer match. *(d)* With premature loss of both maxillary deciduous canines, the midline will not displace.

Premature loss of deciduous incisors and canines

With little space in the anterior region, as in a deciduous dentition without diastemata, deciduous incisors and canines can be lost prematurely with the emergence of an adjacent permanent tooth (Fig 16-1). Trauma is usually the cause of premature loss of maxillary central deciduous incisors. If they are not pushed into the jaw, which can cause displacement and dilaceration of successors, but rather knocked out, the only effect will be delayed emergence of their successors.[24] In addition, maxillary central deciduous incisors do not play a role in the mechanism of distal displacement of lateral deciduous incisors and deciduous canines during the eruption and emergence of the central permanent incisors (Fig 16-2a).

With the eruption and emergence of a maxillary central permanent incisor, the root of the adjacent lateral deciduous incisor can resorb, and the crown can exfoliate (Fig 16-2b). In unilateral premature loss of a maxillary lateral deciduous incisor, the deciduous canine on that side will not displace distally and buccally during the eruption of the central permanent incisor; in bilateral loss, this phenomenon will occur on both sides.

In a comparable way, the eruption of maxillary lateral permanent incisors can lead to premature loss of deciduous canines (Figs 16-2c and 16-2d). If this happens only on one side, the incisors will migrate in that direction. Consequently, insufficient space remains there for the maxillary permanent canine, which will emerge buccally. If both deciduous canines are lost prematurely, both permanent canines will be outside the dental arch.

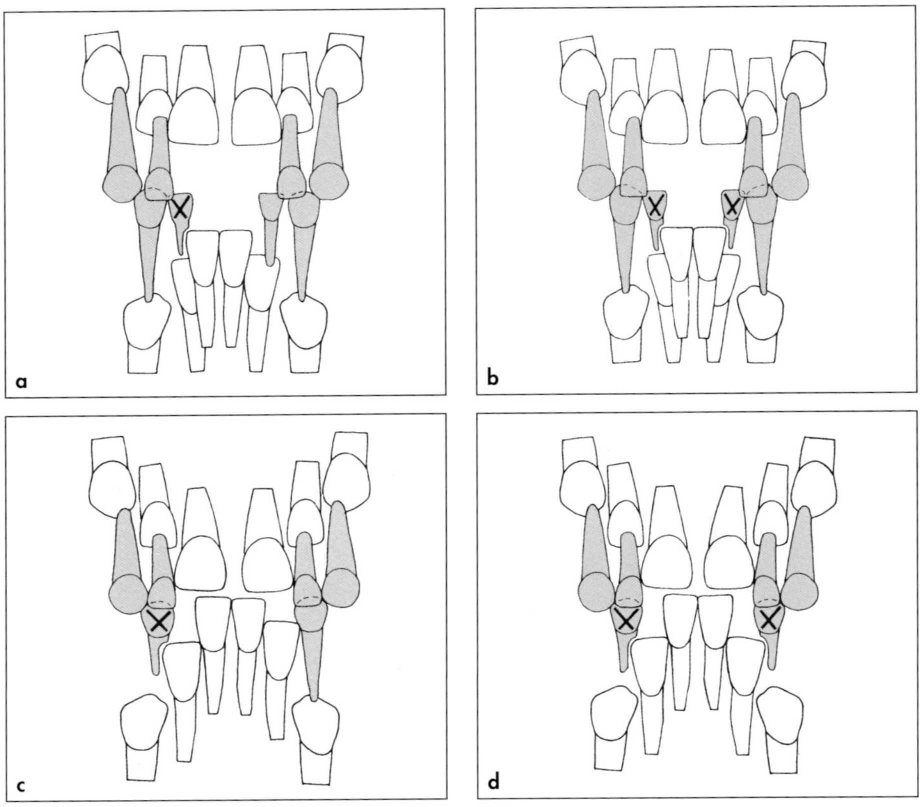

FIG 16-3 Premature loss of mandibular lateral deciduous incisors and deciduous canines. *(a)* Unilateral loss of a mandibular lateral deciduous incisor as can happen with asymmetric positioning and eruption of mandibular central permanent incisors. *(b)* Bilateral loss of mandibular lateral deciduous incisors. *(c)* Unilateral loss of a mandibular deciduous canine, followed by migration of the incisors to that side and shifting of the midline. *(d)* Bilateral loss of mandibular deciduous canines, usually without deviation of the midline.

With asymmetry in location of formation and in eruption of permanent incisors, the premature loss can be unilateral (Figs 16-3a and 16-3c). This occurs more often than bilateral premature loss, particularly in the mandible (Figs 16-3b and 16-3d). Unilateral premature loss of deciduous canines leads to alterations in the angulation of the permanent incisors and to displacement of the midline of the dental arches (Fig 16-4).

In the mandible, premature loss of deciduous incisors has consequences for the increase in intercanine distance. Furthermore, premature loss of mandibular deciduous canines can result in an increase in overjet and overbite.

Premature loss of deciduous molars

Undesirable migrations may or may not result from untimely loss of deciduous molars, and they are less likely to occur with the loss of first than second deciduous molars.[11,13] With the loss of second deciduous molars, the migration is usually limited to mesial displacement of the first permanent molars (Figs 16-5 and 16-6). The mesial displacement of the teeth distal to prematurely lost first deciduous molars is more limited. The teeth mesial of them will tend to migrate distally, but to a lesser extent. With sufficient space and a neutroclusion, problems due to premature loss of a second deciduous molar are rare in the mandible, but common in the maxilla. This difference is due to the three aspects described in the following text.

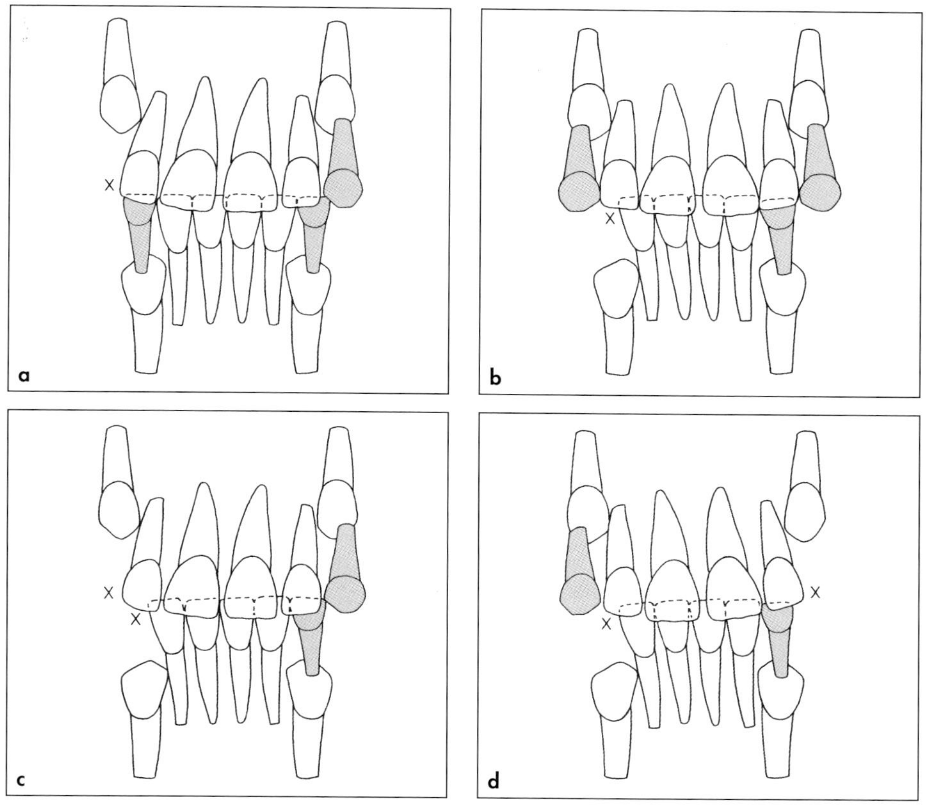

Fig 16-4 Effects of premature loss of deciduous canines on the angulation of permanent incisors and the position of the midline. *(a)* Unilateral loss of a maxillary deciduous canine results in tipping of the permanent incisors and shifting of the midline. *(b)* Unilateral loss of a mandibular deciduous canine has the same results. *(c)* Unilateral loss of opposing deciduous canines leads to tipping of the incisors in the same direction in both jaws. *(d)* With the loss of a deciduous canine in the mandible on one side and in the maxilla on the other side, the maxillary and mandibular permanent incisors will tip in opposite directions.

First, the crown of the mandibular second deciduous molar is usually wider than that of the maxillary second deciduous molar, and in a neutroclusion the terminal plane is generally flush. Under these circumstances, a maxillary second deciduous molar can overerupt after the opposing mandibular tooth is lost and block the mesial migration of the mandibular first permanent molar (Figs 16-7 and 16-8). In premature loss of a maxillary second deciduous molar, the antagonist cannot overerupt, because it also occludes with the maxillary first deciduous molar (Figs 16-9 and 16-10). The maxillary first permanent molar will move mesially. This displacement is not parallel but involves rotation around the axis through the mesiopalatal cusp and the large palatal root. If this cusp occludes with the central fossa of the mandibular first permanent molar, the rotation will be enhanced.

The second aspect relates to the potential to regain space by the eruption and emergence of second premolars. In the maxilla, an erupting maxillary second premolar will diverge palatally, exerting little or no distally directed force on the first permanent molar because of the trapezoid shape of the reduced space between the first permanent molar and the first premolar. The situation is different in the mandible because the reduced space is more rectangular, and the mesial surface of the first permanent molar is perpendicular to the dental arch. (See video clip 50.)

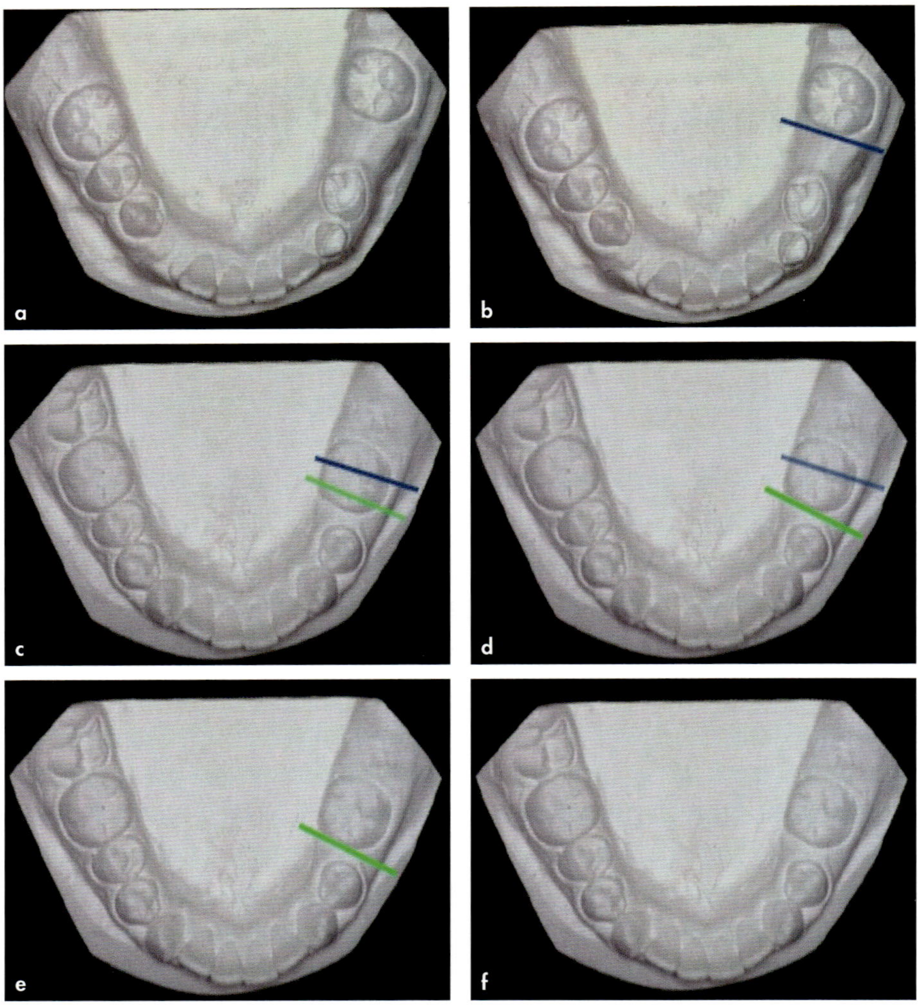

Fig 16-5 Premature loss of a mandibular left second deciduous molar, followed by excessive migration of the first permanent molar. *(a)* In the first weeks after the extraction, migration of the first permanent molar does not occur. *(b)* Its mesial surface is oriented perpendicular to the dental arch. *(c)* Five months later, the first permanent molar has migrated and tipped slightly mesially, but not rotated. *(d)* If the occlusion does not interfere, further migration can take place. *(e)* Tipping will also occur. *(f)* Little space remains for the second premolar.

The third aspect is that the leeway space—the difference between the sum of the mesiodistal crown dimensions of the deciduous canines and first and second deciduous molars and that of their successors—is greater in the mandible than in the maxilla. Therefore, more space can be lost in the mandibular dental arch before a problem arises.

Unilateral premature loss of the mandibular first and second deciduous molars, or premature loss of both on one side and one on the other side, leads to a displacement of the midline of the mandibular dental arch and to an enlargement of the overjet and overbite (Fig 16-11). In a Class III malocclusion with a negative overjet, premature loss of maxillary deciduous molars likewise leads to an increase in the overbite and negative overjet.

Unilateral loss of both second deciduous molars almost always has a negative effect on the development of the dentition (Fig 16-12). The mandibular and maxillary first permanent molars migrate mesially unhindered. Intercuspation of the mesiopalatal cusp of the maxillary first permanent molar in the central fossa of the corresponding mandibular tooth does not present an obstruction to its migration because the latter moves mesially as well.

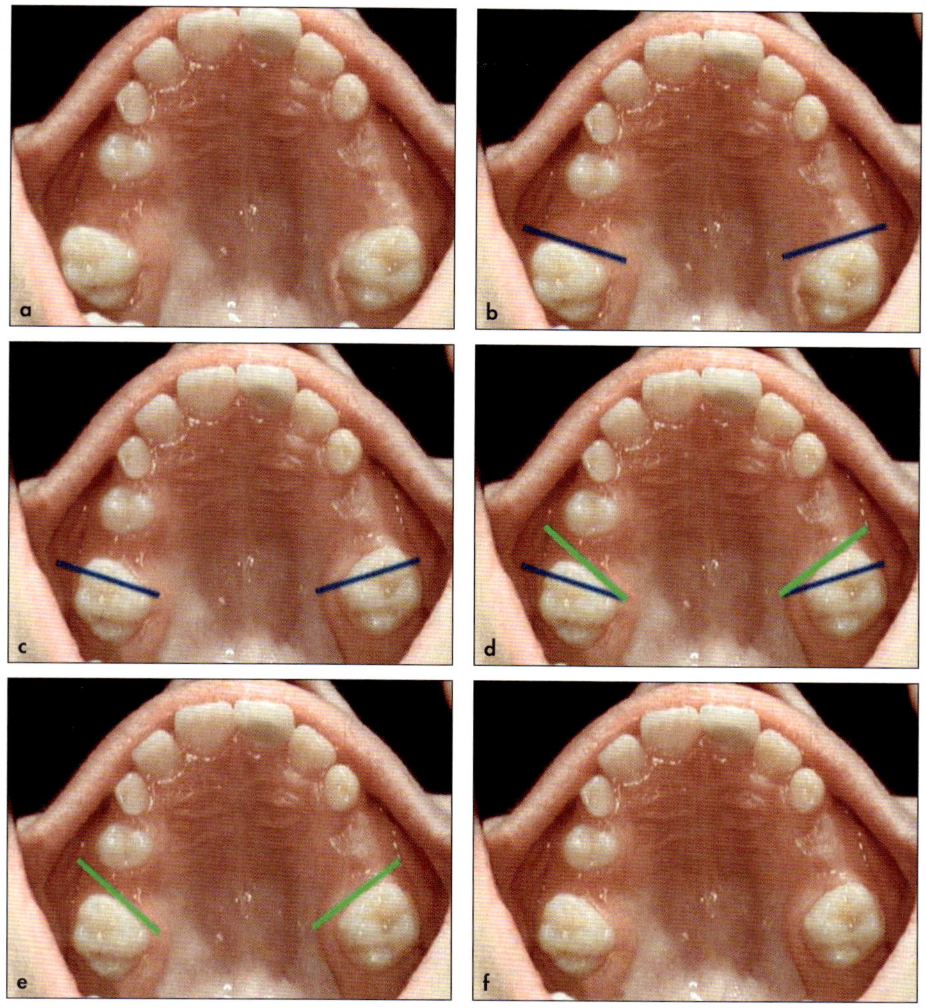

Fig 16-6 Premature loss of both maxillary second deciduous molars, followed by excessive migration. *(a)* In the first 5 weeks after the extraction, the first permanent molars have not moved. *(b)* Their mesial surfaces are oriented perpendicular to the dental arch. *(c)* Six months later, the space is markedly reduced on both sides. *(d)* The first permanent molars have migrated mesially and rotated around the axis through the mesiopalatal cusp and the large palatal root. *(e)* Their mesial surfaces are now at an oblique angle to the dental arch. *(f)* Their migration and rotation interfere with adequate intercuspation.

In Class II, division 1 malocclusions with premature loss of a mandibular second deciduous molar, the opposing maxillary tooth cannot overerupt because it also occludes with the mandibular first deciduous molar. Therefore, mesial migration of the mandibular first permanent molar is not blocked (Figs 16-13 and 16-14). In addition, if the lower lip is positioned behind the maxillary incisors, more pressure is exerted on the mandibular incisors, increasing the likelihood of reduction of space from the mesial. After loss of a maxillary second deciduous molar in a Class II, division 1 malocclusion, mesial migration and rotation of the maxillary first permanent molar also occurs (Figs 16-15 and 16-16).

If in a Class II, division 1 malocclusion opposing second deciduous molars are lost, the adjacent first permanent molars migrate mesially. Premature loss of all four mandibular deciduous molars in a Class II, division 1 malocclusion is extremely adverse, particularly if the lower lip is or becomes positioned behind the maxillary incisors.

In Class II, division 2 malocclusions, the teeth mesial to the premature loss have a strong tendency to move distally. Premature loss of mandibular deciduous molars will lead to further lingual tipping of maxillary and mandibular incisors. Premature loss of deciduous molars and canines in both jaws is particularly adverse.

In Class III malocclusions, the maxillary, but not the mandibular, incisors tend to move palatally with premature loss of deciduous molars (Figs 16-17 and 16-18).

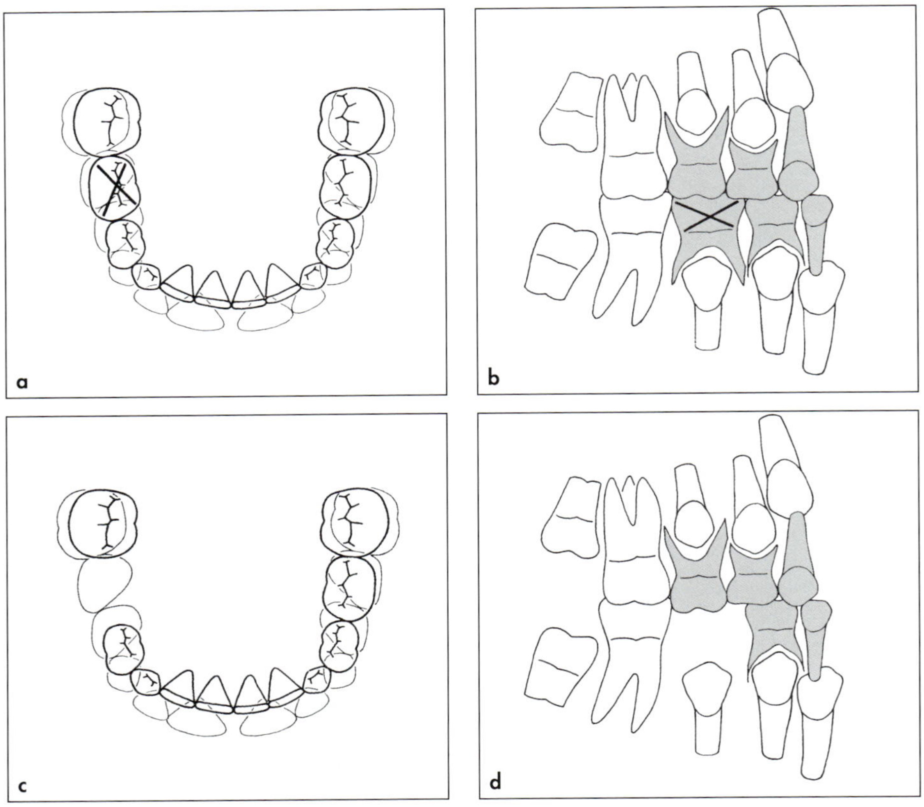

FIG 16-7 Premature loss of a mandibular second deciduous molar in neutroclusion. *(a and b)* The second deciduous molar in the mandible is wider than that in the maxilla. The terminal plane distal of the second deciduous molars is flush or has a small mesial step. *(c and d)* The maxillary second deciduous molar can overerupt and block the mesial migration of the mandibular first permanent molar. The development of the dentition is not affected by this premature loss.

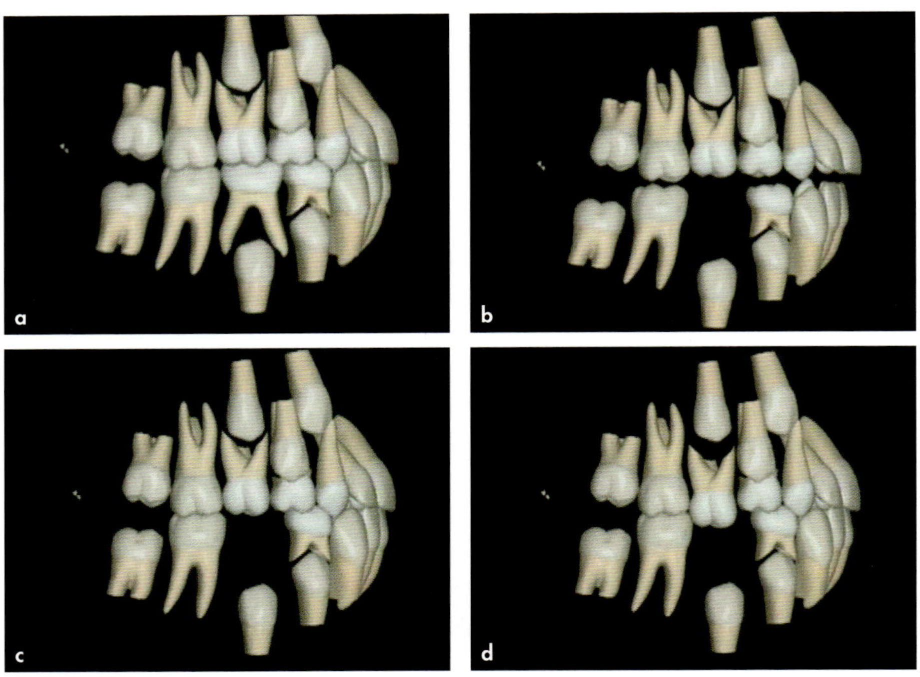

FIG 16-8 Premature loss of a mandibular second deciduous molar in a neutroclusion. *(a)* With a flush terminal plane, the mesial sides of the first permanent molars are aligned. *(b and c)* After loss of the mandibular second deciduous molar, the adjacent first permanent molar tends to migrate to the mesial. *(d)* However, the maxillary second deciduous molar will overerupt and block the mesial migration.

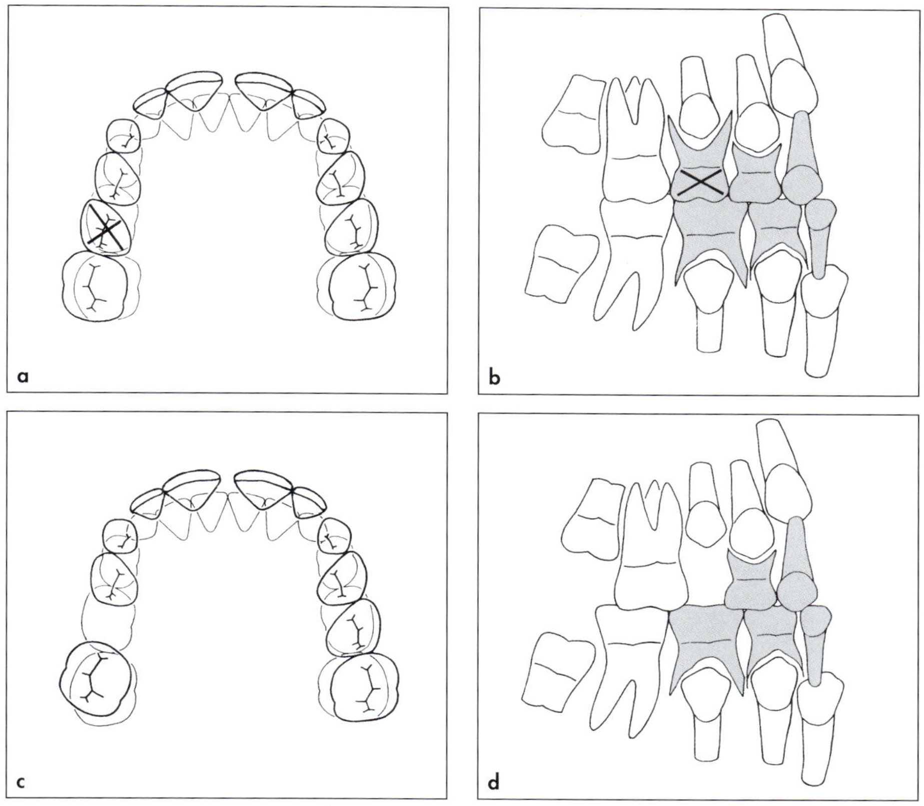

Fig 16-9 Premature loss of a maxillary second deciduous molar in neutroclusion. *(a and b)* The second deciduous molar in the mandible has a wider crown than that in the maxilla. It cannot overerupt because it also occludes with the maxillary first deciduous molar. *(c and d)* The maxillary first permanent molar migrates mesially and rotates around an axis through the mesiopalatal cusp and palatal root. Because of its trapezoid shape, it will occupy more space in the dental arch after mesial rotation.

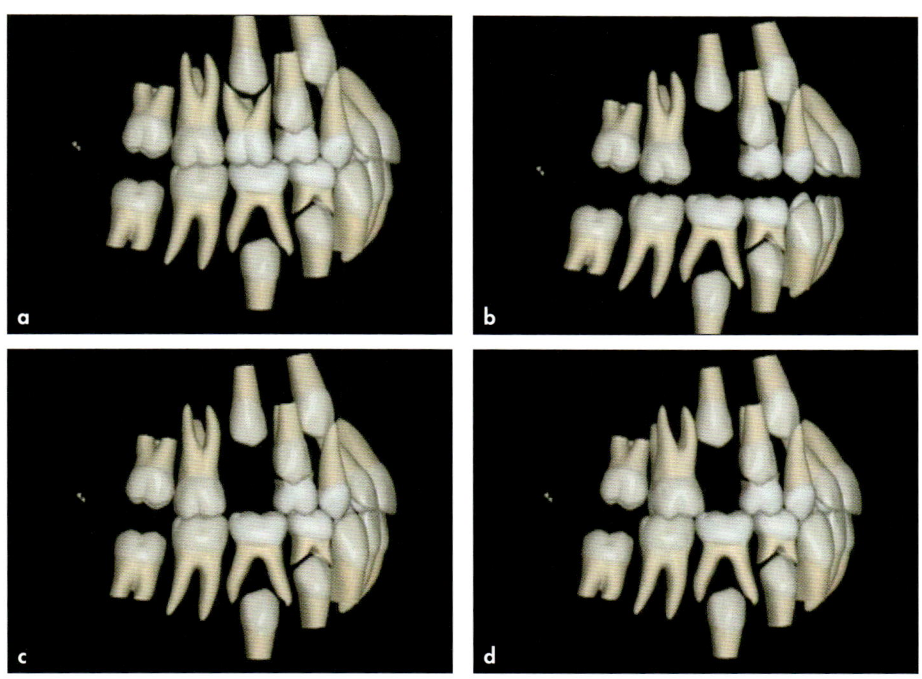

Fig 16-10 Premature loss of a maxillary second deciduous molar in a neutroclusion. *(a and b)* The tooth that is lost is narrower than its antagonist, which also occludes with the maxillary first deciduous molar. *(c)* The mandibular second deciduous molar cannot overerupt. *(d)* The maxillary first permanent molar will migrate and rotate to the mesial.

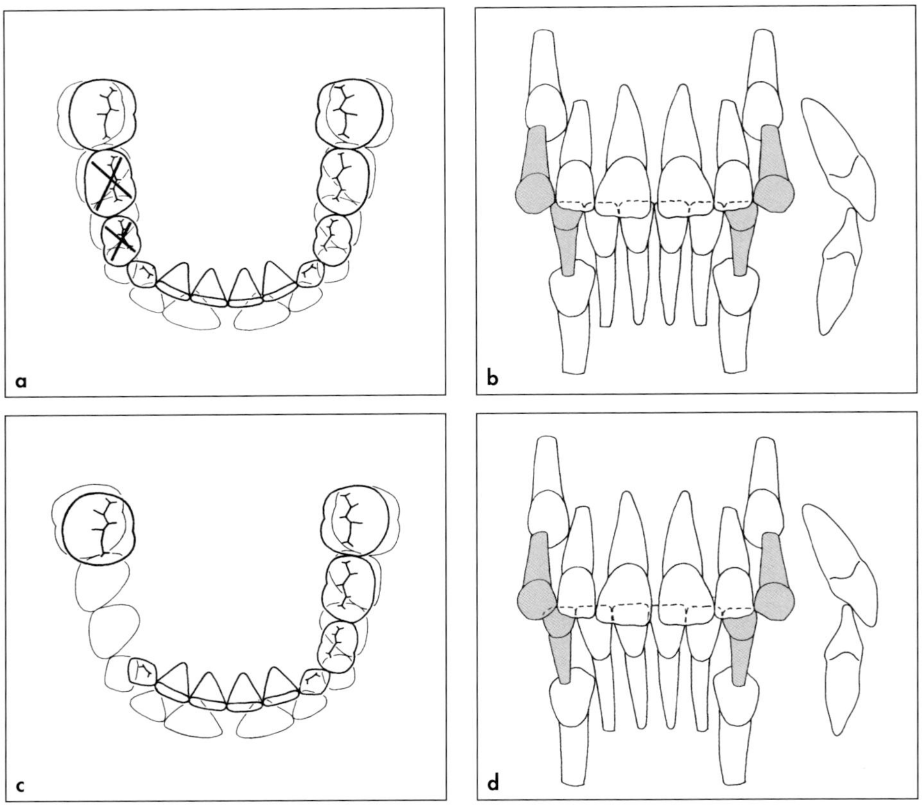

FIG 16-11 Unilateral premature loss of two mandibular right deciduous molars and its effect on the incisors. *(a and b)* Situation at the loss of the deciduous molars. *(c and d)* The mandibular incisors tip lingually, and the midline shifts to the right side. The overjet and overbite increase. The mandibular right permanent molar moves mesially.

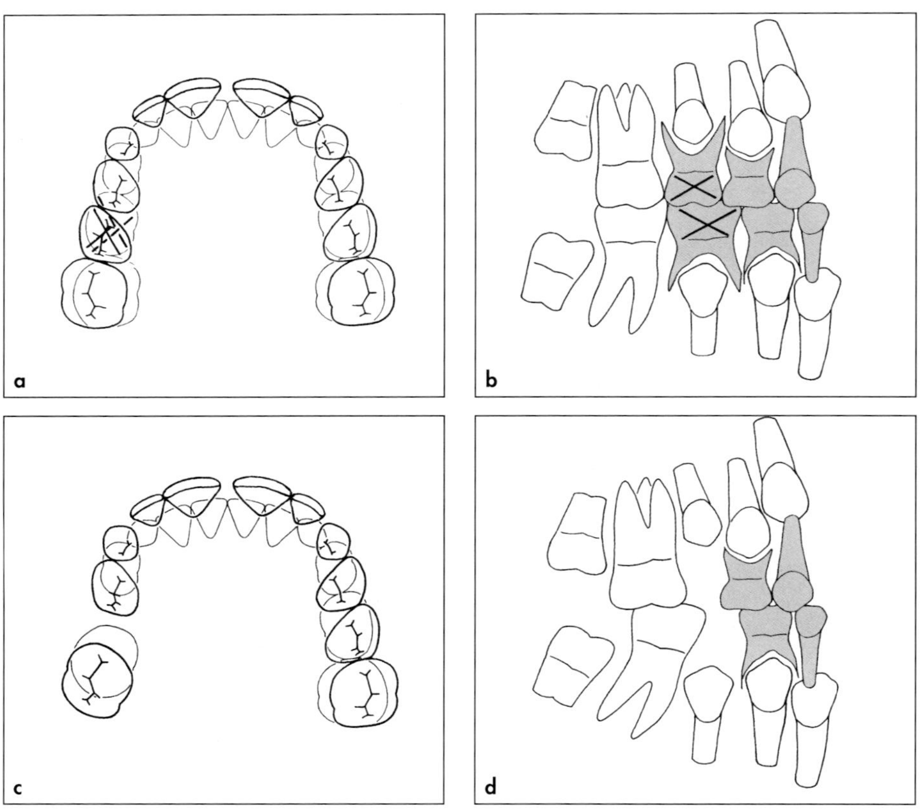

FIG 16-12 Unilateral premature loss of both second deciduous molars in a neutroclusion. *(a and b)* After the loss of two opposing second deciduous molars, there is nothing to block mesial migration. *(c and d)* Both first permanent molars migrate mesially. The migration of the maxillary molar is greater than it would be if the premature loss had not occurred in the mandible. The mesial migration and tipping of the mandibular first permanent molar is sometimes combined with a slight mesiolingual rotation. Mesial migration of first permanent molars leads to accelerated emergence of second permanent molars.

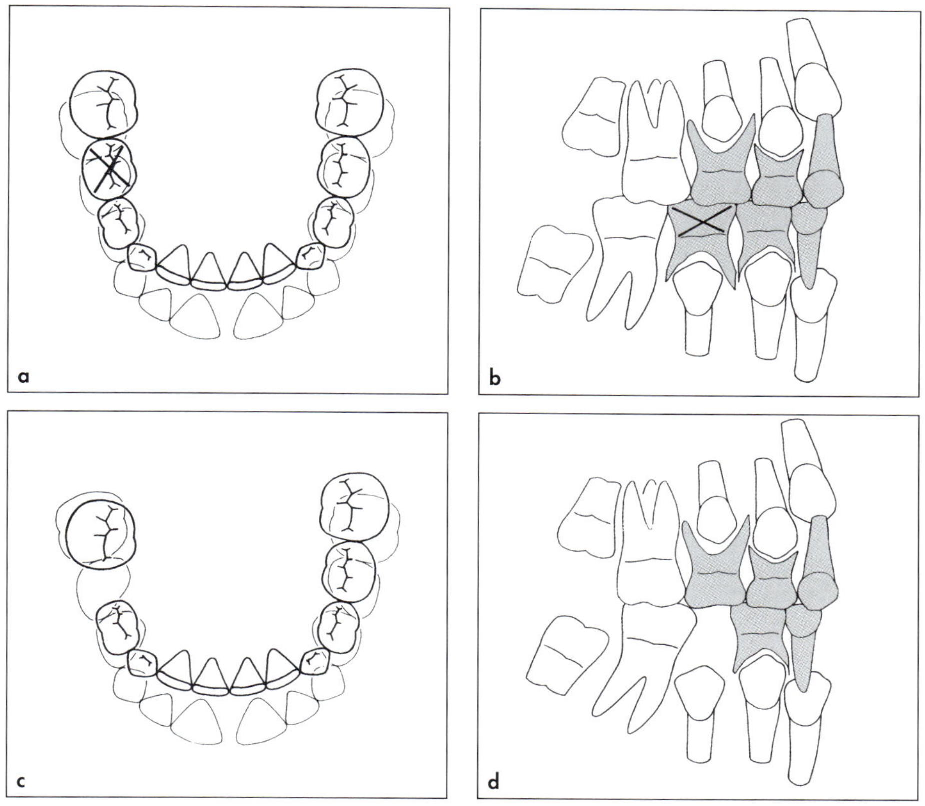

Fig 16-13 Premature loss of a mandibular second deciduous molar in a Class II, division 1 malocclusion. *(a and b)* The maxillary second deciduous molar occludes with both the mandibular first and second deciduous molars. *(c and d)* Because the maxillary second deciduous molar cannot overerupt, the mesial migration of the mandibular first permanent molar is not blocked. If the lower lip is positioned between the mandibular and maxillary incisors, the space created by the premature loss is reduced from the mesial more than it otherwise would be.

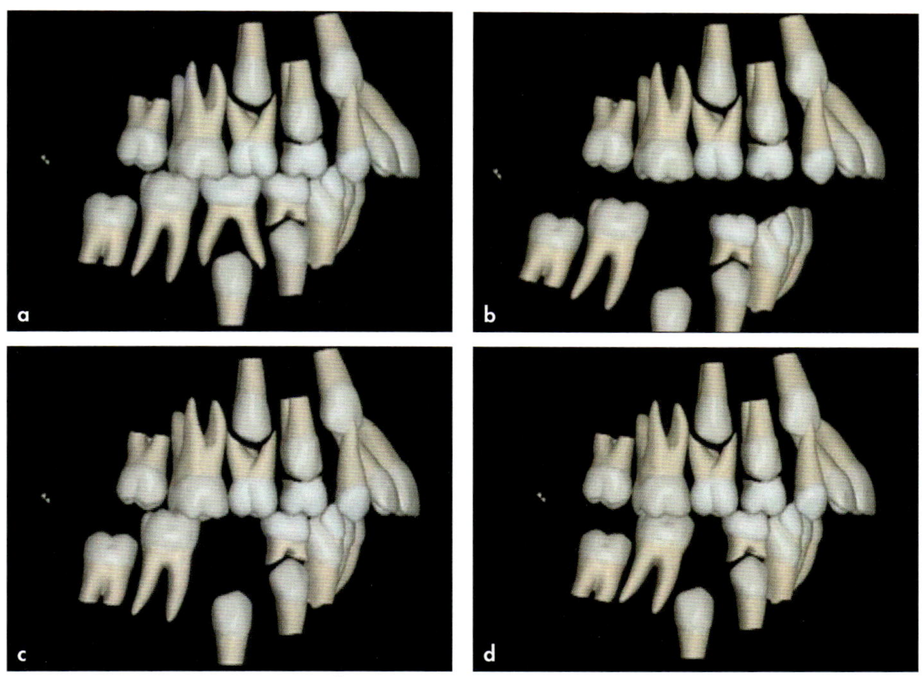

Fig 16-14 Premature loss of a mandibular second deciduous molar in a distoclusion. *(a)* With a distoclusion of one premolar crown width, the maxillary second deciduous molar also occludes with the mandibular first deciduous molar. *(b)* As a result, it will not overerupt after the loss of its antagonist. *(c and d)* The occlusion of the mandibular first permanent molar does not hinder its mesial migration.

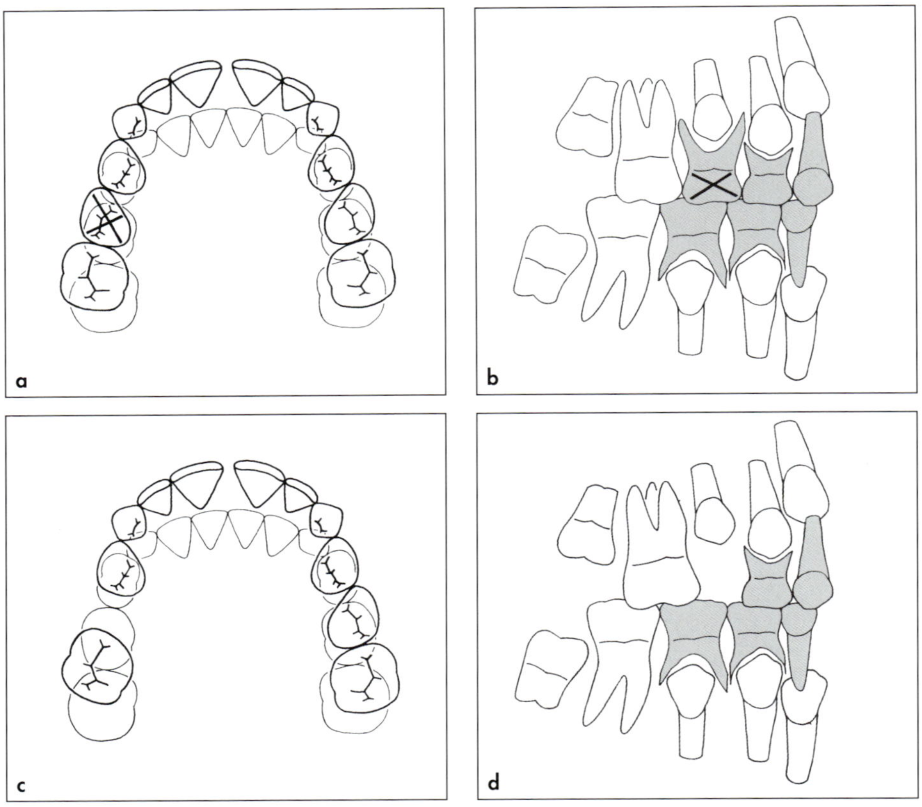

FIG 16-15 Premature loss of a maxillary second deciduous molar in a Class II, division 1 malocclusion. *(a and b)* The wide mandibular second deciduous molar cannot overerupt after loss of its maxillary antagonist. *(c and d)* The maxillary first permanent molar migrates and rotates mesially. Its mesiopalatal cusp does not intercuspate in the central fossa of the mandibular first molar; if it did, this would provide a hindrance to mesial migration.

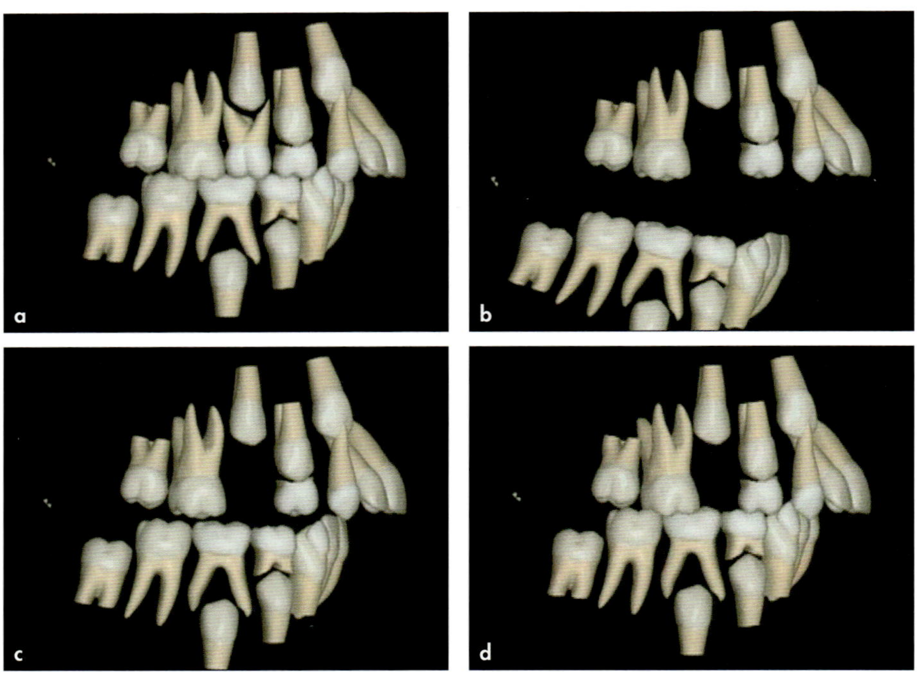

FIG 16-16 Premature loss of a maxillary second deciduous molar in a distoclusion. *(a)* With a distoclusion of one premolar crown width, the mandibular second deciduous molar occludes also with the maxillary first permanent molar. *(b and c)* It cannot overerupt after loss of its antagonist. *(d)* The maxillary first permanent molar will migrate and rotate mesially. In any case, a mandibular second deciduous molar cannot overerupt when only one opposing deciduous tooth is lost, independent of the occlusion; it is only possible if both maxillary deciduous molars are missing.

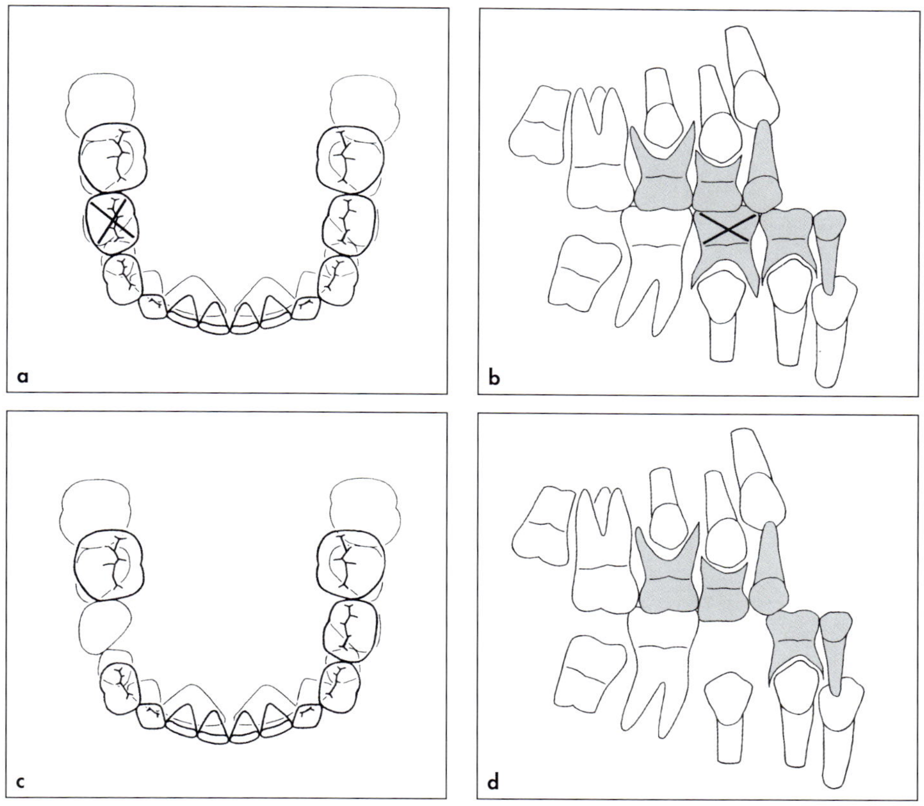

FIG 16-17 Premature loss of a mandibular second deciduous molar in a Class III malocclusion. *(a and b)* The maxillary first deciduous molar can overerupt. *(c and d)* The mandibular first permanent molar will migrate only slightly. The overerupted maxillary first deciduous molar blocks its mesial migration.

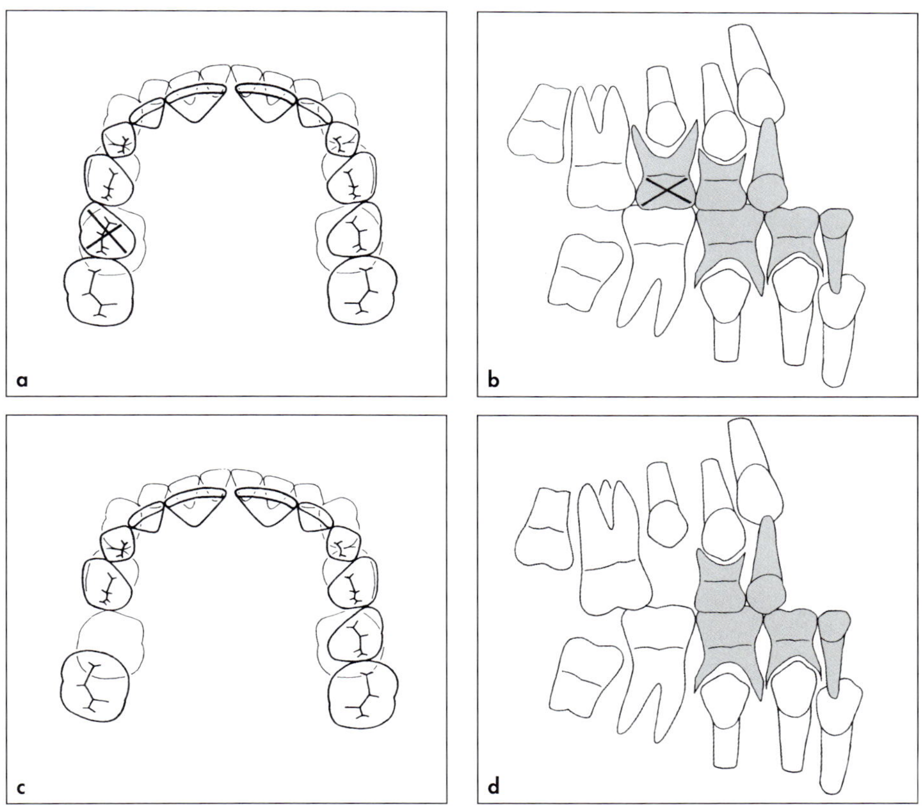

FIG 16-18 Premature loss of a maxillary second deciduous molar in a Class III malocclusion. *(a and b)* There is no possibility for overeruption of a mandibular tooth. *(c and d)* The maxillary first permanent molar migrates and rotates to the mesial.

Box 16-1 Premature loss of second deciduous molars: Factors affecting migration and expected effects

Essential factors
- Crowding/spacing
- Local occlusal relations
- Jaw relationship (Angle classification)
- Relationship of lips to the maxillary and mandibular incisors
- Size of leeway space
- Timing of premature loss

Additional factors
- Midline deviations
- Increase of overjet
- Increase of overbite

Effects of loss of maxillary second deciduous molar
- Always migration of maxillary first permanent molar
- Seldom and little remigration of maxillary first permanent molar

Effects of loss of mandibular second deciduous molar
- Almost always migration of mandibular first permanent molar, although amount is often limited, depending on over-eruption of maxillary second decidous molar and how this tooth contacts the mandibular first permanent molar
- Often partial remigration of the mandibular first permanent molar
- In most cases no permanent undesirable effect

Table 16-1 Effect of premature loss of second deciduous molars on the space available for their successors based on existing occlusion and spacing

	Neutroclusion		Distoclusion			Mesioclusion	
Tooth lost	Spacing	Crowding	Spacing	Crowding	Lower lip*	Spacing	Crowding
Maxillary second deciduous molar	(+)	++	(+)	++	+	(+)	+++
Mandibular second deciduous molar	(+)	+	(+)	++	+++	(+)	(+)
Maxillary and mandibular second deciduous molars	(+)	+++	(+)	+++	+++	(+)	++

*Lower lip behind maxillary incisors
(+), space for successor hardly or not at all restricted; +, space for successors slightly restricted; ++, space for successors considerably restricted; +++, space for successor very restricted.

Loss of a second deciduous molar is more harmful before the emergence of a first permanent molar than after. A not-yet-emerged first permanent molar begins migrating mesially within the jaw if the second deciduous molar is lacking. In addition, the second premolar is still some distance away from the occlusal plane and does not act as an obstacle against migration. If the second deciduous molar is lost prior to the emergence of the second permanent molar, the first molar migrates more mesially than it would if the second molar had already emerged.[21] Furthermore, premature loss of a second deciduous molar advances the emergence of second permanent molars.[25] Box 16-1 and Table 16-1 provide an overview of the sequelae of premature loss of second deciduous molars.

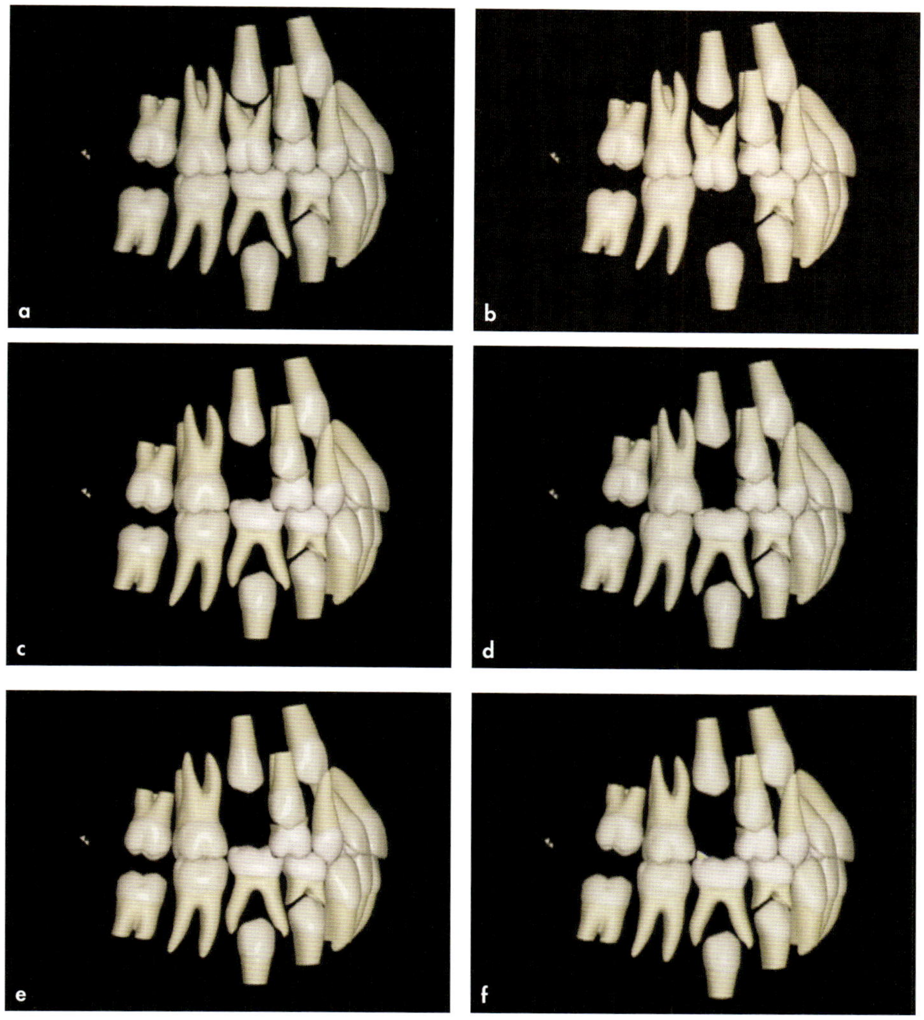

FIG 16-19 Prevention of migration. *(a and b)* In a neutroclusion, when a mandibular second deciduous molar is lost prematurely, the maxillary second deciduous molar can overerupt and block the mesial migration of the mandibular first permanent molar. *(c and d)* However, when a maxillary second deciduous molar is lost prematurely, the mandibular second deciduous molar cannot overerupt. *(e)* As a preventive intervention, a portion of the mesio-occlusal surface of the mandibular second deciduous molar can be removed to allow it to overerupt and subsequently serves as a blockade against mesial migration of the maxillary first permanent molar. *(f)* A comparable result is obtained when a blockade of resin composite is bonded on the occlusal surface of the mandibular second deciduous molar. In deviating sagittal occlusions, the removal of tooth material or placement of resin composite must be carried out at different sites, but the principle remains the same. However, these procedures will not be effective in patients with a posterior open bite or nonocclusion. Deciduous teeth, like permanent teeth, will erupt until occlusal contacts or other factors impede their eruption. Strategic use of this potential provides the possibility of preventing undesirable migration.

Prevention of Migration

In situations where a strategic tooth cannot overerupt due to the occlusion, measures can be taken by the clinician to prevent mesial migration (Fig 16-19). The first method is to remove the part of the crown that hinders eruption to allow overeruption (see Fig 16-19e). Undesirable migration also can be prevented by bonding a blockade of resin composite to the occlusal surface of the tooth opposing the lost tooth (see Fig 16-19f). These two procedures largely eliminate the need for placing space maintainers. Space maintainers are often placed in situations where no negative sequelae are expected.

Deciduous and permanent teeth that lose their occlusal support start to overerupt shortly thereafter. Mesiodistal migration of teeth following the loss of an adjacent tooth takes longer; in fact, it does not occur in the first 4 weeks. This difference in the initiation of eruption and migration plays an essential role in the spontaneous blocking of undesirable migrations after premature loss of a deciduous tooth. Likewise, it is important that preventive techniques such as grinding away a part of an opposing deciduous molar so it can overerupt or applying a blockade of composite are carried out in a timely manner.

References

1. Bjerklin K, Kurol J. Ectopic eruption of the maxillary first permanent molars: Etiologic factors. Am J Orthod 1983;84:147–155.
2. Bjerklin K, Kurol J, Paulin G. Ectopic eruption of maxillary first permanent molars in children with cleft lip and/or palate. Eur J Orthod 1993;15:535–540.
3. Breakspear EK. Further observations on early loss of deciduous molars. Dent Pract (Bristol) 1961;11:233–252.
4. De Boer M. Aspekten van de gebitsontwikkeling bij kinderen tussen vijf en tien jaar [thesis]. Utrecht: Utrecht University, 1970.
5. Hoffding J, Kisling E. Premature loss of primary teeth. I. Its overall effect on occlusion and space in the permanent dentition. ASDC J Dent Child 1978;45:279–283.
6. Northway WM. Anteroposterior Arch Dimension Changes in French-Canadian Children: A Study of the Effects of Dental Caries and Premature Extractions [thesis]. Montreal: University of Montreal, 1977.
7. Ungar AL. Incidence and effects of premature loss of deciduous teeth. Int J Orthod 1938;24:613–621.
8. Bauer WH. Effect of periapical processes of deciduous teeth on the buds of permanent teeth. Am J Orthod Oral Surg 1946;32:232–241.
9. Morningstar CH. Effect of infection of the deciduous molar on the permanent tooth germ. J Am Dent Assoc 1937;24:786–791.
10. Shiere FR, Frankl SN. The effect of deciduous tooth infection on permanent teeth. Dent Prog (Chic) 1961;2:59–64.
11. Brauer JE. A report of 113 early or premature extractions of primary molars and the incidence of closure of space. J Dent Child 1941;8:222–224.
12. Davey KW. Effect of premature loss of deciduous molars on the anteroposterior position of maxillary first permanent molars and other maxillary teeth. J Can Dent Assoc 1966;32:406–416.
13. Helm S, Siersbæk-Nielsen S. Crowding in the permanent dentition after early loss of deciduous molars or canines. Trans Eur Orthod Soc 1973;137–149.
14. Lundström A. The significance of early loss of deciduous teeth in the etiology of malocclusion. Am J Orthod 1955;41:819–826.
15. Owen D. The incidence and nature of space closure following the premature extraction of deciduous teeth. A literature survey. Am J Orthod 1971;59:37–49.
16. Rönnerman A. Early extraction of deciduous molars and canines. Trans Eur Orthod Soc 1965;153–168.
17. Clinch LM. A longitudinal study of the results of premature loss of deciduous teeth between 3-4 and 13-14 years of age. Dent Pract Dent Rec 1959;9:109–128.
18. Richardson ME. The relationship between the relative amount of space present in the deciduous dental arch and the rate and degree of space closure subsequent to extraction of a deciduous molar. Dent Pract Dent Rec 1965;16:111–118.
19. Fanning EA. Effect of extraction of deciduous molars on the formation and eruption of their successors. Angle Orthod 1962;32:44–53.
20. Linder-Aronson S. The effect of premature loss of deciduous teeth. A biometric study in 14- and 15-year olds. Acta Odontol Scand 1960;18:101–122.
21. Prahl-Andersen B, Berendsen WJH. Some consequences of premature loss of the second deciduous molars in the mandible [in Dutch]. Ned Tijdschr Tandheelk 1979;86:89–92.
22. Seipel CM. Prevention of malocclusion. Trans Eur Orthod Soc 1948;203–213.
23. Magnusson TE. The effect of premature loss of deciduous teeth on the spacing of the permanent dentition. Eur J Orthod 1979;1:243–249.
24. Korf SR. The eruption of permanent central incisors following premature loss of their antecedents. ASDC J Dent Child 1965;32:39–44.
25. Rönnerman A. The effect of early loss of primary molars on tooth eruption and space conditions. A longitudinal study. Acta Odontol Scand 1977;35:229–239.

17

Statistical Data

The content of this chapter serves to support the various topics covered in the preceding chapters and to present statistical data in a compact and easily accessible format.

The data in this chapter have been selected and compiled from results of studies carried out mainly in Western countries. The data presentation starts with the formation, eruption, and emergence of the deciduous teeth, followed by that of the permanent teeth. The correlations in crown widths among individual teeth in both dentitions and between the deciduous teeth and their successors are presented. Dental arch dimensions, the size of the overjet and overbite, and molar occlusion are shown from 3 to 18 years of age in tables and graphs. Information on the variation in inclination and angulation of teeth in adults is provided. Finally, the prevalence of agenesis and malocclusions is given.

A comparison of findings from various published studies is complicated by differences in design, data collection, and presentation of results.[1] For example, most information on times of emergence of deciduous teeth is derived from observations in clinics for babies and small children and from notes made by mothers.[2] The data collected in this way are more precise than those derived from annually prepared dental casts. Dental casts have served to provide information not only on times of emergence of permanent teeth but also on changes in dental arch dimensions and occlusion. In some studies only children with normal occlusion were included. In other studies this selection criterion was not or only moderately used.

Annually collected data on times of emergence are based on observations that certain teeth had emerged in the preceding 12 months. Assuming a normal distribution of times of emergence, the calculated average times of emergence should be decreased by 6 months. However, this was not done in any of the studies that dealt with times of emergence. As a result, the data presented in this chapter can be assumed to be 6 months higher than in reality. There is only one investigation in which data were collected every 6 months—the Nijmegen Growth Study. Therefore, the data on times of emergence derived from that study are 3 months too high.

The most valuable information is obtained with longitudinal growth studies, followed by those with overlapping cohorts (mixed longitudinal). Sometimes it is more practical to collect data only once from a very large sample (cross-sectional). The data presented in this chapter come from all three types of studies.

Formation and Emergence of Deciduous Teeth

The progress in formation of deciduous teeth is plotted against age in Table 17-1 and for the mandibular deciduous teeth in Fig 17-1. The average times of emergence of deciduous teeth in five populations is presented in Table 17-2. The results of the longitudinal studies differ only slightly from each other but deviate from those of the cross-sectional study. From the data in Table 17-2, it could be concluded that the average sequence of emergence is the same in all five studies. However, this presentation disguises the large individual variation in time of emergence. In the longitudinal study on 171 children, only 5% had the average sequence in time of emergence.[4]

The average times of emergence of deciduous teeth differ between boys and girls, but the average sequence of emergence does not (Table 17-3; Fig 17-2). In accordance with the large individual variation in time of emergence of deciduous teeth, the standard deviation in times of emergence is high. The range in time of emergence is the smallest for the central incisors (SD, 1.5 months), larger for the lateral incisors and canines (SD, 2.8 months), and the largest for the second molars (SD, 4.1 months). It is remarkable that, in contrast with the permanent teeth, deciduous teeth emerge in boys earlier than in girls, with the exception of the first molars. Another difference between the two dentitions is that the maxillary deciduous teeth emerge before the mandibular ones, with the exception of the central incisor and the second molar.[11,12,13]

Table 17-1 Formation stages of mandibular and maxillary deciduous teeth[3-6]

Age	Start of formation	Start of mineralization	Crown complete	Root(s) complete
6 wk pc	Dental lamina			
8–12 wk pc	I, II, III, IV, V			
5 mo pc		I, II		
6 mo pc		III, IV		
7 mo pc		V		
2–3 mo			I, II	
6 mo			IV	
9 mo			III	
11 mo			V	
2.5 y				I, II
3 y				IV
3.5 y				III, V

pc, postconception; I, central deciduous incisor; II, lateral deciduous incisor; III, deciduous canine; IV, first deciduous molar; V, second deciduous molar.

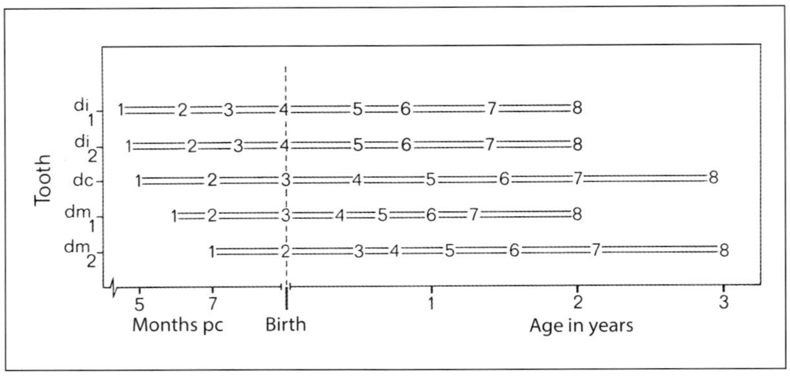

Fig 17-1 The eight formation stages (see Figs 17-3 and 17-4) of mandibular deciduous teeth plotted against age.[7] di_1, central deciduous incisors; di_2, lateral deciduous incisors; dc, deciduous canines; dm_1, first deciduous molars; dm_2, second deciduous molars; pc, postconception.

Table 17-2 Average ages (in months*) of emergence of deciduous teeth in boys and girls combined

Country	USA	Sweden	Sweden	Korea	Korea
Year	1942[8]	1962[4]	1986[9]	1977[10]	2001[11]
n	64*†	171*†	212*†		1,070*‡
+I	9.3	10.2	9.7	9.5	8.7
+II	11.1	11.4	10.8	10.0	9.4
+III	19.5	19.2	19.1	19.0	16.4
+IV	15.8	16.0	15.6	17.0	15.4
+V	28.0	29.1	27.8	26.0	25.5
−I	7.5	8.0	7.7	7.5	6.2
−II	13.4	13.2	13.2	13.0	10.8
−III	19.8	19.7	19.7	19.0	16.9
−IV	15.9	16.3	15.8	18.0	15.5
−V	26.5	27.1	26.3	23.0	24.0

n, sample size; +, maxillary; −, mandibular; I, central deciduous incisor; II, lateral deciduous incisor; III, deciduous canine; IV, first deciduous molar; V, second deciduous molar.
*Decimals indicate tenths of years, not months.
†Longitudinal.
‡Cross-sectional.

Table 17-3 Times of emergence of deciduous teeth for boys and girls (in months*)[12]

Tooth	Boys		Girls	
	Mean	SD	Mean	SD
+I	9.1	1.5	9.6	2.0
+II	10.4	2.4	11.9	2.7
+III	18.9	2.7	20.1	3.2
+IV	16.0	2.3	15.7	2.3
+V	27.6	4.4	28.4	4.3
−I	7.3	1.6	7.8	2.1
−II	13.0	2.8	13.8	3.6
−III	19.3	2.9	20.2	3.4
−IV	16.2	1.9	15.6	2.2
−V	25.9	3.8	27.1	4.2

+, maxillary; −, mandibular; I, central deciduous incisor; II, lateral deciduous incisor; III, deciduous canine; IV, first deciduous molar; V, second deciduous molar.
*Decimals indicate tenths of years, not months.

Formation and Emergence of Permanent Teeth

The progress in formation of permanent teeth in relation to age is shown in Table 17-4. In addition, details are provided for the mandibular permanent teeth in Figs 17-3 to 17-5.

The data on emergence of permanent teeth are presented similarly to those on emergence of deciduous teeth (Figs 17-6 and 17-7 and Tables 17-5 to 17-7). Table 17-5 displays the average times of emergence of permanent teeth in girls. The data were collected in various countries over a period of 40 years. The differences in times of emergence are caused in part by the diversity in the methods of collecting and reporting data and partly by regional and ethnic variability. However, they conform largely in sequence of emergence and also in the phenomenon that mandibular permanent teeth emerge before the maxillary ones. That also applies to the earlier emergence in girls than in boys.

Table 17-6 presents means and standard deviations of times of emergence of permanent teeth derived from the Nijmegen Growth Study.[22] These data also show a significant range in times of emergence for all teeth. Twice the standard deviation on both sides of the average encompasses 95% of the population. That means that in boys an emergence of maxillary central permanent incisors between 5.6 and 8.8 years of age cannot be considered outside the norm. For maxillary permanent canines in boys, the range is between 8.8 and 14.5 years. It has to be remarked that the data of times of emergence of the Nijmegen Growth Study deviate only slightly from those of Hurme[8] in Fig 17-6. It provided slightly younger times of emergence, but that could be because in the Nijmegen study data were collected every 6 months rather than yearly.

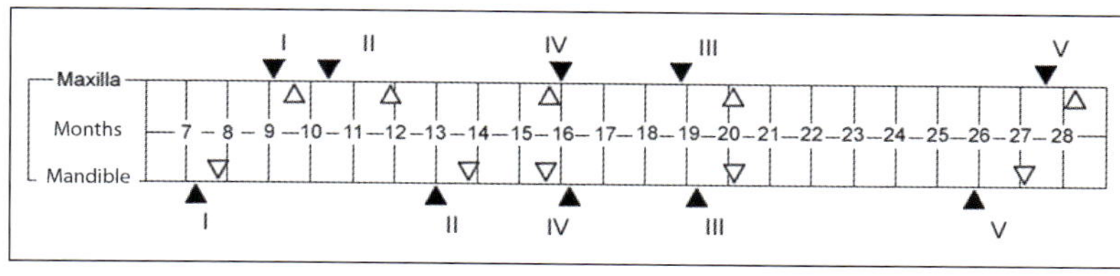

FIG 17-2 Average times of emergence of deciduous teeth in boys *(black triangles)* and girls *(white triangles)*. I, central deciduous incisors; II, lateral deciduous incisors; III, canines; IV, first deciduous molars; V, second deciduous molars.

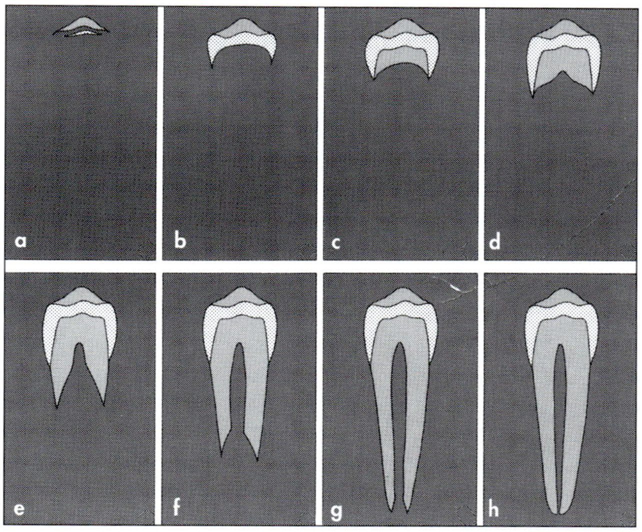

FIG 17-3 *(a to h)* Eight stages of formation of a mandibular first premolar.[7,15]

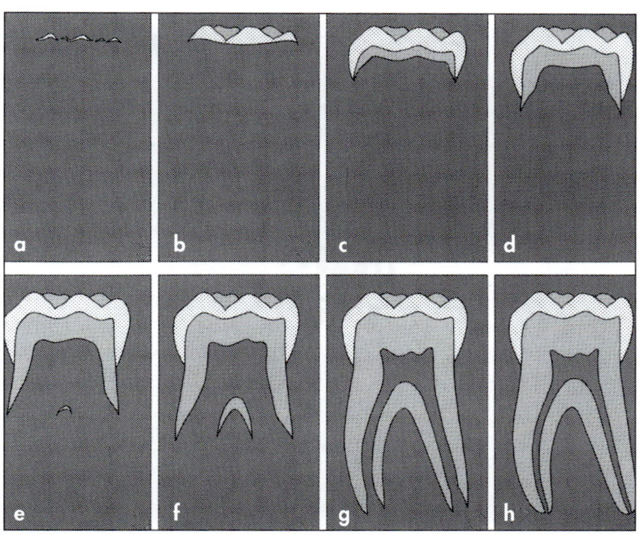

FIG 17-4 *(a to h)* Eight stages of formation of a mandibular first permanent molar.[7,15]

Table 17-4 Formation stages of permanent teeth[3–6,14]

Age	Start of formation	Start of mineralization	Crown complete	Root(s) complete
4 mo pc	6			
5–6 mo pc	1, 2			
7 mo pc	3			
9 mo pc	4	6		
6 mo		−1, +1, −2		
9 mo	5, 7	+2		
12 mo		3		
2.5 y		4		
3 y		5	6	
3.5 y		7		
4 y			1, 2	
6.5 y			3, 4, 7	
7 y			5	
9 y				1, 6
10 y				2
13 y				4
14 y				3, 5
15 y				7

pc, postconception; +, maxillary; −, mandibular; 1, central permanent incisor; 2, lateral permanent incisor; 3, permanent canine; 4, first premolar; 5, second premolar; 6, first permanent molar; 7, second permanent molar.

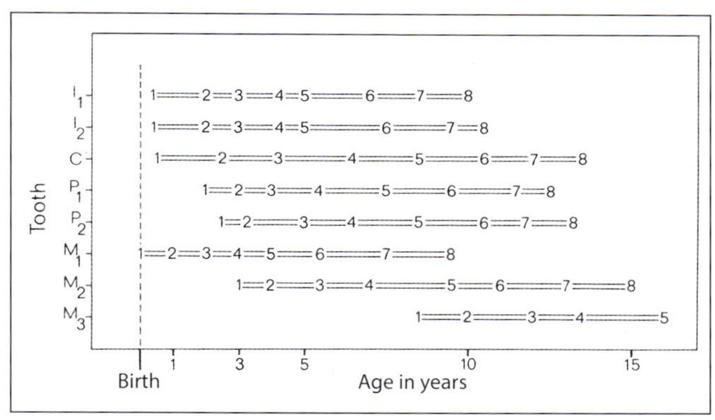

FIG 17-5 The eight formation stages of mandibular permanent teeth, plotted against age.[7] I_1, central incisors; I_2, lateral incisors; C, canines; P_1, first premolars; P_2, second premolars; M_1, first molars; M_2, second molars; M_3, third molars.

Table 17-7 shows variations in the sequence of emergence of permanent teeth. Striking is the large variation found in the population of 174 children; however, in almost all children, the first permanent molar was the first tooth to emerge in both jaws (indicated by a 1 in the 6th place). A larger variation in times of emergence was recorded for the maxilla than for the mandible, particularly for the canines and premolars.

The correlation in times of emergence among mandibular permanent teeth in girls is shown in Table 17-8. The highest correlation in times of emergence is between central and lateral incisors. It is high also between the first and second molars. The rate of eruption after emergence is illustrated on the increase in clinical crown heights (Figs 17-8 and 17-9). The mesiodistal crown dimensions of both dentitions are shown in Table 17-9. There are no differences between boys and girls in the width of deciduous teeth; however, boys have wider permanent tooth crowns than girls, particularly for canines and molars.

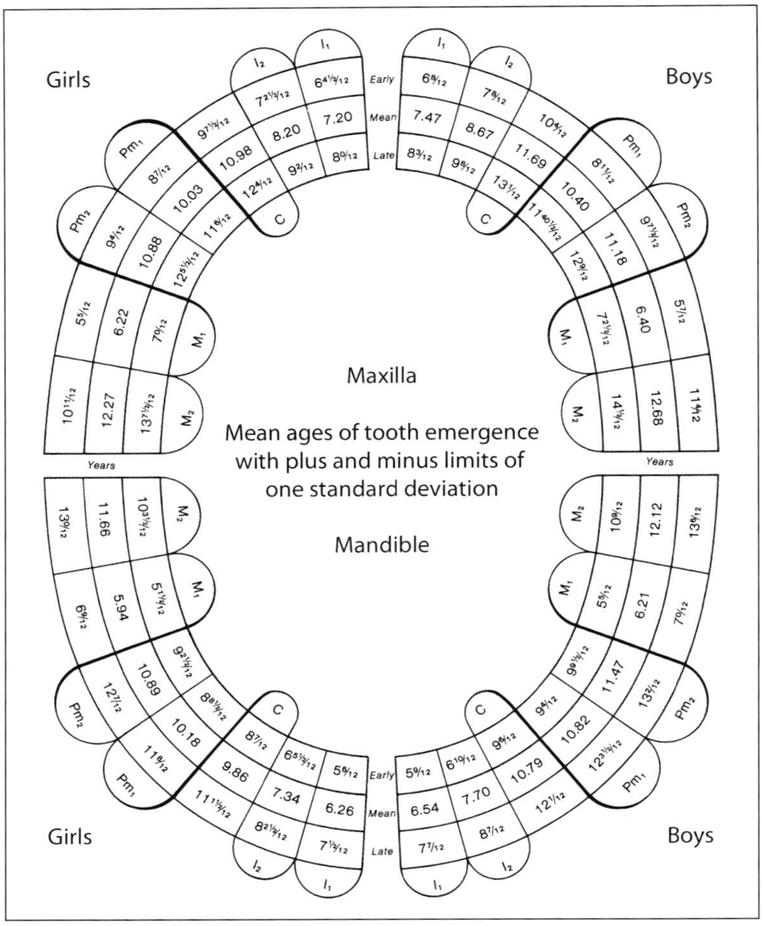

FIG 17-6 Early, mean, and late times of emergence of permanent teeth for girls *(left)* and boys *(right)*. The indicated range in times of emergence is representative of two-thirds of the population. The data are based on 24 publications, together comprising 93,000 children in the United States and Europe. In those data, which cover one century, little difference appeared in times of emergence. It was evident that the mean times of emergence are 5 months earlier in girls than in boys. The range of variation in times of emergence of corresponding teeth did not differ between the two sexes. However, it did differ among various teeth, with the smallest range for the mandibular first permanent molars, a large range for the maxillary second premolars, and the largest range for the mandibular second premolar. However, the latter can be affected by agenesis. I_1, central incisors; I_2, lateral incisors; C, canines; Pm_1, first premolars; Pm_2, second premolars; M_1, first molars; M_2, second molars. (Reprinted from Hurme[8] with permission.)

Table 17-5 Average times of emergence of permanent teeth in girls (in years*)

Country	US	Dominican Republic	Japan	Sweden	Denmark	Finland	N Ireland	Belgium	Iran
Year	1949[8]	1982[16]	1984[17]	1986[9]	1986[18]	1994[19]	1998[20]	2003[21]	2000[21]
n	93,000†	50‡	855†	90‡	371,970†	455†	130‡	2,133†	1,786†
+1	6.9	6.5	7.1	6.8	6.9	7.4	7.1	6.9	7.5
+2	7.9	6.9	8.0	7.9	7.8	8.2	8.1	7.9	8.8
+3	10.9	10.6	10.3	10.8	10.9	11.3	11.0	11.0	12.2
+4	10.3	9.0	9.3	10.3	10.5	10.9	10.5	10.4	11.1
+5	11.1	10.2	10.3	11.0	11.5	11.9	11.2	11.4	12.6
+6	6.2	6.5		6.3	6.0	6.9	6.4	6.2	6.7
+7	11.9	11.6	12.3	12.0	11.8	12.4	12.1	12.0	12.6
−1	6.0	6.4		6.0	6.0	6.6	6.3	6.1	6.5
−2	7.1	7.0	6.9	6.3	7.1	7.5	7.4	7.1	7.9
−3	9.8	9.0	9.2	9.5	9.8	10.1	9.9	9.7	10.2
−4	10.1	10.5	9.7	10.3	10.4	10.8	10.4	10.3	11.1
−5	11.0	11.2	10.4	11.2	11.4	11.5	11.4	11.4	12.6
−6	6.0	6.1		6.1	6.0	6.8	6.3	6.2	6.7
−7	11.2	10.9	11.5	11.6	11.4	11.9	11.9	11.6	12.4

n, sample size; +, maxillary; −, mandibular; 1, central permanent incisor; 2, lateral permanent incisor; 3, permanent canine; 4, first permanent premolar; 5, second permanent premolar; 6, first permanent molar; 7, second permanent molar.
*Decimals indicate tenths of years, not months.
†Cross-sectional.
‡Longitudinal.

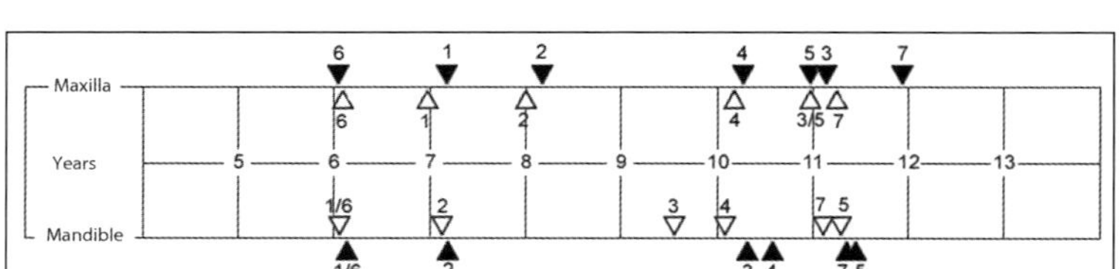

FIG 17-7 Average times of emergence of permanent teeth in boys *(black triangles)* and girls *(white triangles)*. 1, central incisors; 2, lateral incisors; 3, canines; 4, first premolars; 5, second premolars; 6, first molars; 7, second molars.

Table 17-6 Times of emergence of permanent teeth for boys and girls (in years*)[22]

Tooth	Boys			Girls		
	Mean	SD	n	Mean	SD	n
+1	7.20	0.80	166	6.94	0.73	224
+2	8.22	0.88	166	7.97	0.96	222
+3	11.16	1.68	172	10.89	1.16	250
+4	10.27	1.38	172	10.20	1.32	250
+5	10.96	1.36	172	10.88	1.52	249
+6	6.06	0.92	161	6.10	0.64	210
+7	11.87	1.08	172	11.35	2.22	250
−1	6.21	0.72	166	6.13	0.64	221
−2	7.36	0.73	166	7.21	0.75	224
−3	10.34	1.05	172	9.56	0.98	250
−4	10.55	1.73	172	10.09	1.38	250
−5	11.44	1.87	172	11.35	1.77	247
−6	6.21	0.68	166	6.10	0.60	215
−7	11.31	1.79	172	11.13	1.97	250

+, maxillary; −, mandibular; 1, central permanent incisor; 2, lateral permanent incisor; 3, permanent canine; 4, first premolar; 5, second premolar; 6, first permanent molar; 7, second permanent molar.
*Decimals indicate tenths of years, not months.

Table 17-7 Variation in sequence* of emergence of permanent teeth[23]

Boys				Girls			
Maxilla	n	Mandible	n	Maxilla	n	Mandible	n
2-3-6-4-5-1-7	9	1-3-4-5-6-2-7	9	2-3-5-4-6-1-7	12	1-3-4-5-6-2-7	21
2-3-4-4-5-1-6	4	1-3-4-5-7-2-6	6	2-3-6-4-5-1-7	9	1-3-4-5-7-2-6	9
1-3-4-6-5-2-7	4	1-2-3-4-5-1-6	4	2-3-4-5-6-1-7	9	2-3-4-5-6-1-7	6
2-3-5-4-6-1-7	4	1-3-6-4-5-2-7	4	1-3-5-4-6-2-7	7	1-2-3-4-5-1-6	5
2-3-4-5-6-1-7	3	2-3-4-5-6-1-7	4	2-3-4-4-5-1-6	5	1-3-5-4-6-2-7	5
2-3-5-4-4-1-6	3	2-3-4-5-7-1-6	4	2-3-4-5-7-1-6	5	2-3-5-4-6-1-7	5
2-3-5-4-6-1-6	3	1-2-4-5-6-3-7	2	2-3-5-4-7-1-6	5	2-3-4-5-7-1-6	4
2-3-6-4-7-1-5	3	1-3-4-4-5-2-6	2	1-2-5-3-4-1-6	4	1-3-4-4-5-2-6	3
1-2-5-3-4-1-6	2	1-3-5-4-7-2-6	2	2-3-4-4-4-1-5	4	1-3-4-6-5-2-7	3
2-3-4-4-6-1-5	2	2-3-4-4-5-1-6	2	2-3-5-6-4-1-7	4	1-2-3-4-5-1-4	2
2-3-4-5-5-1-6	2			2-3-5-4-5-1-6	3	1-2-3-4-5-2-6	2
2-3-4-5-6-1-6	2			2-3-7-5-4-1-6	3	1-2-3-4-6-1-5	2
2-3-4-5-7-1-6	2			1-3-6-4-5-2-7	2	1-2-5-3-4-1-6	2
2-3-5-4-5-1-6	2			2-3-5-4-4-1-6	2	1-3-4-6-7-2-5	2
2-3-5-4-7-1-6	2			2-3-6-4-7-1-5	2	2-2-3-4-6-1-5	2
				2-3-7-4-5-1-6	2		
Unique†	20	Unique†	30	Unique†	27	Unique†	24
Total	67	Total	69	Total	105	Total	97

*Sequence: central incisor, lateral incisor, canine, first premolar, second premolar, first molar, second molar. Numbers indicate sequence of emergence. When two teeth emerged in the same period, both teeth were given the same number; therefore, the number 7 is missing.
†Sequence that occurred only once in the group.

Table 17-8 Correlations among times of emergence of mandibular permanent teeth in girls[24]

	2	3	4	5	6	7
1	0.85	0.78	0.64	0.43	0.59	0.44
2		0.83	0.70	0.53	0.62	0.58
3			0.78	0.59	0.56	0.58
4				0.65	0.55	0.58
5					0.48	0.64
6						0.76

1, central permanent incisor; 2, lateral permanent incisor; 3, permanent canine; 4, first premolar; 5, second premolar; 6, first permanent molar; 7, second permanent molar.

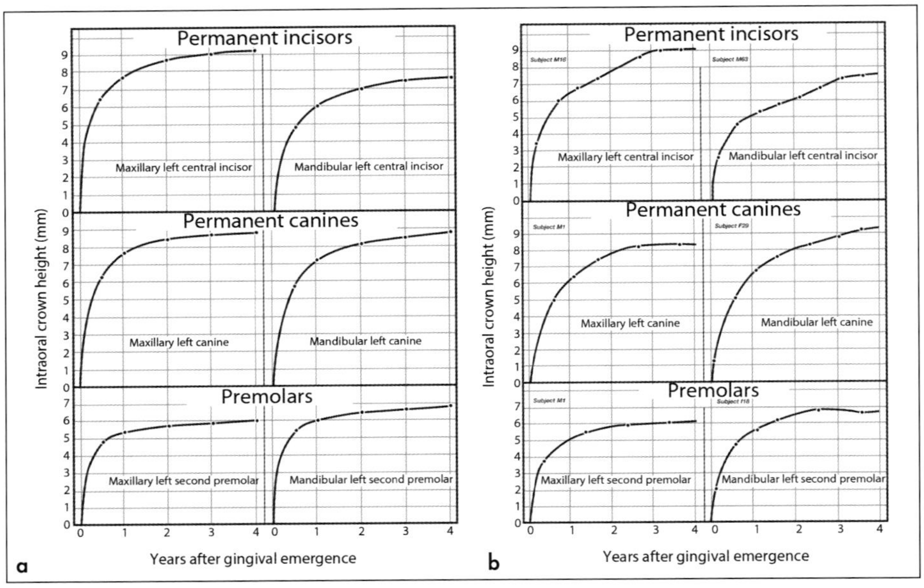

FIG 17-8 Average *(a)* and sample individual *(b)* increases in visible crown height in six erupting permanent teeth. The graphs are based on longitudinal observations of 50 children. In the first 6 months after emergence, there is a rapid increase in clinical crown height. In the second 6 months, it tapers off. In the second year after emergence, there is still some increase in height; in the subsequent years there is little increase. (Reprinted from Giles et al[25] with permission.)

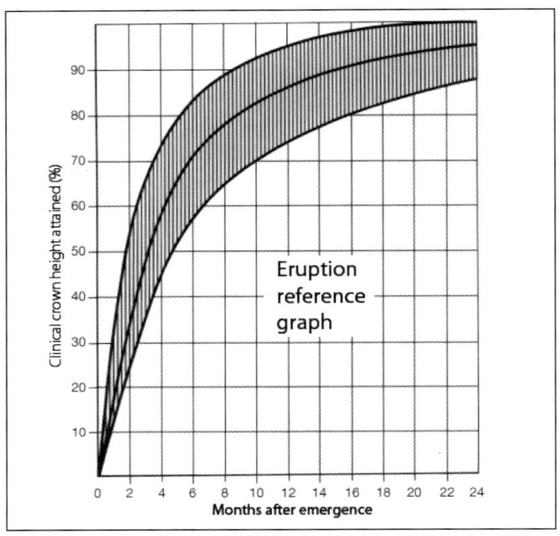

FIG 17-9 Generalized increase in clinical crown height. This graph is based on a compilation of data obtained on the increase in clinical crown height of central incisors, canines, and second premolars in both jaws. The percentage of the maximally attained crown height during the first 24 months after emergence is plotted. The width of the shaded area between the outer curves represents the range of time in which 80% of the children had attained the indicated level of crown height. (Reprinted from Giles et al[25] with permission.)

Table 17-9 Mesiodistal crown dimensions (mm) of deciduous and permanent teeth[26]

	Boys			Girls				Boys			Girls		
	M	SD	n	M	SD	n		M	SD	n	M	SD	n
+I	6.41	0.43	166	6.48	0.43	169	+1	8.91	0.59	212	8.67	0.57	189
+II	5.26	0.37	189	5.29	0.43	175	+2	6.88	0.64	201	6.78	0.64	172
+III	6.76	0.34	212	6.63	0.35	194	+3	7.99	0.42	152	7.49	0.36	125
+IV	6.74	0.49	214	6.61	0.49	195	+4	6.76	0.47	157	6.60	0.46	122
+V	8.84	0.53	213	8.74	0.47	196	+5	6.67	0.37	132	6.50	0.46	99
							+6	10.58	0.56	216	10.18	0.58	192
							+7	9.50	0.71	121	8.79	0.73	80
–I	4.06	0.35	144	4.10	0.31	144	–1	5.54	0.32	214	5.46	0.34	196
–II	4.64	0.43	182	4.68	0.40	171	–2	6.04	0.37	208	5.92	0.34	189
–III	5.84	0.33	213	5.82	0.65	193	–3	6.96	0.40	170	6.58	0.34	148
–IV	7.82	0.47	209	7.71	0.46	195	–4	6.89	0.63	159	6.78	0.70	134
–V	9.90	0.52	214	9.73	0.48	196	–5	7.22	0.47	132	7.07	0.46	100
							–6	10.71	0.60	215	10.29	0.74	191
							–7	9.98	0.61	115	9.50	0.59	92

M, mean; +, maxillary; –, mandibular; I, central deciduous incisor; II, lateral deciduous incisor; III, deciduous canine; IV, first deciduous molar; V, second deciduous molar; 1, central permanent incisor; 2, lateral permanent incisor; 3, permanent canine; 4, first premolar; 5, second premolar; 6, first permanent molar; 7, second permanent molar.

Table 17-10 Correlation coefficients for mesiodistal crown dimensions among deciduous and permanent teeth*[27]

	+1	+2	+3	+4	+5	+6	+7
+I	0.63	0.36	0.35	0.33	0.31	0.40	0.28
+II	0.32	0.31	0.29	0.27	0.22	0.19	0.25
+III	0.27	0.26	0.29	0.42	0.31	0.25	0.35
+IV	0.34	0.25	0.35	0.34	0.41	0.36	0.45
+V	0.32	0.26	0.23	0.39	0.38	0.51	0.39
	–1	–2	–3	–4	–5	–6	–7
–I	0.43	0.41	0.32	0.24	0.29	0.28	0.26
–II	0.42	0.44	0.39	0.15	0.24	0.35	0.32
–III	0.30	0.30	0.26	0.25	0.36	0.25	0.34
–IV	0.29	0.38	0.44	0.47	0.51	0.45	0.42
–V	0.24	0.37	0.35	0.39	0.41	0.53	0.43

Table 17-11 Correlation coefficients among the sums of mesiodistal crown dimensions of corresponding groups of deciduous and permanent teeth[28]

	Boys		Girls	
Groups of teeth	r ± SDr	n	r ± SDr	n
+I and +II / +1 and +2	+0.31 ± 0.11	62	+0.55 ± 0.09	58
+III, +IV, and +V / +3, +4, and +5	+0.45 ± 0.10	62	+0.55 ± 0.09	58
–I and –II / –1 and –2	+0.39 ± 0.11	58	+0.44 ± 0.10	61
–III, –IV, and –V / –3, –4, and –5	+0.57 ± 0.09	58	+0.59 ± 0.08	61

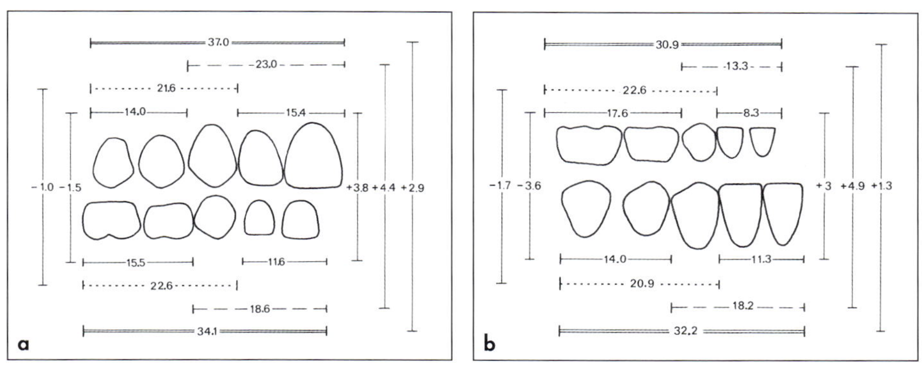

Fig 17-10 *(a and b)* Comparison of the average sums of mesiodistal crown widths of corresponding deciduous and permanent teeth. The data are derived from Nance[29] and differ slightly from those in Table 17-9. According to Nance, a central and lateral permanent incisor are together wider than their predecessors by 3.8 mm in the maxilla and 3.0 mm in the mandible. When a canine is included, the differences become 4.9 and 4.4 mm, respectively. A first and second premolar are together narrower than their predecessors by 1.5 mm in the maxilla and 3.6 mm in the mandible. When a canine is included, the three teeth together are smaller than their predecessors by 1.0 mm in the maxilla and 1.7 mm in the mandible.

Correlations in Crown Widths

Correlation coefficients among crown widths of deciduous and permanent teeth are gathered in Table 17-10, which shows that, except for the maxillary central incisors, there is only a moderate correlation in crown width among deciduous teeth and their successors. Small deciduous teeth can be replaced by large permanent teeth and vice versa. In Table 17-11, correlation coefficients are displayed for crown dimensions of corresponding groups of deciduous and permanent teeth. It reveals that the teeth involved in the first transition differ more in combined width than those involved in the second transition. In addition, the average sums of corresponding deciduous and permanent teeth are illustrated in Fig 17-10.

Dental Arch Width, Overjet and Overbite, and Molar Occlusion

Changes in arch width dimensions, overjet and overbite, and occlusion can be presented in two ways: *(1)* based on chronologic age and *(2)* according to a developmental characteristic in the dentition, such as the time of emergence of a mandibular central permanent incisor. The chronologically arranged data facilitates comparison with results from other studies. The advantage of using dental developmental parameters to arrange growth data is explained in Fig 17-11 and demonstrated for the increase in the intercanine distance in Figs 17-12 and 17-13.

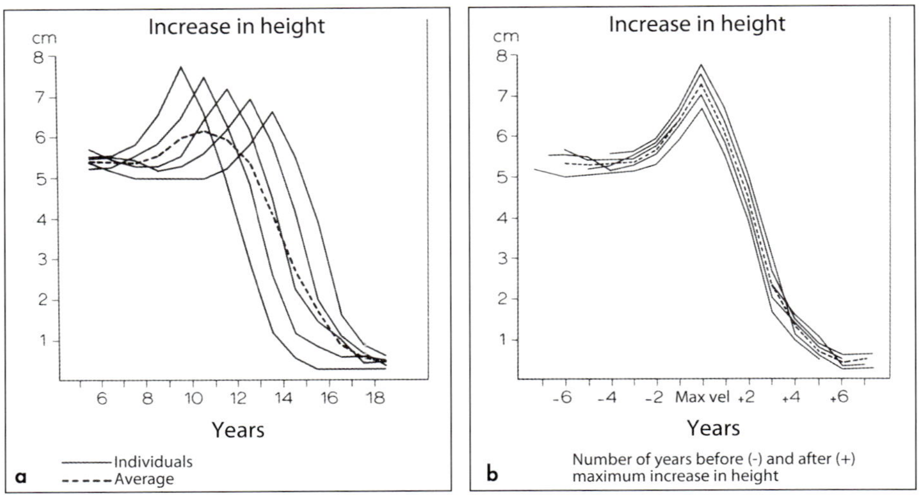

Fig 17-11 Arrangement of growth curves on a developmental parameter. *(a)* When the adolescence growth spurts of five girls are plotted based on chronologic age, the average maximum value becomes reduced and the curve smoothed *(dotted line)*. *(b)* When the growth spurts are superpositioned on the highest points of the curves, the course of the growth spurt of the five girls is almost identical. This approach was published by Shuttleworth[30] in 1939. Moorrees et al introduced it for the analysis of data on the development of the dentition.[31] Max vel, maximum velocity. (Reprinted from Shuttleworth[30] with permission.)

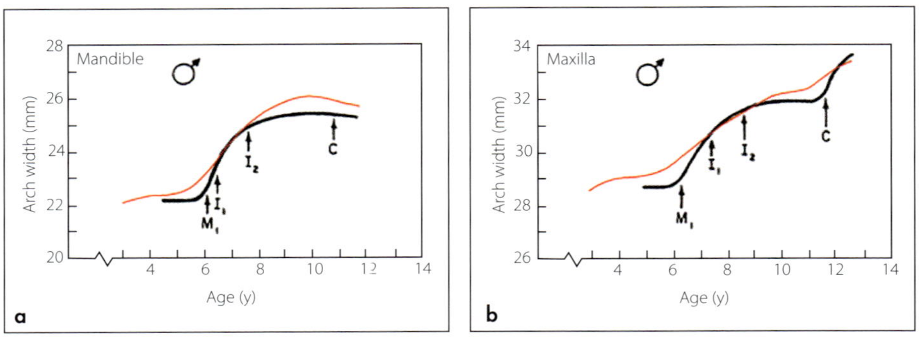

Fig 17-12 Average enlargement of the intercanine distance. When the averages of the longitudinally collected data of 84 boys were plotted on the chronologic age scale (red curve), the increase in intercanine width was spread out over 7 years. When they were plotted on a dental developmental age scale, based on the emergence of the mandibular central permanent incisor (black curve), the increase was spread out over 2 years for the mandible *(a)* and 3 years for the maxilla *(b)*. I_1, central incisor; I_2, lateral incisor; C, canine; M_1, first molar. (Reprinted from Moorrees and Reed[32] with permission.)

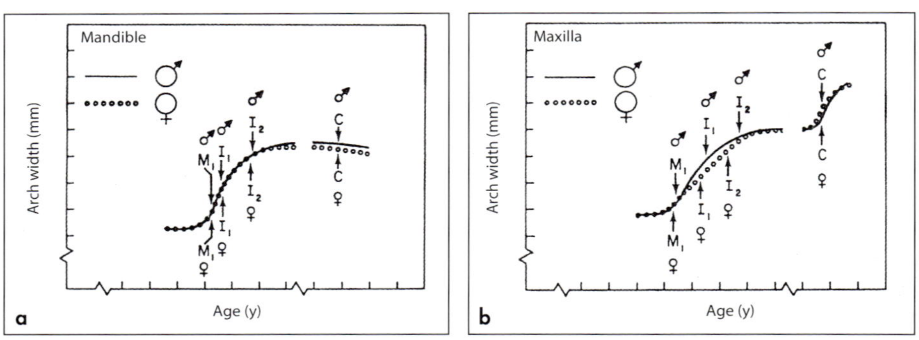

Fig 17-13 Superposition of the average intercanine distances for boys and girls on dental developmental age. *(a)* No differences between the sexes are seen for the mandible. *(b)* There is only a slight difference between the sexes for the maxilla. The intercanine distance increases in the maxilla with the emergence of the permanent canines, but this does not occur in the mandible. The crown of the maxillary permanent canine is substantially bigger than that of the deciduous canine. The difference is less marked in the mandible. In addition, the registration point of the maxillary permanent canine, which was the crown tip, is more buccal than that of its predecessor. (Reprinted from Moorrees and Reed[32] with permission.)

Changes in arch width, overjet and overbite, and molar occlusion are presented numerically and graphically in Tables 17-12 to 17-29. Tables 17-12 to 17-15 are based on data from the Nijmegen Growth Study.[22] Tables 17-16 to 17-29 and the superpositions of dental arches in Figs 17-14 and 17-15 are based on data from the University of Michigan Elementary and Secondary School Study.[26] In both studies, calculated centers of tooth crowns, rather than cusp tips, were used for measuring arch widths. For that purpose, dental casts were digitized three-dimensionally.[33–35]

Table 17-12 Arch width (in mm) at the mandibular canines based on chronologic age[22]

Age (y)	Boys M	Boys SD	Boys n	Girls M	Girls SD	Girls n
4.0	23.64	1.46	29	23.19	1.70	35
4.5	23.52	1.34	35	22.81	1.43	26
5.0	23.84	1.65	26	23.39	1.66	34
5.5*	23.98	1.69	59	23.32	1.74	59
6.0	24.11	1.90	59	23.61	1.91	59
6.5	24.73	2.09	56	24.47	2.14	57
7.0	25.31	2.09	89	24.90	2.32	105
7.5	26.07	2.00	130	25.56	2.18	130
8.0*	26.52	1.93	124	25.92	2.06	125
8.5**	26.86	2.09	120	25.97	2.04	127
9.0**	26.48	1.70	98	25.62	1.83	97
9.5**	26.32	1.97	137	25.65	1.87	173
10.0**	26.68	1.88	135	25.68	1.73	169
10.5**	26.52	1.91	132	25.63	1.64	167
11.0**	26.43	2.02	132	25.63	1.74	168
11.5**	26.54	1.98	133	25.65	1.73	166
12.0**	26.58	1.97	98	25.73	1.69	121
12.5	26.10	1.81	61	25.65	1.87	88
13.0	26.11	1.87	59	25.79	1.93	83
13.5	26.17	1.88	59	25.86	1.90	83
14.0	26.35	2.00	59	25.88	1.92	83

*Significant difference at 5% level (P ≤ .05).
**Significant difference at 1% level (P ≤ .01).
-III, mandibular deciduous canines; -3, mandibular permanent canines

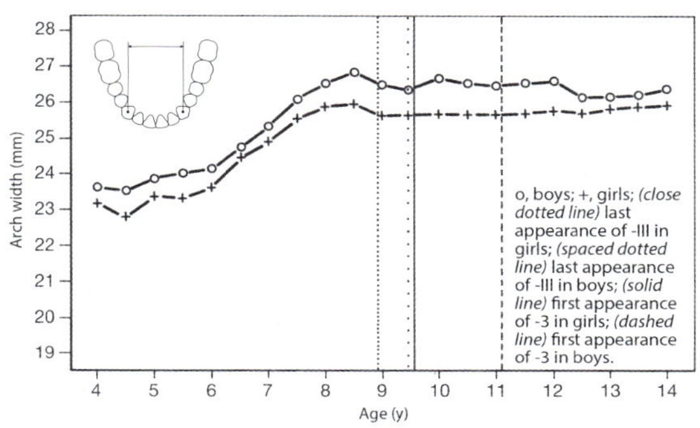

Table 17-13 Arch width (in mm) at the maxillary canines based on chronologic age[22]

Age (y)	Boys M	Boys SD	Boys n	Girls M	Girls SD	Girls n
4.0	28.71	2.20	29	28.12	1.89	35
4.5*	28.80	1.40	35	27.94	1.42	27
5.0	28.94	2.24	26	28.23	1.87	34
5.5*	28.84	1.88	59	28.03	1.69	60
6.0*	28.82	1.94	59	28.15	1.75	59
6.5	29.63	2.10	56	28.90	1.99	58
7.0*	30.26	2.30	90	29.61	2.10	107
7.5*	30.71	2.16	131	30.07	2.03	135
8.0**	31.21	2.11	127	30.44	2.08	130
8.5**	31.42	2.06	124	30.43	2.10	131
9.0**	31.38	1.98	100	30.16	1.99	97
9.5**	31.58	2.02	135	30.78	2.11	157
10.0**	32.20	2.11	129	31.36	1.95	154
10.5**	32.25	2.21	121	31.43	1.98	154
11.0**	32.78	2.36	125	31.91	2.03	158
11.5**	33.17	2.32	125	32.21	2.37	157
12.0**	33.93	2.30	93	32.67	2.18	114
12.5**	34.05	2.13	60	32.77	2.19	83
13.0**	34.26	2.13	58	33.02	2.39	80
13.5**	34.46	2.25	59	33.08	2.47	81
14.0**	34.63	2.11	59	33.08	2.14	82

*Significant difference at 5% level (P ≤ .05).
**Significant difference at 1% level (P ≤ .01).
+III, maxillary deciduous canines; +3, maxillary permanent canines

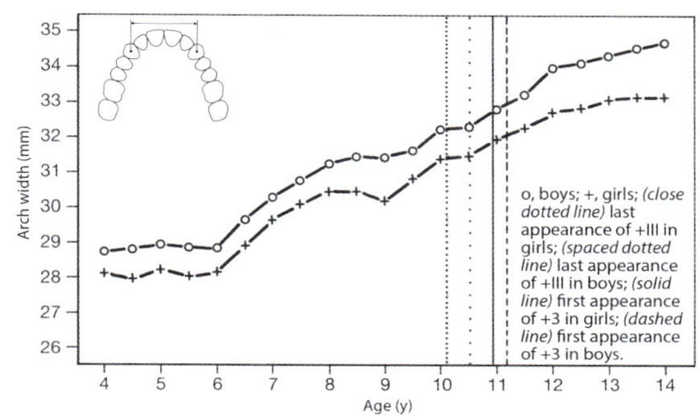

Table 17-14 Arch width (in mm) at the mandibular first molars based on chronologic age[22]

Age (y)	Boys M	Boys SD	Boys n	Girls M	Girls SD	Girls n
7.0	39.94	3.24	87	39.71	3.18	107
7.5**	41.16	2.61	125	40.14	2.37	139
8.0**	41.38	2.19	124	40.37	2.32	137
8.5**	41.68	2.32	127	40.67	2.41	138
9.0**	41.49	2.52	106	40.43	2.24	105
9.5**	41.34	2.53	146	40.26	2.41	173
10.0**	41.82	2.61	141	40.68	2.45	169
10.5**	41.85	2.54	135	40.76	2.45	168
11.0**	41.86	2.56	133	40.83	2.46	165
11.5**	41.90	2.78	133	40.96	2.44	163
12.0**	42.41	2.75	97	41.32	2.44	116
12.5**	42.84	2.62	58	41.60	2.44	84
13.0*	42.72	2.44	56	41.60	2.52	79
13.5**	42.66	2.45	56	41.49	2.39	79
14.0**	42.63	2.42	56	41.43	2.50	79

*Significant difference at 5% level (P ≤ .05).
**Significant difference at 1% level (P ≤ .01).
-6, mandibular permanent first molar

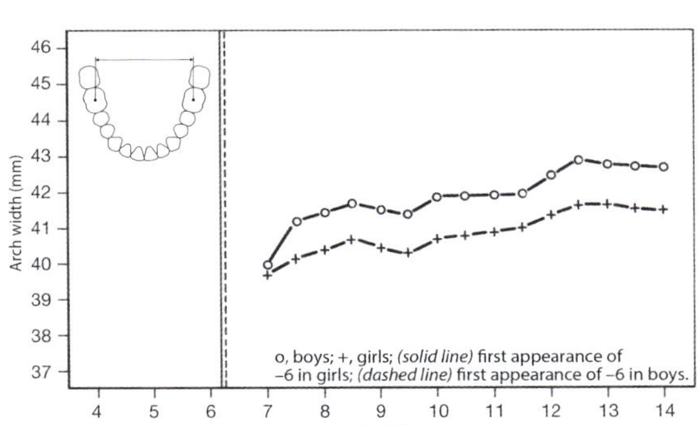

Table 17-15 Arch width (in mm) at the maxillary first molars based on chronologic age[22]

Age (y)	Boys M	Boys SD	Boys n	Girls M	Girls SD	Girls n
7.0	42.41	2.56	90	42.32	2.38	107
7.5*	43.86	2.59	133	43.01	2.24	138
8.0*	44.41	2.19	129	43.34	2.29	137
8.5*	44.51	2.16	128	43.43	2.25	139
9.0*	44.67	2.24	107	43.61	2.28	104
9.5*	45.15	2.50	146	43.94	2.32	172
10.0*	45.04	2.55	140	43.90	2.40	168
10.5*	45.31	2.57	129	44.09	2.46	160
11.0*	45.39	2.61	126	44.19	2.43	158
11.5*	45.45	2.61	125	44.29	2.44	156
12.0*	45.72	2.47	95	44.32	2.26	111
12.5*	45.59	2.50	56	44.13	2.10	77
13.0*	45.80	2.59	54	44.28	2.12	74
13.5*	45.89	2.56	54	44.37	2.12	75
14.0*	45.87	2.73	55	44.43	1.96	76

*Significant difference at 5% level (P ≤ .05).
+6, maxillary permanent first molar

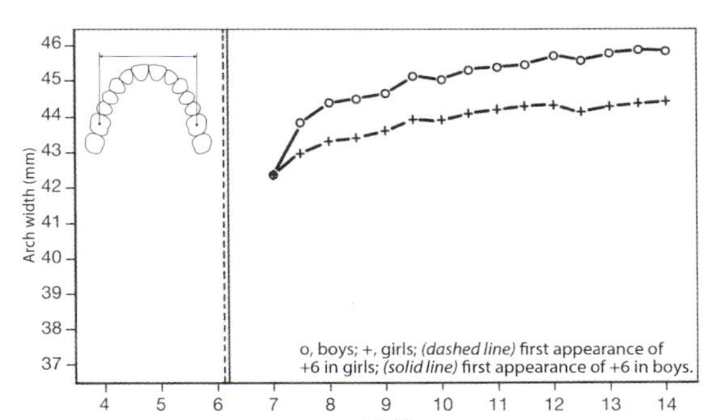

Table 17-16 Arch width (in mm) at the mandibular canines, based on chronologic age[26]

	At deciduous canines						At permanent canines					
	Boys			Girls			Boys			Girls		
Age (y)	M	SD	n	M	SD	n	M	SD	n	M	SD	n
3	22.27	0.72	4	21.39	0.79	6	–	–	0	–	–	0
4	21.58	1.22	33	21.75	1.32	31	–	–	0	–	–	0
5	21.87	1.28	53	21.75	1.26	55	–	–	0	–	–	0
6	22.33	1.57	82	22.19	1.57	77	–	–	0	–	–	0
7	23.36	1.76	93	22.97	1.82	85	–	–	0	23.93	–	1
8	24.31	1.89	82	23.95	1.70	88	–	–	0	24.00	–	1
9*	24.93	1.66	76	24.24	1.66	59	–	–	0	24.24	1.61	4
10	24.55	1.56	53	24.06	1.26	29	24.97	1.32	2	24.70	0.93	16
11*	24.62	1.43	22	23.42	1.28	8	24.84	1.96	20	24.86	1.54	29
12	25.72	0.85	7	23.95	–	1	25.14	1.73	35	24.81	1.42	43
13	–	–	0	–	–	0	24.88	1.56	54	24.70	1.12	46
14	–	–	0	–	–	0	24.73	1.45	48	24.39	1.14	31
15	–	–	0	–	–	0	24.82	1.64	39	24.15	1.48	33
16	–	–	0	–	–	0	24.66	1.68	44	23.90	1.76	23
17	–	–	0	–	–	0	24.54	1.53	31	23.93	1.53	19
18*	–	–	0	–	–	0	24.81	1.27	13	23.08	2.01	6

*Significant difference at 5% level ($P \leq .05$).

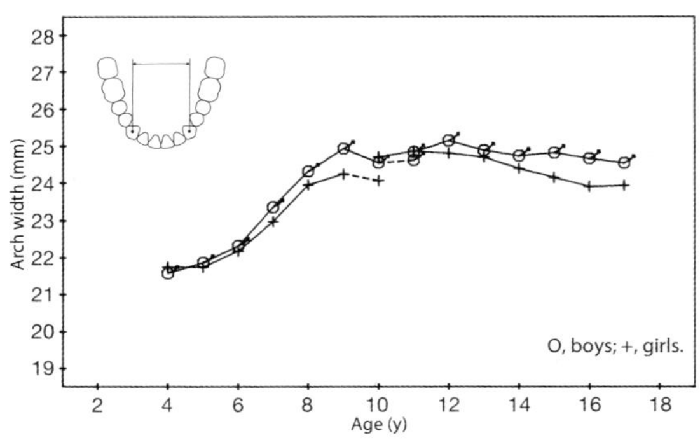

Table 17-17 Arch width (in mm) at the maxillary canines, based on chronologic age[26]

	At deciduous canines						At permanent canines					
	Boys			Girls			Boys			Girls		
Age (y)	M	SD	n	M	SD	n	M	SD	n	M	SD	n
3	27.45	0.53	4	26.73	1.01	6	–	–	0	–	–	0
4	26.83	1.33	35	36.37	1.48	32	–	–	0	–	–	0
5**	27.24	1.36	56	26.51	1.55	56	–	–	0	–	–	0
6*	27.53	1.58	84	26.88	1.78	81	–	–	0	–	–	0
7*	28.70	2.05	96	27.99	2.04	87	–	–	0	32.03	–	1
8*	29.70	2.12	89	29.06	1.90	94	–	–	0	31.48	–	1
9**	30.36	1.87	91	29.56	1.83	76	–	–	0	30.50	–	1
10*	30.47	1.96	74	29.77	1.79	59	–	–	0	32.00	1.20	2
11**	30.46	1.90	51	29.24	1.78	29	33.30	3.14	4	32.47	0.42	3
12	29.97	1.60	18	30.38	1.42	7	32.54	1.48	20	31.52	1.89	25
13**	32.27	1.84	3	–	–	0	32.46	1.41	34	31.24	1.81	31
14**	–	–	0	–	–	0	32.45	1.55	42	31.30	1.36	31
15**	–	–	0	–	–	0	32.37	1.98	39	31.21	1.44	32
16	–	–	0	–	–	0	32.25	1.84	45	31.43	1.62	24
17*	–	–	0	–	–	0	32.00	1.94	33	31.00	1.09	19
18	–	–	0	–	–	0	32.31	1.66	13	31.18	2.45	6

*Significant difference at 5% level ($P \leq .05$).
**Significant difference at 1% level ($P \leq .01$).

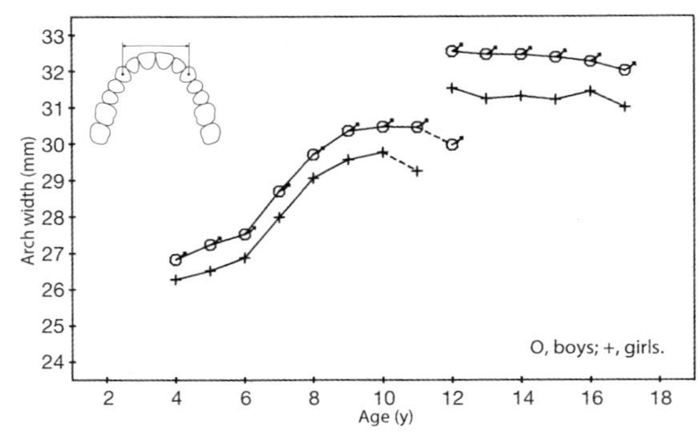

Table 17-18 Arch width (in mm) at the mandibular first molars, based on chronologic age[26]

	Boys			Girls		
Age (y)	M	SD	n	M	SD	n
5	–	–	0	43.40	–	1
6	40.15	1.83	4	39.96	2.11	11
7	40.20	1.78	41	39.94	1.91	45
8	40.93	1.93	68	40.33	1.91	72
9**	41.28	1.96	80	40.44	1.88	73
10	41.47	2.01	86	40.98	1.88	73
11	41.79	1.85	85	41.17	2.15	63
12	42.08	1.90	64	41.80	2.04	53
13	42.18	2.04	65	41.87	2.50	46
14*	42.13	2.27	52	41.11	2.58	38
15*	42.64	2.38	40	41.29	2.37	33
16*	42.77	2.62	45	41.46	2.11	25
17**	43.36	2.67	32	41.30	2.43	19
18	42.96	2.30	13	41.68	2.32	6

*Significant difference at 5% level ($P \leq .05$).
**Significant difference at 1% level ($P \leq .01$).

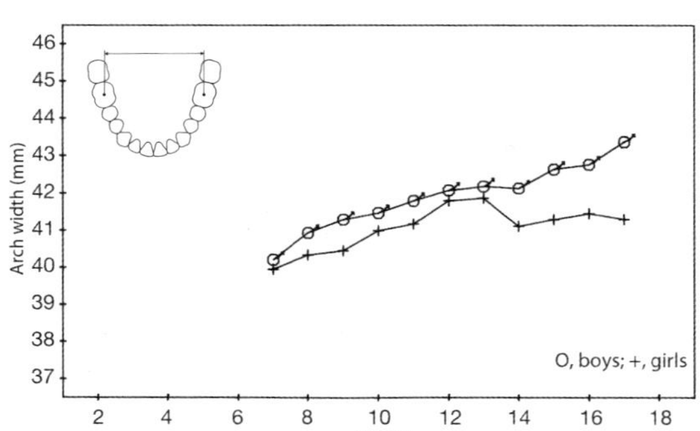

Table 17-19 Arch width (in mm) at the maxillary first molars, based on chronologic age[26]

	Boys			Girls		
Age (y)	M	SD	n	M	SD	n
5	39.71	–	1	39.12	0.27	2
6	41.85	1.89	7	41.34	2.37	17
7	42.37	2.25	49	41.54	2.60	52
8	43.12	2.41	73	42.38	2.83	74
9**	44.02	2.32	87	42.87	2.73	77
10*	44.46	2.55	86	43.52	2.51	80
11**	44.90	2.32	86	43.77	2.51	65
12	45.34	2.27	68	44.64	2.23	56
13*	45.63	2.25	64	44.66	2.68	47
14**	45.86	2.53	54	44.32	2.47	37
15**	46.39	2.74	41	44.61	2.57	33
16*	46.63	2.87	46	45.01	2.65	25
17**	47.06	2.82	33	44.33	2.27	19
18	46.69	2.58	13	43.94	4.19	6

*Significant difference at 5% level ($P \leq .05$).
**Significant difference at 1% level ($P \leq .01$).

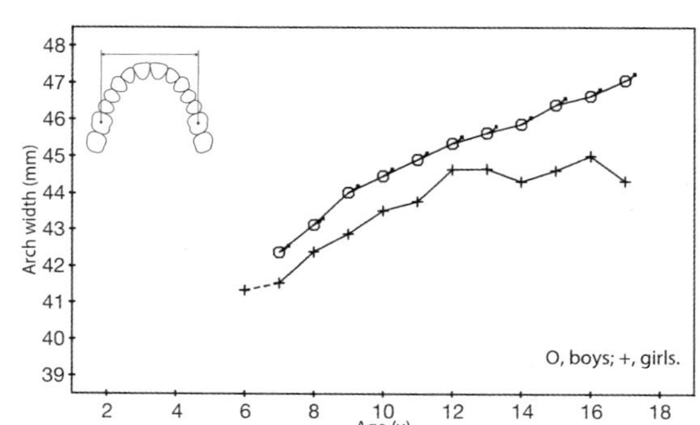

Table 17-20 Arch width (in mm) at the mandibular canines, based on the time of emergence of the mandibular central permanent incisor[26]

	At deciduous canines						At permanent canines					
	Boys			Girls			Boys			Girls		
DA†	M	SD	n	M	SD	n	M	SD	n	M	SD	n
−5	–	–	0	19.40	–	1	–	–	0	–	–	0
−4	22.19	1.16	4	20.83	0.90	2	–	–	0	–	–	0
−3	21.56	1.29	20	21.62	1.13	18	–	–	0	–	–	0
−2	21.62	1.17	40	21.69	1.31	39	–	–	0	–	–	0
−1	21.88	1.40	65	21.64	1.39	70	–	–	0	–	–	0
0	22.99	1.70	64	22.55	1.55	69	–	–	0	–	–	0
+1	24.14	1.93	56	23.60	1.71	64	–	–	0	–	–	0
+2	24.82	1.65	47	24.07	1.52	61	–	–	0	–	–	0
+3	24.89	1.68	39	24.20	1.24	33	–	–	0	25.10	–	1
+4	24.86	1.67	23	24.75	0.88	3	25.90	–	1	24.53	0.96	13
+5	25.68	0.75	5	–	–	0	25.26	1.25	13	24.57	1.29	32
+6	–	–	0	–	–	0	25.00	1.45	27	24.54	1.26	31
+7	–	–	0	–	–	0	24.80	1.10	27	24.42	1.27	26
+8	–	–	0	–	–	0	24.78	1.25	22	24.12	1.61	20
+9	–	–	0	–	–	0	24.77	1.53	21	23.77	1.80	13
+10	–	–	0	–	–	0	25.04	1.65	14	23.58	1.91	11

DA, developmental age.
†Years before and after the emergence of the mandibular central permanent incisor.

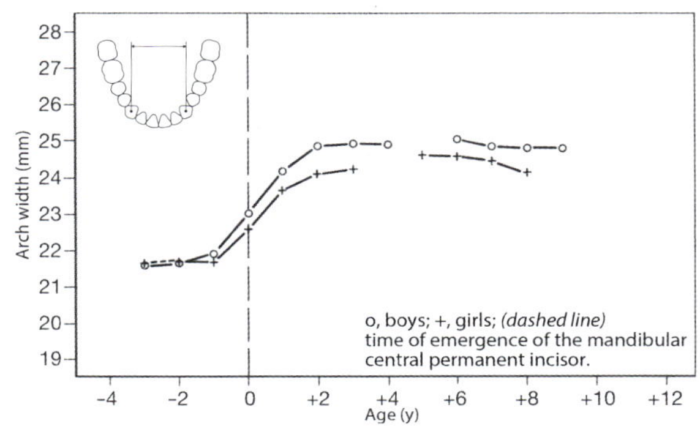

Table 17-21 Arch width (in mm) at the maxillary canines, based on the time of emergence of the mandibular central permanent incisor[26]

	At deciduous canines						At permanent canines					
	Boys			Girls			Boys			Girls		
DA†	M	SD	n	M	SD	n	M	SD	n	M	SD	n
−5	–	–	0	24.60	–	1	–	–	0	–	–	0
−4	26.93	1.55	4	25.82	1.55	2	–	–	0	–	–	0
−3	26.43	1.22	21	26.43	1.49	19	–	–	0	–	–	0
−2*	26.99	1.26	42	26.26	1.44	40	–	–	0	–	–	0
−1**	27.14	1.50	67	26.47	1.49	72	–	–	0	–	–	0
0*	27.88	1.64	66	27.25	1.72	71	–	–	0	–	–	0
+1*	29.29	1.92	59	28.57	1.84	65	–	–	0	–	–	0
+2	30.11	1.87	53	29.43	1.90	65	–	–	0	–	–	0
+3*	30.32	1.97	52	29.48	1.87	50	–	–	0	–	–	0
+4	30.17	1.80	40	29.31	1.86	32	–	–	0	–	–	0
+5	30.41	1.79	21	29.66	2.46	7	32.11	0.15	2	32.66	2.24	6
+6*	–	–	0	–	–	0	32.57	1.69	13	30.99	2.22	22
+7*	–	–	0	–	–	0	32.25	1.24	23	31.29	1.41	22
+8	–	–	0	–	–	0	32.26	1.78	21	31.43	1.40	21
+9	–	–	0	–	–	0	32.38	2.28	21	31.19	1.68	13
+10	–	–	0	–	–	0	32.24	2.37	15	31.12	1.53	12

DA, developmental age.
†Years before and after the emergence of the mandibular central permanent incisor.
*Significant difference at 5% level ($P \leq .05$).
**Significant difference at 1% level ($P \leq .01$).

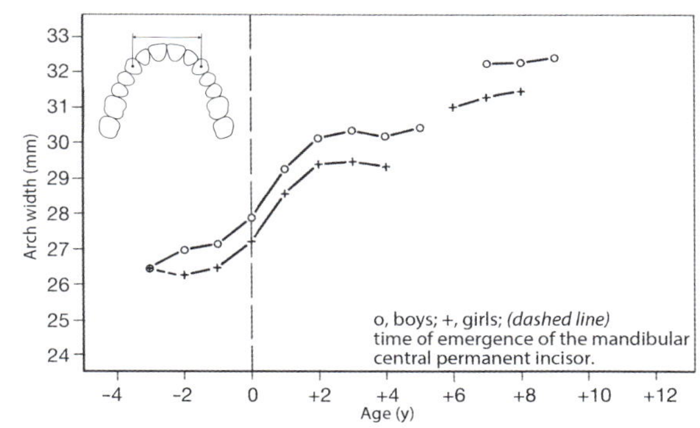

Table 17-22 Arch width (in mm) at the mandibular first permanent molars, based on the time of emergence of the mandibular central permanent incisor[26]

	Boys			Girls		
DA†	M	SD	n	M	SD	n
−2	–	–	0	–	–	0
−1	–	–	0	38.20	–	1
0	39.72	–	1	38.32	1.00	2
+1	40.47	2.22	25	39.94	2.09	27
+2	40.96	1.82	42	40.34	1.74	49
+3	41.32	1.88	49	40.76	1.81	53
+4	41.83	1.87	47	41.05	2.12	44
+5	41.91	1.81	43	41.52	2.13	43
+6	42.47	1.97	37	41.75	2.17	32
+7	42.46	2.18	27	41.46	2.91	26
+8**	42.63	2.22	23	40.52	2.73	22
+9*	42.87	2.42	21	40.93	1.79	14
+10*	43.74	2.45	15	41.48	1.95	12

DA, developmental age.
†Years before and after the emergence of the mandibular central permanent incisor.
*Significant difference at 5% level ($P \leq .05$).
**Significant difference at 1% level ($P \leq .01$).

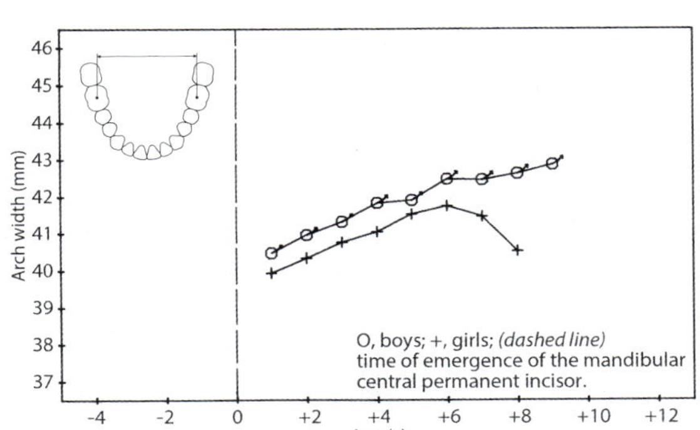

Table 17-23 Arch width (in mm) at the maxillary first permanent molars, based on the time of emergence of the mandibular central permanent incisor[26]

	Boys			Girls		
DA†	M	SD	n	M	SD	n
−2	–	–	0	–	–	0
−1	–	–	0	36.71	–	1
0	41.77	2.48	3	37.26	4.31	2
+1	42.31	1.97	28	41.23	2.62	32
+2*	43.60	2.05	44	42.54	2.75	52
+3**	44.39	2.26	51	43.22	2.31	56
+4**	44.86	2.38	46	43.48	2.43	48
+5	45.10	2.45	45	44.25	2.31	43
+6	45.77	2.10	35	44.69	2.49	34
+7*	46.07	2.49	28	44.27	2.72	25
+8**	46.65	2.37	23	44.36	2.64	22
+9*	47.01	2.61	21	44.87	2.41	14
+10*	47.40	2.81	15	45.18	2.24	12

DA, developmental age.
†Years before and after the emergence of the mandibular central permanent incisor.
*Significant difference at 5% level ($P \leq .05$).
**Significant difference at 1% level ($P \leq .01$).

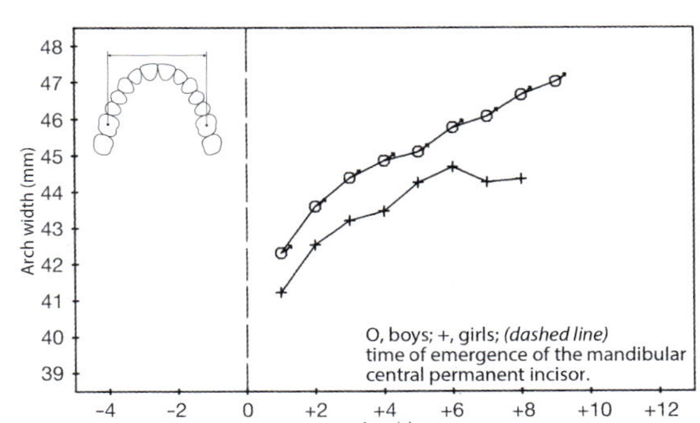

Table 17-24 Overjet (in mm), based on chronologic age[26]

Age (y)	Deciduous teeth Boys M	SD	n	Deciduous teeth Girls M	SD	n	Permanent teeth Boys M	SD	n	Permanent teeth Girls M	SD	n
3	3.06	2.02	4	4.18	2.78	6	–	–	0	–	–	0
4	2.73	1.59	34	3.41	2.24	29	–	–	0	–	–	0
5	2.74	1.51	52	3.23	2.04	47	–	–	0	–	–	0
6	2.96	1.63	44	2.73	2.02	39	6.48	–	1	3.15	–	1
7	3.07	1.81	8	3.59	2.10	10	3.90	1.38	12	2.64	2.19	8
8	–	–	0	–	–	0	3.99	2.27	38	3.32	1.94	40
9	–	–	0	–	–	0	4.08	2.05	76	3.70	2.41	64
10*	–	–	0	–	–	0	4.01	1.99	90	3.24	2.10	82
11	–	–	0	–	–	0	4.08	1.88	86	3.49	1.95	66
12	–	–	0	–	–	0	3.91	1.83	68	3.27	1.84	54
13*	–	–	0	–	–	0	3.79	1.78	65	2.98	1.61	46
14	–	–	0	–	–	0	3.48	1.49	51	2.97	1.50	36
15	–	–	0	–	–	0	3.67	1.85	39	3.07	1.64	32
16	–	–	0	–	–	0	3.14	1.83	45	2.97	1.69	22
17	–	–	0	–	–	0	3.55	1.21	33	2.95	1.53	17
18	–	–	0	–	–	0	3.16	1.05	12	2.45	2.60	5

*Significant difference at 5% level ($P \leq .05$).

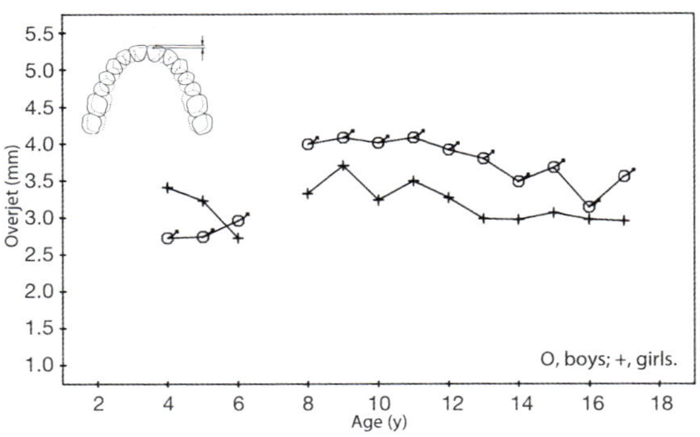

Table 17-25 Overjet (in mm), based on the time of emergence of the mandibular central permanent incisor[26]

DA†	Deciduous teeth Boys M	SD	n	Deciduous teeth Girls M	SD	n	Permanent teeth Boys M	SD	n	Permanent teeth Girls M	SD	n
−5	–	–	0	2.99	–	1	–	–	0	–	–	0
−4	1.73	2.66	4	6.11	–	1	–	–	0	–	–	0
−3	2.63	1.48	21	3.45	1.99	19	–	–	0	–	–	0
−2	2.72	1.47	41	3.49	2.21	36	–	–	0	–	–	0
−1	2.90	1.47	56	3.03	2.07	64	–	–	0	–	–	0
0	2.92	1.76	6	1.66	1.89	4	–	–	0	–	–	0
+1	–	–	0	–	–	0	3.90	1.99	8	3.55	1.84	8
+2	–	–	0	–	–	0	4.08	2.29	36	3.25	2.12	45
+3	–	–	0	–	–	0	4.00	1.94	54	3.69	2.47	55
+4	–	–	0	–	–	0	3.81	1.70	49	3.68	2.16	51
+5	–	–	0	–	–	0	3.64	1.77	45	3.38	1.88	41
+6*	–	–	0	–	–	0	4.04	1.60	35	3.09	1.94	34
+7	–	–	0	–	–	0	3.30	1.19	26	2.94	1.50	26
+8	–	–	0	–	–	0	3.21	1.46	21	3.15	1.04	20
+9	–	–	0	–	–	0	3.16	1.58	21	3.34	1.18	12
+10	–	–	0	–	–	0	3.15	1.21	14	3.32	1.09	11

DA, developmental age.
†Years before and after the emergence of the mandibular central permanent incisor.
*Significant difference at 5% level ($P \leq .05$).

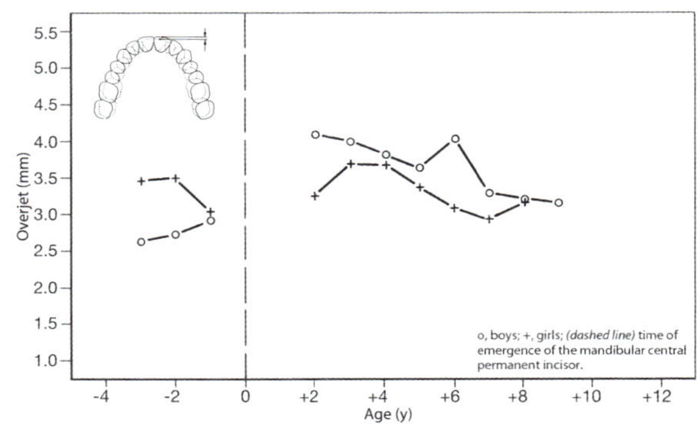

Table 17-26 Overbite (in mm), based on chronologic age[26]

Age (y)	Deciduous teeth Boys M	SD	n	Deciduous teeth Girls M	SD	n	Permanent teeth Boys M	SD	n	Permanent teeth Girls M	SD	n
3	0.92	0.99	4	0.78	1.58	5	–	–	0	–	–	0
4	1.06	1.77	34	0.26	2.09	29	–	–	0	–	–	0
5	1.03	1.68	46	0.92	1.59	46	–	–	0	–	–	0
6	1.14	1.73	43	0.52	1.69	38	−3.45	2.19	2	−3.50	–	1
7	1.49	1.23	7	1.48	1.76	10	2.60	2.04	12	1.12	2.18	9
8	–	–	0	–	–	0	2.62	2.06	39	1.71	2.28	38
9	–	–	0	–	–	0	2.87	1.78	75	2.46	1.95	63
10	–	–	0	–	–	0	3.13	1.79	90	2.83	1.61	83
11	–	–	0	–	–	0	3.33	1.79	81	3.02	1.62	65
12	–	–	0	–	–	0	3.45	1.73	69	3.13	1.32	53
13	–	–	0	–	–	0	3.48	1.82	66	3.25	1.49	45
14	–	–	0	–	–	0	3.45	1.71	51	2.87	1.48	37
15	–	–	0	–	–	0	3.15	1.87	41	2.92	1.57	33
16	–	–	0	–	–	0	2.83	2.02	43	2.97	1.54	24
17	–	–	0	–	–	0	3.02	2.09	31	3.62	1.55	18
18	–	–	0	–	–	0	3.05	1.55	11	3.03	1.69	6

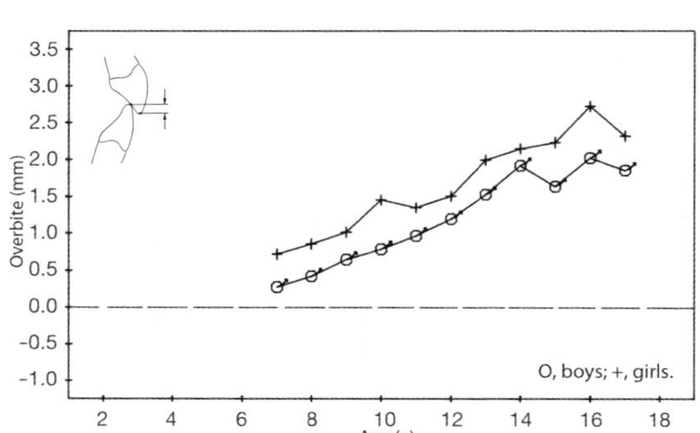

Table 17-27 Overbite (in mm), based on the time of emergence of the mandibular central permanent incisor[26]

DA†	Deciduous teeth Boys M	SD	n	Deciduous teeth Girls M	SD	n	Permanent teeth Boys M	SD	n	Permanent teeth Girls M	SD	n
−5	–	–	0	0.90	–	1	–	–	0	–	–	0
−4	1.40	1.36	4	1.85	3.46	2	–	–	0	–	–	0
−3	1.01	1.68	20	0.54	1.95	17	–	–	0	–	–	0
−2	0.99	1.69	39	0.27	1.72	37	–	–	0	–	–	0
−1	1.16	1.65	52	0.94	1.75	61	–	–	0	–	–	0
0	1.07	2.35	6	0.05	1.38	4	–	–	0	–	–	0
+1	–	–	0	–	–	0	1.97	2.60	8	1.07	4.06	8
+2	–	–	0	–	–	0	2.73	1.79	38	2.33	2.23	42
+3	–	–	0	–	–	0	2.87	1.89	53	2.76	1.70	56
+4	–	–	0	–	–	0	3.04	1.49	49	2.94	1.85	48
+5	–	–	0	–	–	0	3.27	1.48	46	3.16	1.53	40
+6	–	–	0	–	–	0	3.59	1.55	36	3.05	1.19	33
+7	–	–	0	–	–	0	3.57	1.04	26	3.02	1.34	25
+8	–	–	0	–	–	0	2.89	1.54	23	2.99	1.35	20
+9	–	–	0	–	–	0	2.90	1.48	20	3.26	1.07	14
+10	–	–	0	–	–	0	2.85	1.69	14	3.39	0.99	11

DA, developmental age.
†Years before and after the emergence of the mandibular central permanent incisor.

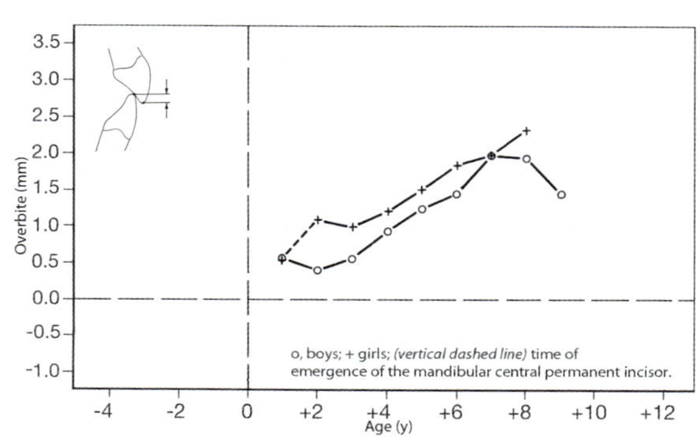

Table 17-28 Sagittal relationship of first permanent molars (in mm), based on chronologic age[26]

Age (y)	Boys M	Boys SD	Boys n	Girls M	Girls SD	Girls n
5	–	–	0	-1.39	–	1
6	-0.75	2.86	9	-0.49	2.13	13
7	0.28	1.52	65	0.72	1.75	62
8	0.42	1.72	84	0.86	1.75	91
9	0.65	1.51	97	1.01	1.68	84
10*	0.79	1.65	95	1.45	1.62	85
11	0.97	1.55	89	1.35	1.64	69
12	1.20	1.45	70	1.51	1.62	56
13	1.53	1.83	65	2.00	1.53	49
14	1.92	1.70	53	2.15	1.70	38
15	1.64	2.07	41	2.23	1.78	34
16	2.02	2.07	46	2.72	1.83	24
17	1.86	2.26	33	2.32	1.29	19
18	1.86	2.56	13	2.90	3.07	5

*Significant difference at 5% level ($P \leq .05$).

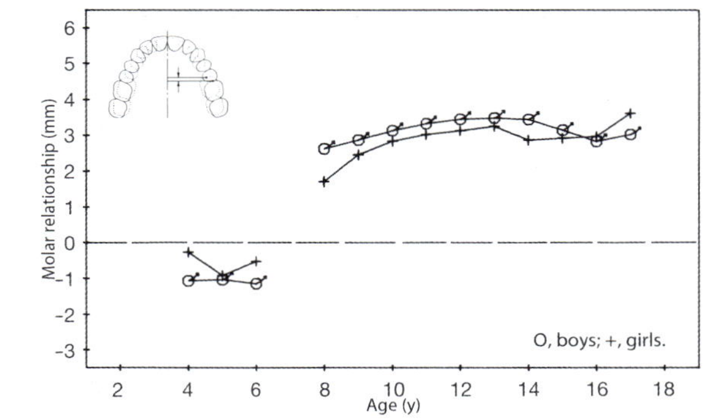

Table 17-29 Sagittal relation of first permanent molars (in mm), based on the time of emergence of the mandibular central permanent incisor[26]

DA[†]	Boys M	Boys SD	Boys n	Girls M	Girls SD	Girls n
-3	–	–	0	–	–	0
-2	–	–	0	–	–	0
-1	-6.08	–	1	–	–	0
0	-2.17	–	1	1.60	–	1
+1	0.58	1.59	28	0.51	1.46	30
+2*	0.40	1.66	51	1.08	1.65	61
+3	0.56	1.55	57	0.99	1.45	57
+4	0.94	1.40	51	1.18	1.61	53
+5	1.24	1.54	46	1.49	1.57	44
+6	1.44	1.17	36	1.84	1.75	35
+7	1.97	1.41	28	1.95	1.24	27
+8	1.94	1.74	23	2.31	1.44	22
+9	1.44	1.98	21	2.49	0.91	13
+10*	1.23	2.32	15	2.92	1.03	12

DA, developmental age.
†Years before and after the emergence of the mandibular central permanent incisor.
*Significant difference at 5% level ($P \leq .05$).

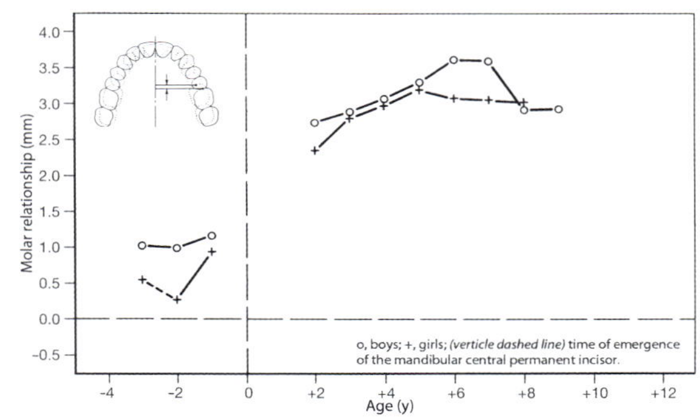

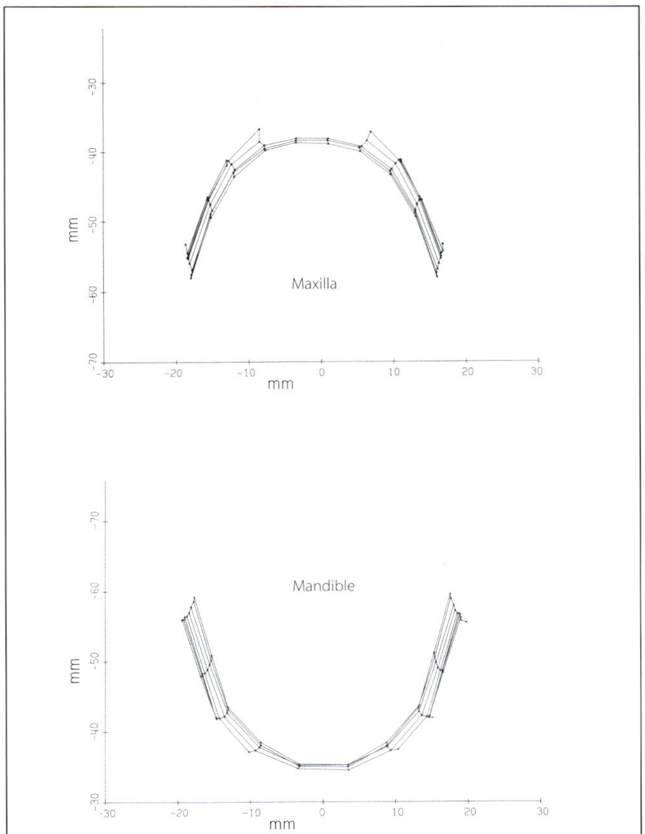

Fig 17-14 Superposition of the deciduous dental arches, based on the centers of the tooth crowns, arranged by the emergence of the mandibular central permanent incisor.[26]

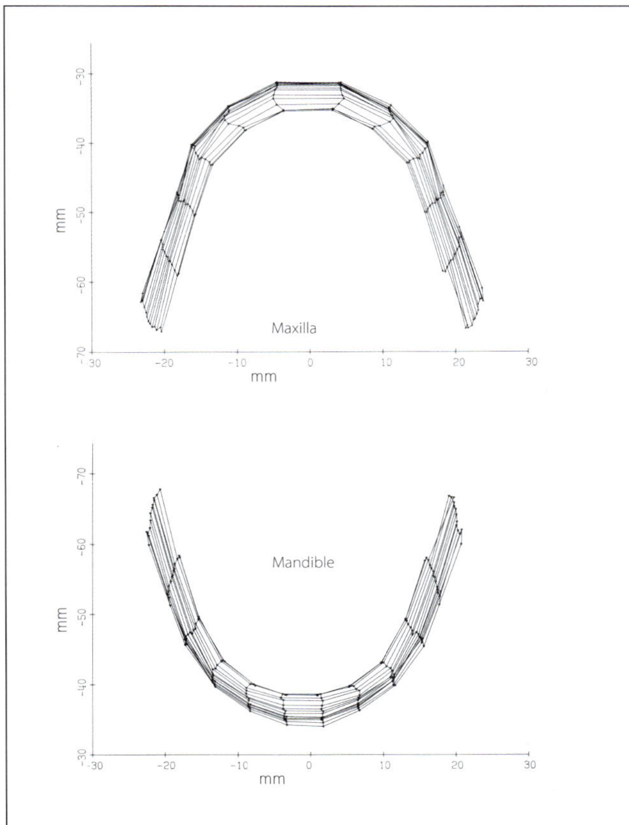

Fig 17-15 Superposition of the dental arches of the permanent dentition, based on the centers of the tooth crowns, arranged by chronologic age.[26]

Table 17-30 Inclination and angulation of permanent teeth, measured on 11 skulls*[36]

Root	Average inclination (degrees)	Average deviation	Average angulation (degrees)	Average deviation	Measured roots† (n)
+1	2	5	29.0	4.1	22
+2	16	6	29.0	3.4	22
+3	6	14	20.6	3.2	22
+4L	3	22	9.6	3.2	12
+4P	8	20	10.4	3.4	12
+5	19	36	8.6	3.6	22
+6MB	-2	46	10.4	3.9	22
+6DB	-28	35	13.0	4.6	22
+6P	45	30	13.0	4.9	22
+7MB	0	78	9.6	3.9	16
+7DB	28	66	9.3	2.8	16
+7P	61	44	10.7	3.2	20
+8MB	72	39	11.6	5.5	7
+8DB	89	40	11.3	4.6	7
+8P	103	42	12.3	3.9	11
-1	2	15	19.3	7.5	22
-2	17	10	21.2	6.4	22
-3	13	27	14.6	6.4	22
-4	14	35	9.8	3.9	22
-5	-34	54	10.1	3.4	22
-6D	-58	23	16.8	4.0	22
-6M	-58	36	12.8	5.6	22
-7D	-53	18	28.0	3.4	22
-7M	-51	19	25.4	4.6	22
-8D	-51	16	38.5	8.0	9
-8M	-53	15	32.6	4.5	10

+, maxillary; –, mandibular; L, labial; P, palatal; MB, mesiobuccal; DB, distobuccal; M, mesial; D, distal; 1, central permanent incisor; 2, lateral permanent incisor; 3, permanent canine; 4, first premolar; 5, second premolar; 6, first permanent molar; 7, second permanent molar; 8, third permanent molar.
*The data are based on the orientation of long needles placed in the root canals of the teeth of 11 adult skulls with normal occlusion. *Inclination* refers to buccolingual orientation; *angulation* refers to mesiodistal orientation.
†If the number of roots is less than 22, the roots were fused and not included in the table. Agenesis of third molars also resulted in reduction of the number of roots.

Inclination and Angulation of Permanent Teeth

The inclination and angulation of permanent teeth varies considerably, not only in orthodontic malocclusions but also in normal occlusions (Table 17-30). Frequently not all teeth are formed (agenesis); in particular, third molars are often missing. The percentages in Table 17-31 are based on 8,694 panoramic radiographs of 9- to 10-year-old schoolchildren in Zürich. The mandibular second premolar was most often not formed (4.37%), followed by the maxillary second premolar (1.72%). The maxillary lateral incisor was also sometimes missing (1.67%), but this was a rarer occurrence for the two mandibular incisors (0.45%). Very rarely one of the other permanent teeth was missing, but the maxillary central incisors were never missing. In this study the prevalence of agenesis of third molars could not be assessed because the children were too young. Another study has revealed that in Western Europe about 20% of third molars are not formed.[38]

Prevalence of Agenesis and Malocclusions

An ideal arrangement of teeth and occlusion does not occur often. In most cases there is a slight to moderate deviation from the ideal situation. Studies on prevalence of normal and abnormal occlusions and arrangement of teeth are difficult to compare because the criteria and definitions used vary. In some studies the occlusion was categorized using the Angle classification. In others, the size of the overjet was used. Nevertheless, it is clear that ethnic and regional differences exist in the prevalence of orthodontic malocclusions.

Table 17-31 Prevalence (%) of agenesis of permanent teeth*[37]

Tooth	Boys (n = 4,438)	Girls (n = 4,256)	Boys and girls (n = 8,694)
+1	0	0	0
+2	1.19	2.18	1.67
+3	0.15	0.09	0.12
+4	0.20	0.21	0.20
+5	1.26	2.20	1.72
+6	0.09	0.16	0.12
+7	0.06	0.18	0.12
−1	0.33	0.58	0.46
−2	0.33	0.56	0.44
−3	0.02	0.04	0.03
−4	0.11	0.11	0.11
−5	4.21	4.53	4.37
−6	0.04	0.02	0.03
−7	0.22	0.39	0.31

+, maxillary; −, mandibular; 1, central permanent incisor; 2, lateral permanent incisor; 3, permanent canine; 4, first premolar; 5, second premolar; 6, first permanent molar; 7, second permanent molar.

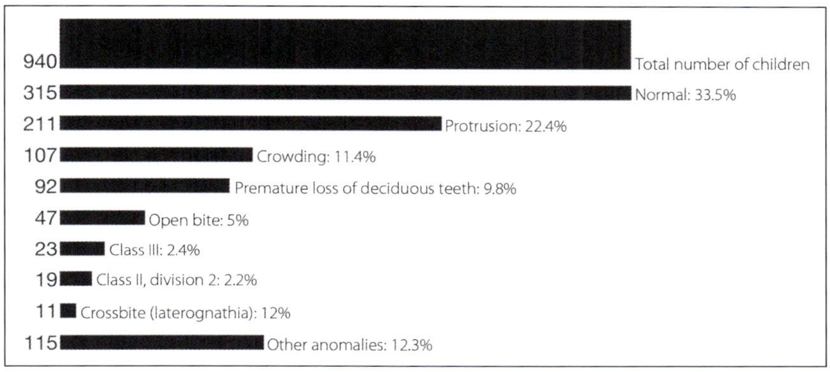

Fig 17-16 Occlusal conditions of 940 schoolchildren selected from 30 schools (each 15th child). The sample can be considered to be representative for the city of Groningen, the Netherlands. Class II, division 1 malocclusions are labeled as protrusion. (Reprinted from Bijlstra[44] with permission.)

Large surveys in the United States have provided the most data.[39–41] They showed an age difference in the prevalence of malocclusions. In about half of the children between 8 and 11 years of age, the incisors were well aligned. After emergence of the other permanent teeth, crowding of the mandibular incisors occurred more often. Only 34% of the adults had well-aligned mandibular incisors. In the children, 23% had an overjet of more than 5 mm, in the adolescents 15%, and in the adults 13%. About half of them had a neutroclusion with abnormalities in the dental arches, 15% had a distoclusion, and 1% had a mesioclusion with a negative overjet.[41,42]

Asymmetries are quite common in the United States. About 25% of the population has a difference in molar occlusion between the left and right side. In about 20%, the midlines of the dental arches deviate more than 2 mm. In 12% is a noticeable asymmetry of the face.[43] Studies in northwest Europe provided a larger percentage of Class II, division 1 malocclusions than in the United States—about 25%[44–46] (Fig 17-16). Malocclusions also occur in the deciduous dentition, but not so often and not in such a severe form. In Brazil, 12% of the children have been reported to have a unilateral crossbite and 1% a bilateral crossbite.[47]

References

1. Parner ET, Heidmann JM, Kjær I, Væth M, Poulsen S. Biological interpretation of the correlation of emergence times of permanent teeth. J Dent Res 2002;81:451–454.
2. Lumbau A, Sale S, Chessa G. Ages of eruption: Study on a sample of 204 Italian children aged 6 to 24 months. Eur J Paediatr Dent 2008;9:76–80.
3. Logan WHG, Kronfeld R. Development of the human jaws and surrounding structures from birth to the age of fifteen years. J Am Dent Assoc 1933;20:379–427.

4. Lysell L, Magnusson B, Thilander B. Time and order of eruption of the primary teeth. Odontol Revy 1962;13:217–234.
5. Schroeder HE. Orale Strukturbiologie. 4. Stuttgart: Thieme Verlag, 1992.
6. Van Waes HJM, Stöckli PW. Kinderzahnmedizin. Stuttgart: Thieme Verlag, 2001.
7. Prahl-Andersen B, Van der Linden FPGM. The estimation of dental age. Trans Eur Orthod Soc 1972;535–541.
8. Hurme VO. Ranges of normalcy in the eruption of permanent teeth. J Dent Child 1949;16:11–15.
9. Hägg U, Taranger J. Timing of tooth emergence. A prospective longitudinal study of Swedish urban children from birth to 18 years. Swed Dent J 1986;10:195–206.
10. Cho YH. The study on the eruption timing of primary teeth [in Korean]. J Korean Pediatr Dent Assoc 1977;4:7–17.
11. Choi NK, Yang KH. A study on the eruption timing of primary teeth in Korean children. J Dent Child 2001;68:244–249.
12. Robinow M, Richards TW, Anderson M. The eruption of deciduous teeth. Growth 1942;6:27–133.
13. Lunt RC, Law DB. A review of the chronology of calcification of deciduous teeth. J Am Dent Assoc 1974;89:599–606.
14. Proffit WR. Contemporary Orthodontics, ed 4. St Louis: Mosby, 2008.
15. Demirjian A, Goldstein H, Tanner JM. A new system of dental age assessment. Hum Biol 1973;45:211–227.
16. Garcia-Godoy F, Diaz AN, del Valle JM, Arana EJ. Timing of permanent tooth emergence in a Southeastern Dominican schoolchildren population sample. Community Dent Oral Epidemiol 1982;10:43–46.
17. Höffding J, Maeda M, Yamaguchi K, et al. Emergence of permanent teeth and onset of dental stages in Japanese children. Community Dent Oral Epidemiol 1984;12:55–58.
18. Heidmann J. Comparison of different methods for estimating human tooth-eruption time on one set of Danish national data. Arch Oral Biol 1986;31:815–817.
19. Virtanen J, Bloigu RS, Larmas MA. Timing of eruption of permanent teeth: Standard Finnish patient documents. Community Dent Oral Epidemiol 1994;22:286–288.
20. Kochhar R, Richardson A. The chronology and sequence of eruption of human permanent teeth in Northern Ireland. Int J Paediatr Dent 1998;8:243–252.
21. Leroy R, Bogaerts K, Lesaffre E, Declerck D. The emergence of permanent teeth in Flemish children. Community Dent Oral Epidemiol 2003;31:30–39.
22. Van der Linden FPGM, Boersma H, Prahl-Andersen B. Development of the dentition. In: Prahl-Andersen B, Kowalski CJ, Heydendael PHJ (eds). A Mixed-Longitudinal Interdisciplinary Study of Growth and Development. New York: Academic Press, 1979:521–536.
23. Savara BS, Steen JC. Timing and sequence of eruption of permanent teeth in a longitudinal sample of children from Oregon. J Am Dent Assoc 1978;97:209–214.
24. Moorrees CFA, Kent RL. Patterns of dental maturation. In: McNamara JA Jr (ed). The Biology of Occlusal Development, monograph 7, Craniofacial Growth Series. Ann Arbor: University of Michigan, 1977:25–41.
25. Giles NB, Knott VB, Meredith HV. Increase in intraoral height of selected permanent teeth during the quadrennium following gingival emergence. Angle Orthod 1963;33:195–206.
26. Moyers RE, Van der Linden FPGM, Riolo ML, McNamara JA Jr. Standards of Human Occlusal Development, monograph 5, Craniofacial Growth Series. Ann Arbor: University of Michigan, 1976.
27. Moorrees CFA, Reed RB. Correlations among crown diameters of human teeth. Arch Oral Biol 1964;9:685–697.
28. Moorrees CFA, Chadha JM. Crown diameters of corresponding tooth groups in the deciduous and permanent dentition. J Dent Res 1962;41:466–470.
29. Nance HN. The limitations of orthodontic treatment. I. Mixed dentition diagnosis and treatment. Am J Orthod 1947;33:177–223.
30. Shuttleworth FK. The physical and mental growth of girls and boys age six to nineteen in relation to age at maximum growth. Monogr Soc Res Child Dev 1939;4(3):1–291.
31. Moorrees CFA, Fanning EA, Grön AM, Lebret L. The timing of orthodontic treatment in relation to tooth formation. Trans Eur Orthod Soc 1962;87–101.
32. Moorrees CFA, Reed RB. Changes in dental arch dimensions expressed on the basis of tooth eruption as a measure of biologic age. J Dent Res 1965;44:129–141.
33. Van der Linden FPGM. A new method to determine tooth positions and dental arch dimensions. J Dent Res 1972;51:1104.
34. Van der Linden FPGM, Boersma H, Zelders T, Peters KA, Raaben JH. Three-dimensional analysis of dental casts by means of the Optocom. J Dent Res 1972;51:1100.
35. Van der Linden FPGM, Miller RL. Quality control of digitized data and inclusion of essential and meaningful checkpoints. J Dent Res 1971;50:982.
36. Dempster WT, Adams WJ, Duddles RA. Arrangement in the jaws of the roots of the teeth. J Am Dent Assoc 1963;67:779–797.
37. Bachmann H. Die Häufigkeit von Nichtanlagen bleibender Zähne (ausgenommen der Weisheitszähne). Ergebnisse der Auswertung von 8694 Orthopantogrammen 9-10 jähriger Schulkinder aus Zürich [thesis]. Zürich: University of Zürich, 1974.
38. Bredy E, Erbring C, Hübenthal B. The incidence of hypodontia with the presence and absence of wisdom teeth [in German]. Dtsch Zahn Mund Kieferheilkd Zentralbl 1991;79:357–363.
39. El-Mangoury NH, Mostafa YA. Epidemiologic panorama of dental occlusion. Angle Orthod 1990;60:207–214.
40. Emrich RE, Brodie AG, Blayney JR. Prevalence of Class I, Class II, and Class III malocclusions (Angle) in an urban population. An epidemiological study. J Dent Res 1965;44:947–953.
41. Proffit WR, Fields HW Jr, Moray LJ. Prevalence of malocclusion and orthodontic treatment need in the United States: Estimates from the NHANES III survey. Int J Adult Orthodon Orthognath Surg 1998;13:97–106.
42. Brunelle JA, Bhat M, Lipton JA. Prevalence and distribution of selected occlusal characteristics in the US population, 1988-91. J Dent Res 1996;75:706–713.
43. Sheats RD, McGorray SP, Musmar Q, Wheeler TT, King GJ. Prevalence of orthodontic asymmetries. Semin Orthod 1998;4:138–145.
44. Bijlstra KG. Frequency of dentofacial anomalies in school children and some aetiologic factors. Trans Eur Orthod Soc 1958;34:231–236.
45. Helm S. Prevalence of malocclusion in relation to development of the dentition. An epidemiological study of Danish school children. Acta Odontol Scand 1970;28(suppl 58).
46. Thilander B, Myrberg N. The prevalence of malocclusion in Swedish schoolchildren. Scand J Dent Res 1973;81:12–21.
47. da Silva Filho OG, Santamaria M Jr, Capelozza Filho L. Epidemiology of posterior crossbite in the primary dentition. J Clin Pediatr Dent 2007;32:73–78.

Index

Page numbers followed by "f" indicate figures; those followed by "t" indicate tables; those followed by "b" indicate boxes

D

E

F

G

H

I

J

L

M

N

O

P

R

S

T

U

W

Y